NEUROBLASTOMA

Carl Pochedly, M.D.
Director, Pediatric Hematology-Oncology
Nassau County Medical Center
East Meadow, L.I., N.Y.
Associate Professor of Pediatrics
School of Medicine
State University of New York
at Stony Brook

RC280
NH
NH8
1976

Publishing Sciences Group, Inc.
Acton, Massachusetts
a subsidiary of CHC Corporation

Distributed in

Canada
   McAinsh & Company, Ltd.
   1835 Yonge Street
   Toronto, Ontario M4S 1L6
   Canada

Australia and New Zealand
   Butterworths Pty. Ltd.
   586 Pacific Highway
   Chatswood, NSW 2067
   Australia

Asia
   Toppan Company Ltd.
   5, 1-Chome, Taito-Ku
   Tokyo 110
   Japan

   Toppan Company, Ltd.
   No. 38 Liu Fang Road
   Jurong Town
   Singapore-22

India and Sri Lanka
   Affiliated East-West Press Pvt. Ltd.
   9 Nizamuddin East
   New Delhi 110013
   India

United Kingdom and Europe
South Africa
   Medical and Technical Publishing Co., Ltd.
   P. O. Box 55
   St. Leonardgate
   Lancaster LA1 1PE
   England

Printed in the United States of America.

International Standard Book Number: 0-88416-117-X

Library of Congress Catalog Card Number: 75-18337

CONTRIBUTORS

Carl Pochedly, M.D.
Director, Pediatric Hematology-
Oncology
Nassau County Medical Center
East Meadow, N.Y.
Associate Professor of Pediatrics
Health Sciences Center
SUNY at Stony Brook

Dvorah Balsam, M.D.
Pediatric Radiologist
Department of Radiology
Nassau County Medical Center
East Meadow, N.Y.

Laura Bertani Dziedzic, Ph.D.
Research Assistant Professor
Department of Medicine
Mount Sinai School of Medicine
City University of New York
New York, N.Y.

Stanley W. Dziedzic, Ph.D.
Associate in Medicine
Department of Medicine
Mount Sinai School of Medicine
City University of New York
New York, N.Y.

Stanley E. Gitlow, M.D.
Clinical Professor of Medicine
Department of Medicine
Mount Sinai School of Medicine
City University of New York
New York, N.Y.

Jordan U. Gutterman, M.D.
Assistant Professor of Medicine
Section of Immunology
Department of Developmental
Therapeutics
M.D. Anderson Hospital and
Tumor Institute
Houston, Texas

Evan M. Hersh, M.D.
Associate Professor of Medicine
Chief, Section of Immunology
Department of Developmental
Therapeutics
M.D. Anderson Hospital and
Tumor Institute
Houston, Texas

Giora M. Mavligit, M.D.
Assistant Professor of Medicine
Section of Immunology
Department of Developmental
Therapeutics
M.D. Anderson Hospital and
Tumor Institute
Houston, Texas

Anthony Shaw, M.D.
Chief, Pediatric Surgery
Medical Center
Professor of Surgery and Pediatrics
School of Medicine
University of Virginia
Charlottesville, Virginia

Lotte Strauss, M.D.
Professor of Pathology
Mt. Sinai School of Medicine
City University of New York
Department of Pathology
Mt. Sinai Medical Center
New York, N.Y.

Melvin Tefft, M.D.
Attending Radiotherapist
Memorial Sloan-Kettering Cancer
Center
Professor of Radiology
Cornell Medical School
New York, N.Y.

John T. Truman, M.D.
Chief, Pediatric Hematology Unit
Massachusetts General Hospital
Assistant Professor of Pediatrics
Harvard Medical School
Boston, Massachusetts

CONTENTS

Preface vii
Carl Pochedly, M.D.

1 **Neuroblastoma in Infancy** 1
Carl Pochedly, M.D.

2 **Neuroblastoma in the Head and Central
Nervous System** 35
Carl Pochedly, M.D.

3 **Neuroblastoma in the Neck, Chest, Abdomen,
and Pelvis** 59
Carl Pochedly, M.D.

4 **Neuroblastoma in the Skeletal System** 93
Carl Pochedly, M.D.
Dvorah Balsam, M.D.

5 **Catecholamine Metabolism in Neuroblastoma** 115
Stanley E. Gitlow, M.D.
Laura Bertani Dziedzic, Ph.D.
Stanley W. Dziedzic, Ph.D.

6 **Histogenesis and Pathology of Neuroblastoma** 155
Carl Pochedly, M.D.
Lotte Strauss, M.D.

7 **Biology of the Neuroblastoma Cell** 181
Carl Pochedly, M.D.

8   **Immunology of Neuroblastoma**   205
Giora M. Mavligit, M.D.
Jordan U. Gutterman, M.D.
Evan M. Hersh, M.D.

9   **Ganglioneuroma**   217
Carl Pochedly, M.D.

10   **Surgical Management of Neuroblastoma**   237
Anthony Shaw, M.D.

11   **Radiotherapeutic Management of Neuroblastoma**   251
Melvin Tefft, M.D.

12   **Chemotherapy of Neuroblastoma**   263
John T. Truman, M.D.

13   **Prognosis: The Biological Vagaries of Neuroblastoma**   273
Carl Pochedly, M.D.

Index   307

Although neuroblastomas have been intensively studied and have fascinated clinical investigators for more than 100 years, they still remain an enigma as far as effective treatment. Except for acute leukemia and brain tumors, neuroblastoma is the most common malignancy in children. Neuroblastoma is a tumor of early life; its incidence is highest during the first two years and decreases rapidly thereafter. More than 80 percent of cases occur before the age of five years. There is no predilection for either sex or for any race.

Neuroblastomas originate from primitive sympathetic neuroblasts of the neural crests. Recognition of the wide distribution of these primitive sympathetic cells in the embryo helps to explain the widely variable clinical behavior of this tumor. The tumors may arise from any site where one would normally find elements of the sympathetic nervous system. Thus, the spectrum of clinical manifestations of neuroblastoma is vast.

In spite of the fact that neuroblastoma in its usual behavior is the most malignant of human cancers, it also shows the highest rate of spontaneous regression. This peculiarity of frequent spontaneous regression has tantalized and frustrated several generations of clinical investigators.

In 1864 Virchow described a "glioma" in a child with a malignant abdominal tumor. In 1880 Parker described a similar case and called it a "congenital sarcoma." In 1885 Dalton described a child with an abdominal tumor with similar histology who also had massive metastases to the liver. Marchand in 1891 pointed out the relationship between the sympathetic nervous system and adrenal medullary tumors. Pepper in 1901 and Hutchison in 1907 described their famous syndromes which we now know were neuroblastomas with differing patterns of metastasis. But neither clinically nor anatomically are these eponymic designations justified. It was not until 1910 that Wright demonstrated convincingly that neuroblastomas originate from embryonal sympathetic neuroblasts; this conception of the histogenesis is now the accepted one. In 1927 Cushing and Wolbach described their case of neuroblastoma which subsequently showed complete maturation to a histologically proven ganglioneuroma.

In this book I have tried to organize the extensive literature on neuroblastoma into a workable and easily understood scheme. It is recognized, of course, that for such a vast and complex literature, any one scheme of presentation may not be appropriate for the most lucid discussion of all aspects of this disease. One chapter is devoted to neuroblastomas in infancy, since the neonatal manifestations of this tumor are particularly intriguing. Following this are chapters on the various clinical and laboratory manifestations. For convenience, the clinical discussions deal with each region of the body separately. There are also discussions of catecholamine metabolism in neuroblastoma and the various histopathological patterns of this tumor. The in vitro behavior and immunological phenomena associated with this tumor are discussed in separate chapters. Another chapter is devoted to ganglioneuroma, which is a closely related tumor. Finally, extensive discussions are devoted to the various modes of therapy and to the interpretation of the several parameters used in assessing prognosis. Hopefully, these discussions will enable the modern pediatrician and oncologist to see possibilities where his predecessors saw only doom.

The author is grateful to Dr. G. J. D'Angio, Chairman of the Department of Radiotherapy at the Memorial Sloan-Kettering Cancer Center, for critical review of several of the chapters. Dr. Audrey Evans, Director of Oncology at the Children's Hospital of Philadelphia, kindly reviewed the chapter on prognosis. Mr. Nicholas Levycky, Director of Medical Illustration at Nassau County Medical Center, prepared the illustrations. The many superb line drawings and the cover design were done by Mr. Gregory Guiteras. Deep appreciation is extended to the several authors who contributed excellent chapters in their areas of special competence. Finally, thanks are owed to the many pediatricians and pediatric surgeons on the staff of Nassau County Medical Center who, over the years, referred their patients to my service.

Carl Pochedly, M.D.

1 Neuroblastoma in Infancy

Carl Pochedly, M.D.

Introduction
1. Locations of primary tumors and metastases
2. Differential diagnosis
3. Neuroblastoma in the fetus
4. Peculiarities of neuroblastomas in infancy
   a. Skin metastases
   b. High incidence of liver metastases
   c. High rate of spontaneous cure
5. Role of nerve growth factor in neuroblastoma regression
6. Neuroblastoma in situ
7. Familial neuroblastoma
8. Neuroblastoma in animals
   Summary and conclusions

Neuroblastoma is probably the most fascinating tumor of childhood. The unique and intriguing features of this tumor are mainly those manifested when the tumor occurs in children during the first few months of life.

Neuroblastoma is not uncommon in the neonate—more than 60 such cases have been described.[1,2,3] Neuroblastomas present at birth differ in certain respects from those that appear later in childhood, and a larger proportion of infants are cured of their disease. The location of "metastases" varies in the infant, with liver and subcutaneous involvement more commonly found.[4,5]

According to classical descriptions, abdominal neuroblastomas occur in two types. The *Pepper* type[6] (adrenal-hepatic) is characterized by distension of the abdomen from enlargement of the liver, mesenteric lymph node metastases, rapid loss of weight and strength, and anemia (Figure 1). Metastases to the bones of the skull are

1

seldom seen. This type occurs almost exclusively in children less than 6 months of age. The *Hutchison* type[7] (adrenal-skeletal-orbital) is characterized by the peculiar onset of ecchymosis of the eyelids, proptosis, and enlargement of the preauricular, submaxillary, and upper cervical lymph nodes on the same side. These symptoms are caused by metastases in the bones of the skull, which have an unexplained predilection for the region of the orbit. Cases with the Hutchison type almost always occur in children *over* 6 months of age. But on close examination, many patients have features suggestive of both the Pepper and Hutchison types. Thus, these terms, although hallowed by tradition, are of little clinical use. The new staging system, to be described later, offers a more meaningful classification and description of children with neuroblastoma. The terms Pepper type and Hutchison type should be considered obsolete.

The clinical diagnosis of neuroblastoma in infancy is often difficult because the primary tumor may be inconspicuous, and the symptoms are mainly determined by the localization of metastases. X-ray examination is often very useful. But the diagnosis can be made only on the basis of the histological picture of these tumors, in combination with the results of assay of urinary catecholamines[8,9,10] and cystathionine.[11,12]

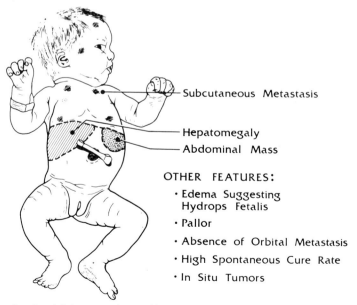

Subcutaneous Metastasis

Hepatomegaly

Abdominal Mass

OTHER FEATURES:
- Edema Suggesting Hydrops Fetalis
- Pallor
- Absence of Orbital Metastasis
- High Spontaneous Cure Rate
- In Situ Tumors

Figure 1. Special features of neuroblastomas in infancy.

The newborn infant with neuroblastoma may be edematous, jaundiced, anemic, and have a distended abdomen.[13,14] Thus, many cases of congenital neuroblastoma resemble severe erythroblastosis fetalis. Similarities in the gross and histological appearance of the placenta in congenital neuroblastoma and in erythroblastosis fetalis are also present.[15]

LOCATIONS OF PRIMARY TUMORS AND METASTASES

Neuroblastoma can arise from sympathetic nervous system tissue in any area of the body. In all age groups, the adrenal gland is the most common site of origin of neuroblastoma. It may, however, be a slightly more frequent site in the newborn than in older children. In 1,303 children of all ages with neuroblastoma, 65.5 percent of the tumors arose from the adrenal; 72.1 percent of neuroblastomas in neonates were of adrenal origin[2] (Table 1). In 7 newborns, tumor was found within both adrenals. This represents metastases from one adrenal to the other, or multiple sites of origin. The frequency of neuroblastoma arising in the thorax or pelvis is the same in all age groups.[1,16]

Prognosis in congenital neuroblastoma is related to the location of the primary tumor. In one series of 10 cases in which the primary tumors were both extra-adrenal and extra-abdominal in location, all survived.[3] But it is doubtful whether this is true for all age groups, since neonates have special "metastases" (i.e., the stage IV-S distribution).[17]

Table 1
Primary sites of Neuroblastomas in Neonates
Compared with the Incidence in Children of All Ages

Location	Percent in Neonate	Percent for All ages
Head*	3.0	0.2
Neck	3.0	3.2
Chest	10.3	14.6
Abdomen	72.1	65.5
Pelvis	8.6	4.5
Unknown	3.0	12.0
Total cases reviewed	68	1303

Source: References 1, 2, 15, 19, 21–23, 25–27, 29, 32, 39, 41, 76, 83.
* Doubtful true neuroblastomas.

In series which include children of all ages, 60 to 70 percent will have metastases at the time of diagnosis. The location of metastases is different in the neonate, about half of whom have disseminated lesions at diagnosis. In cases of congenital neuroblastoma liver metastases are present in 64 percent, subcutaneous metastases in 32 percent, and bony metastases in only 3 percent. In children older than neonates but below 2 years of age, bony metastases are found in 35 percent.[2,18] Bony metastases occur in 66 percent of children over 2 years of age.[18] Subcutaneous metastases seem to be a method of spread unique to the newborn. Hepatic metastases are also more common in the young infant.

In recent reports neuroblastomas in newborn infants have been associated with paraplegia,[19] tumor of the vagus nerve,[20] retroorbital tumor,[21] hypoglycemia,[22,23,24] mass in the scrotum,[25] homocysteinuria,[26] cervical mass,[27] and periumbilical mass.[28]

DIFFERENTIAL DIAGNOSIS

Neuroblastomas often become manifest in the first year of life, and particularly in the neonatal period. In addition they often present as an abdominal mass which may represent either the primary tumor or frequently a liver enlarged by metastases. Thus, the problem in diagnosis lies in distinguishing the mass from other causes of a palpable abdominal tumor.

Three conditions need to be considered in the differential diagnosis: First, kidney enlargement not due to tumor, such as hydronephrosis and cystic kidney. Second, *liver* enlargement not due to tumor, such as that caused by hemolytic disease, congenital syphilis, and congestive cardiac failure due to congenital heart disease. The additional clinical features, serological tests for syphilis, and demonstration of Rh or other blood group incompatibility are obvious aids in distinguishing these conditions. The occasional occurrence of jaundice and, more frequently, a moderate degree of anemia in congenital neuroblastoma may cause initial confusion, especially when the peripheral blood smear shows many normoblasts that may be misinterpreted as evidence of hemolytic disease when seen in association with anemia, jaundice and hepatomegaly. The third condition in the differential diagnosis is *other abdominal tumors* of infancy, including Wilms' tumor, lymphosarcoma, and splenomegaly due to congenital leukemia. Blood and bone marrow examination will help to differentiate leukemia,[29] although disseminated tumor cells in the bone marrow smear may be misinterpreted and lead to an erroneous diagnosis of leukemia. The differentiation among leukemic blasts, neuroblasts, and nonmalignant lymphoblasts may be extremely difficult. Erroneous diagnoses of acute leukemia are commonly made in these children.[30] Roentgen diagnostic maneuvers including I.V.P. and arteriogram may be virtually diagnostic, but tissue biopsy is needed to diagnose the other tumors. Massive hemorrhage into the adrenal gland of a neonate may produce a radiographic picture suggesting neuroblastoma.[31]

NEUROBLASTOMA IN THE FETUS

Since neuroblastomas can develop in utero, it might be supposed that, if much neuroblastomous tissue was present in the fetus, catecholamines might be released which could pass into the maternal circulation and affect the mother. If this occurred, it would be possible to recognize neuroblastoma in the unborn child. In one study there were signs and symptoms in six mothers in whose fetuses neuroblastomas had developed.[32] Sweating, pallor, tingling in the fingers, headaches, palpitations, and hypertension appeared during the last weeks of pregnancy. The symptoms exhibited by the mothers during pregnancy suggest that neuroblastomas within the fetuses secreted catecholamines which were responsible for the observed clinical effects. No one else has reported these findings in women who later delivered infants with congenital neuroblastoma.

Neuroblastoma in the fetus may show multiple sites of origin. A mature stillborn fetus was described in which a small, well-encapsulated neuroblastoma of the left adrenal gland was the only gross finding. Microscopic examination, however, revealed diffuse neoplastic involvement of the liver, adrenals, spleen, kidneys, and lungs. It appears that multicentric proliferation of undifferentiated sympathetic cell groups occurred in these organs.[33] Neuroblastoma may be the cause of antenatal death.[34,35]

Four cases of placental involvement by congenital metastasizing neuroblastoma have been reported. The diagnoses were made upon histological examination of the placenta. Numerous emboli with malignant cells were found in the vessels of the chorionic villi of the placenta. The primary neuroblastomas were located in the adrenal glands with massive spread to the liver in all cases.[14,15] While transplacental metastasis of tumor cells from mother to fetus is known to occur, the reverse has not been encountered. In one case of congenital neuroblastoma and placental metastases, fetal red blood cells were found in the maternal circulation. It is possible in this case that fetal tumor cells entered the maternal circulation via the placenta, although the mother was found to be well one year post-partum.[15] The explanation for this failure of metastases from the fetus to become established in the mother is probably related to immunological mechanisms.[14]

PECULIARITIES OF NEUROBLASTOMAS IN INFANCY

Nodular Skin Lesions

Neuroblastoma with subcutaneous metastases occurs most frequently in the neonatal period.[8,23,36] The appearance and characteristic feel of the subcutaneous lesions may be described by the term "blueberry muffin." This term, usually associated with the rubella syndrome, is borrowed to describe the infant's appearance. Similar skin lesions may be seen in congenital leukemia.[37]

Subcutaneous nodules are observed in nearly one-third of neonates with congenital neuroblastoma. The nodules are usually scattered randomly over the entire body and vary from a few millimeters to several centimeters in diameter. The nodules are firm, nontender, bluish-tinged and mobile within the subcutaneous tissue. These nodules represent disseminated disease but are not necessarily associated with a fatal prognosis, as with bony metastases. Presence of nodules should not alter the usual methods of treatment.[23] In fact, aggressive chemotherapy, X-ray therapy, or deforming surgery may be both unnecessary and dangerous in these cases.[38]

Persistent blanching in and around the cutaneous metastases of a neuroblastoma was observed in a newborn infant with neuroblastoma.[39] The skin had many firm, blue subcutaneous nodules approximately 0.5 to 1 cm in diameter located over the thorax, abdomen, and lower extremities. When palpated, these lesions initially became erythematous for 2 to 3 minutes; the lesions and a circle of the surrounding skin, 2 to 3 cm in diameter, then blanched and remained blanched for 30 to 60 minutes. Catecholamines were demonstrated in the tumor cells from a skin metastasis by electron microscopy and fluorescence histochemistry. The blanching is believed to result from local vasoconstriction following release of catecholamines from the tumor cells. The blanching phenomenon may be a useful diagnostic sign characteristic of the skin metastases of neuroblastoma.[39]

High Incidence of Liver Metastases

The distribution of liver metastases in the infantile type of neuroblastoma (Figures 2 and 3) may be explained on the basis of the anatomy of the fetal circulation.[40] Tumor emboli have less opportu-

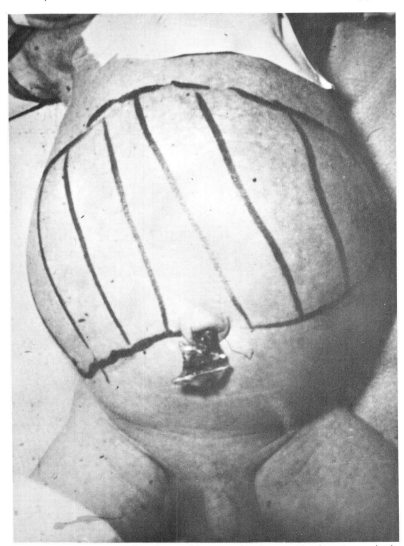

Figure 2. Neonate with adrenal neuroblastoma showing massive hepatomegaly due to liver metastases. (Courtesy of Dr. Alan H. Bennett)

nity of reaching the lung in the fetus because the foramen ovale and ductus arteriosus shunt blood past the lungs (Figure 4). Tumor emboli readily pass through the coarse filter presented by the placenta and re-enter the fetal circulation. The dictus venosus carries a large proportion of the blood directly to the liver, accounting for the greater incidence of hepatic metastases in any neoplasm in the fetus or young infant. Cases with the infantile type usually occur in infants less than 6 months of age. This mechanism does not, however, explain the occurrence of subcutaneous metastases, which are also peculiar to infants with neuroblastoma.

In metastasis of cancer the importance of mechanics is shown by the routes of spread, which determine to a great extent the location of metastases. Generally, hemic metastasis begins in the venous part of the circulatory system. It may be postulated that the spread of cancer cells ends in the capillaries of the organs, which would act, to a great extent, as filters for tumor emboli. So the "linkage" of the organs in the circulatory system plays a decisive part in hemic metastasis. In this respect conditions before and after birth differ vastly. This might result in the peculiarities of metastasis seen in fetal tumors.[40]

There are three important differences between the vascular anatomy before and after birth (Figure 4).

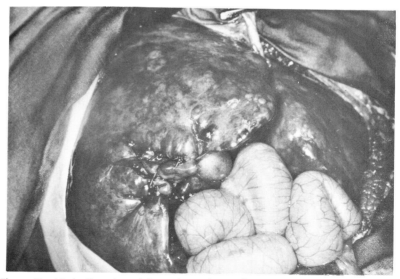

Figure 3. Markedly enlarged liver of an infant with neuroblastoma showing numerous focal metastases. X-ray therapy and chemotherapy resulted in prolonged survival. (Courtesy of Dr. Martin Winnick)

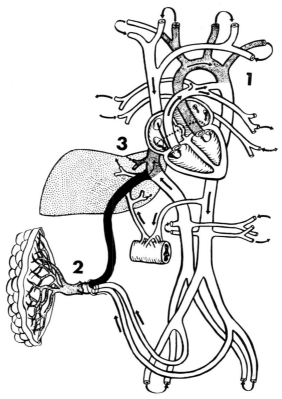

Figure 4. Diagram showing anatomy of the fetal circulation. (1) Bypassing the lungs through the foremen ovale and ductus arteriosis minimizes the likelihood of pulmonary metastases, (2) coarse filtration of the systemic blood through the placenta makes placental metastases rare, and (3) allows circulating tumor cells to lodge mainly in the liver.

1. Short circuits of the pulmonary circulation via foramen ovale and ductus arteriosus These short circuits can convey tumor emboli directly from the venous into the arterial part of the systemic circulation, thus avoiding arrest in the lungs. The ductus arteriosis reaches the aorta distal to the branches to myocardium, head, neck, and arms. Therefore, these parts of the body receive "unfiltered" blood only via the foramen ovale, whereas trunk, intestines, legs, and placenta receive unfiltered blood via both short circuits. In this connection it is of importance to know what percentage of the blood in the inferior vena cava (coming from adrenal glands, liver, placenta, and other organs) passes outside the "lung-filter" into the descending aorta and has therefore a chance of reaching the umbilical arteries. In the fetus it is estimated that at least half the blood from the inferior vena cava passes unfiltered into the descending aorta.[40]

2. The fetal placental circulation The pressure in the umbilical arteries at the end of pregnancy varies from 50 to 80 mm Hg and the pressure in the umbilical vein from 30 to 50 mm Hg, roughly a drop from 2 to 1. In all other organs the drop from arterial to venous blood pressure is approximately from 100 to 1. Thus, mechanical resistance in the placenta is exceptionally slight. Owing to wide connections between its arteries and veins, the placenta must be considered to be at most a very coarse filter for cellular constituents of the fetal blood.

3. The ductus venosus Through this vessel a part of the blood from the placenta passes outside the liver directly to the inferior vena cava. The part that goes through the liver increases relatively during fetal life, so that this finally amounts to more than half.

From these considerations it may be deduced that fetal malignant tumors originating in organs with venous drainage to the inferior vena cava have little chance of giving rise to metastases in the lungs. Via the short circuits of the pulmonary circulation tumor emboli may easily be conveyed to the descending aorta. Once in the aorta they have a good chance of passing through the placenta to the liver. Metastases in this organ will, in turn, have a strong tendency to metastasize to the liver, because the hepatic vein is one of the branches of the inferior vena cava. Compared with metastasis after birth, fetal dissemination may be expected to be characterized by extensive hepatic metastases, especially if the primary tumor is located in the drainage area of the inferior vena cava.[40]

The pathological picture of the infantile type of neuroblastoma can be explained by the mechanical influences of fetal circulatory conditions in hemic metastasis.[40] The importance of mechanical factors in hemic metastasis, especially of the anatomy of the vascular system, must be stressed. Because the fetal vascular system shows several important differences from conditions after birth, fetal metastasis must show properties different from spread with the blood after birth. These properties are deduced from what is known of the fetal circulation. A tendency to extensive metastasis in the liver, especially in tumors draining into the inferior vena cava, is considered to be predominant. It would thus appear that the characteristic features of the infantile type of neuroblastoma may be due to fetal hemic metastasis, rather than due to biological differences in the tumor.[40] But this conclusion may be disputed by reference to the concept of stage IV-S neuroblastoma. Neuroblastomas of infants often do appear to be biologically different from neuroblastomas in older children.

In many ways, the Wieberdink hypothesis seems to be an over-simplification of a complex problem. Predominance of liver metastases is not seen in Wilms' tumors in infants, in which the same hemic hydrodynamics are present. In addition, older neuroblastoma patients—that is, those beyond the neonatal period or older—seldom develop pulmonary metastases, as are frequently seen in Wilms' tumor. The Wieberdink hypothesis also fails to explain the common occurrence of skin metastases. In any event, liver metastases in neonatal neuroblastoma are not all that common.

High Rate of Spontaneous Cure

The occurrence of spontaneous cures of large neuroblastomas in young infants has been known for years.[41,42] Partial excision and chemotherapy (or no therapy) have resulted in many cures. In a study of pooled data, there is a recorded survival rate of 39.9 percent in infants under two years of age, as opposed to 7.5 percent in the older age groups. Of the newborns who had some therapy directed to the neuroblastoma, 62 percent survived.[2] Thus, the age of the patient at the onset of symptoms or at diagnosis is one of the most important factors in assessing prognosis. In general, the younger the patient, the better the chance of survival.[43] But Breslow and McCann have shown that prognosis is inversely related to age *and* stage, both being in-dependent variables.[44]

In neuroblastomas presenting in the newborn, reviews of pooled data show a cure rate varying from 62 to 70 percent.[45] In neuroblastomas presenting within the first year of life, cure rates of 56 and 72 percent are reported.[38,45] The survival rate dropped to 19 and 28 percent in the second year of life and to 5 and 12 percent in neuroblastomas presenting after two years of age (Figure 5).[38,45]

Of the 29 cases of spontaneously regressing neuroblastoma in one series, 21 were detected in infants under six months of age.[45] Their mean age was three months. Of 16 reported cases of neuroblastoma showing histologically documented, regressive maturation to ganglioneuroma that were reviewed, 11 first presented under six months of age.[45] Of this group 9 infants under three months of age manifested the disease, with 4 presenting in the newborn period. Although the primary tumor site, degree of histodifferentiation, type of therapy, and the presence of metastases, particularly to bone, obviously influence survival, age may be the overriding factor. Even the presence of skin, liver, and bony metastases does not eliminate the possibility of cure in the infant with neuroblastoma.[46] Thus, there may be regression or maturation of the metastatic lesions even in the presence of skeletal metastases. In time there may be transformation in persisting subcutaneous metastatic nodules to ganglioneuroma.[45]

Neuroblastomas seem to regress in three ways: First, there may be maturation or transformation to benign ganglioneuroma.[45] Second, there may be massive cytolysis of tumor cells resulting in hemorrhage and necrosis and eventually followed by fibrosis and/or dystrophic calcification. Finally, the tumor may completely cytolyze, leaving no recognizable residua. The probable fate of other instances of neuroblastoma in situ includes adrenal cysts, focal calcific scars, pheochromocytoma, and ganglioneuroma. It should be emphasized that maturation is by far the rarest of the three mechanisms of regression of neuroblastomas.

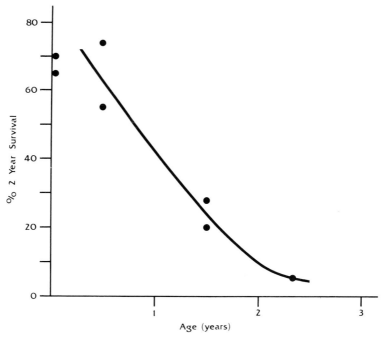

Figure 5. Relation of two-year survival rates to age of children with neuroblastoma. (Data from reported series[38,45]).

Regression of disseminated neuroblastomas Many of the clinical vagaries of neuroblastomas, such as their tendency to undergo spontaneous "maturation" and regression, are well known. Less well appreciated is the possibly related fact that certain patterns of organ involvement, almost invariably lethal in other neoplastic diseases, are associated with a good prognosis with this tumor. Specifically, patients with multiple subcutaneous nodules or with liver metastases have a surprisingly good survival experience despite the fact that malignant cells may also be present in the bone marrow.[38]

The clinical data of 100 children with neuroblastoma in one series were reviewed in detail. Various criteria thought to be of prognostic importance were tested against survival and the following staging system was evolved:[17,38]

Stage I	Tumor confined to the organ or structure of origin.
Stage II	Tumor extending in continuity beyond the organ or structure of origin but not crossing the midline. Regional lymph nodes on the ipsilateral side may be involved.
Stage III	Tumor extending in continuity beyond the midline. Regional lymph nodes may be involved bilaterally.
Stage IV	Remote disease involving the skeleton, organs, soft tissue and distant lymph node groups.
Stage IV-S	(Special category) Patients who would otherwise be stage I or II but who have remote disease confined to liver, skin, or bone marrow, and who have no radiographic evidence of bone metastases on complete skeletal survey.

These staging criteria are schematized in Figures 6 and 7.

Children with widespread neuroblastoma are generally thought to have a poor prognosis. Thus, of 131 patients with stage IV disease only 7 survived two years or longer. In sharp contrast, there was a prolonged survival rate of 84 percent of those children (21 out of 25) with stage IV-S disease; these children also had diffuse neoplastic involvement, but the metastases were limited to soft tissues.[38,47] This paradox is not observed in any other childhood malignancy.

Stage IV-S: an oncological paradox Why do stage IV-S patients show a high cure rate? Their unexpectedly good survival makes one ask if the widespread metastatic lesions are truly neoplastic foci. Their distribution, in tissues not expected to produce a neuroblastoma, favors their being metastases rather than multifocal sites of primary involvement. The frequent identification of free-floating

14

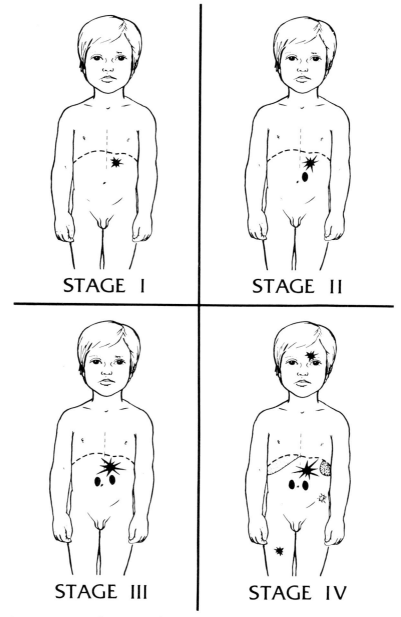

Figure 6. Criteria for staging of neuroblastomas (see text).

tumor cells and clumps in the bone marrow of children with neuroblastoma indicates that neoplastic cells are circulating throughout the
body and supports the contention that the lesions are neoplastic. But
it is still possible that the tumors represent multiple independent foci
of neuroblastoma. There are no known specific anlage in the skin or
liver, but two possible mechanisms for the development of neuroblastoma in these sites can be postulated. First, there might be an abnormal
distribution of neural crest cells during embryonic life. Alternatively, the
cells might undergo abnormal differentiation—for example, a primordial cell of neural crest origin destined to become a skin melanoblast
could aberrantly shift to a nerve-cell pattern of differentiation.[38]

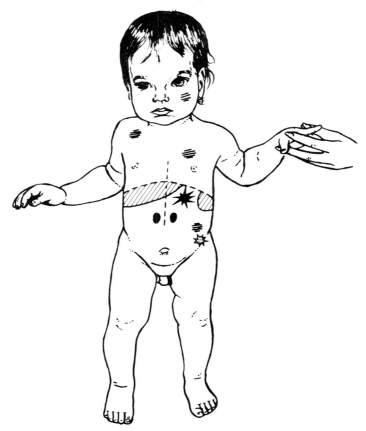

Figure 7. A 10-month old child with stigmata of stage IV-S neuroblastoma. There are metastases to liver, lymph nodes, subcutaneous tissues, and bone marrow.

Normally when a patient has neoplastic disease all through the liver and all biopsies indicate a malignant lesion, the chances for survival are nil. In stage IV-S neuroblastoma, however, the survival rate is extremely good. This has led some to wonder whether this is, in fact, metastatic disease. Is this special category of neoplasia truly dissemination of tumor or is it a multifocal origin of tumor that appears under influences not yet clearly understood? Is it possible embryologically that neuroblasts could migrate to the skin and liver and give rise to tumors there rather than being manifestations of metastatic disease?[48]

Stage IV-S patients have remote disease confined to the liver, skin, or bone marrow, or any combination of these three sites, but without radiographic evidence of bone metastases on skeletal survey. Fetal development, particularly the embryology of derivates of the neural crest, may help explain some of the observations to be made in these children.

At the very early stage in embryonic development, the primordium of the nervous system arises from the ectoderm layer. The mid-dorsal ectoderm thickens to form the neural plate. The lateral edges of this plate elevate as neural folds and finally meet in the midline where they fuse, forming the neural tube. Neural crest cells come from the ectoderm at the junction of the neural tube and epidermal areas. As the neural tube forms, they can be seen as columns of cells which extend down the length of the embryo in the "corners" dorsolateral to the neural tube (Figure 8). These neural crest cells then migrate to many different places and give rise to many different types of cells in the embryo. Of course, a number of them

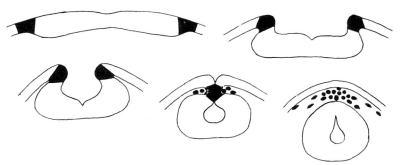

Figure 8. Stages in the formation of the neural plate and neural tube (transverse sections). Neural crest cells are in black. (Courtesy of Dr. B.I. Balinski and W.B. Saunders Company[84])

aggregate lateral to the spinal cord or the posterior part of the brain to give rise to the sensory ganglion cells. Others migrate further down to the area of the dorsal mesentery to give rise to autonomic ganglion cells. Still others migrate even further than that. For example, many embryologists agree that the melanocytes in the skin migrate from the neural crest: neural crest cells migrate along developing nerves to form Schwann cells and so on. There are, therefore, many different derivatives which migrate quite widely in the body.[48]

The neuroblastoma localized in the skin could be either neural crest cells which were unspecified at an early stage or autonomic ganglion cells which got on to the wrong migratory pathway. Everything is very close together at the stage when their migrating begins and they may migrate out to where the dermis of the skin will be instead of to the ganglion locations. On the other hand, it is quite likely that differentiation at this early time, or even later than this, is not very well fixed, so that cells are very easily influenced by environmental factors. They may be switched from melanocyte differentiation to differentiating neuroblastoma or to the nerve-cell type of pathway.[48]

One can make the same hypothesis about the liver. In other words, when the gut primordium starts to develop, there is still a great deal of mesenchyme in the dorsal mesentery. Everything is very close together so it is possible that neural crest cells infiltrate the liver itself along with autonomic cells going to adjacent structures. There is no specific neural crest derivative for the liver as in the case of the skin. However, when the liver first starts to develop as a diverticulum of the gut, it is then so close to the region where the autonomic ganglia, etc., are located that neural crest cells could be easily misdirected in their pathway.[48]

The various neural crest derivatives have been studied in culture situations. Spinal ganglia at a slightly later stage when the ganglion cells have aggregated, and even to the stage where nerve cell differentiation is beginning, will, under certain types of culture conditions, differentiate to pigment cells which really have melanin in them from presumptive spinal ganglion cells. This suggests that there is a great possibility of switching of pathways of differentiation by a number of different environmental factors.[48]

There has been no specific primordium in bone marrow except that as the mesenchyme develops a skeletal system everything is fairly close together; there are nerve and Schwann cells, which normally could migrate in proximity, if not right into the bone marrow in such numbers. In this way, one might postulate how bone marrow may be involved by neuroblastoma cells, similar to involvement of liver and skin, from the embryologic derivation of neural crest tissue.[48]

Thus, in stage IV-S neuroblastoma, the tumor behaves in a benign manner; it often behaves as though it were not neoplasm at all, but undeveloped nerve tissue. There is evidence to suggest that those wandering cells could explain all of the signs we have seen in patients with stage IV-S disease, and that the same factors that cause them to go to the wrong place could maintain them in a relatively underdeveloped status.[48] It is as though in the process of migration cells derived from the neural crest "set up housekeeping" in the wrong place.

The reasons for spontaneous regression of neuroblastomas remain speculative, but there can be no doubt that it exists and that it must be credited, in large part, for the survival of these patients. Laboratory evidence of tumor-host interaction is being accumulated, but it remains to be shown why children with neuroblastoma develop especially potent mechanisms for tumor regression. In fact it can only be speculated that factors of this kind are indeed responsible for tumor disappearance.

It appears that a certain grace period exists during fetal life and early infancy during which the organism is relatively resistant to the development or progression of malignant disease. Increased cancer resistance might further be reflected by higher survival rates or a greater tendency toward spontaneous regression or maturation, or both, in potentially malignant tumors present at birth or appearing in the very young infant.[45]

Role of immunology in neuroblastoma regression Children in whom neuroblastoma is diagnosed before the age of two years have a good prognosis compared with older patients. Reports of neuroblastoma "in situ" (microscopic tumor in the adrenal glands found at necropsy in children under three months old dying of other causes), spontaneous remissions, and unexpectedly favorable responses to therapy in infants suggest that an immune mechanism may be involved. Neuroblastoma cells can be inhibited in vitro by a patient's own lymphocytes or by lymphocytes from the mother. Furthermore, there appears to be a serum factor associated with growing tumor which, in vitro, blocks the cytotoxic effect of the lymphocyte.[49]

A hypothesis has been offered to explain the age-dependent cure rate in neuroblastoma[49] (Figure 9). When tumor develops in the fetus, tumor antigens sensitize fetal lymphocytes but do not yet give rise to the blocking factor. This possibility is strengthened by the demonstration of delayed hypersensitivity to tuberculin from B.C.G. vaccination and dinitrofluorobenzene at birth. Ability to produce blocking factor develops only after birth, analogous to the delayed production of 7S gamma globulins. These same tumor antigens may be released and cross the placenta to the maternal circulation, where both sensitized lymphocytes and blocking factors are produced. The maternal blocking factor alone crosses the placenta and inhibits fetal-lymphocyte

BEFORE BIRTH

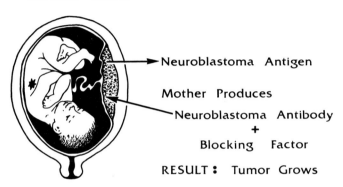

Neuroblastoma Antigen

Mother Produces
Neuroblastoma Antibody
+
Blocking Factor

RESULT: Tumor Grows

AFTER BIRTH

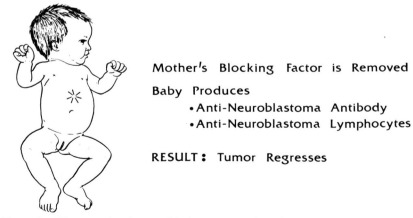

Mother's Blocking Factor is Removed

Baby Produces
• Anti-Neuroblastoma Antibody
• Anti-Neuroblastoma Lymphocytes

RESULT: Tumor Regresses

Figure 9. Diagrams showing possible immunological mechanism causing regression of neuroblastomas during infancy.

anti-tumor activity. Consequently, growth of the fetal tumor is uncontrolled until after birth, when the level of maternal blocking factor declines, allowing autologous sensitized lymphocytes to assume their appropriate activity.[49]

Neuroblastoma "in situ," then, may be explained by the persistence of effective maternal tumor-blocking-factor titers up to three months of age, after which its natural decline would be associated with autologous, lymphocyte-mediated tumor destruction. If tumor growth in utero and in the early months of life was extensive enough to be clinically evident, the decline of maternal blocking factor could be manifested either by "spontaneous cures" or by cures assisted by chemotherapy, surgery, or radiotherapy. Cure would be decreasingly likely as the infant became able to synthesize effective levels of blocking factor.[49]

Experimental models and in vitro colony-inhibition studies with serum and tumor from very young children with neuroblastoma might be applied to test this hypothesis. The clinical implications are that therapy in neuroblastoma might be directed toward reducing the blocking factor and tumor mass without suppressing the cell-mediated immune reaction.[49]

It appears that in infants with stage IV-S neuroblastoma the full development or progression of neuroblastomas is modified or suppressed. Translated into cellular terms, it is suggested that specific repressive influences are exerted in certain infants on the expression of an inborn cancer genome. The net effects on the tumor cell could be either lytic, antimitotic, or cytodifferentiative. At some later point in development, derepression of the cancer genome would permit the full emergence and progression of a malignancy. Investigations into what mechanisms might be involved in this early repression of cancer could be of paramount importance in furthering the understanding and treatment of neoplasms at all ages.[45]

ROLE OF NERVE GROWTH FACTOR IN NEUROBLASTOMA REGRESSION

The nerve growth factor (NGF) is a protein which selectively stimulates the growth of sympathetic and embryonic spinal sensory ganglia. In vivo, NGF induces in the ganglionic neurons a considerable increase in size and a profuse outgrowth of fibers, a relatively moderate increase in cell numbers, and an accelerated differentiation. In vitro, a similar cellular hypertrophy and fiber outgrowth are observed.[50] A fundamental attribute of NGF is its high cell specificity—no tissues other than the sympathetic and spinal sensory ganglia have been found, thus far, to be affected. Evidence for a physiologic and essential requirement for NGF was provided by the extensive destruction of the sympathetic system in animals injected with rabbit anti-NGF antiserum. Similarly, in vitro, ganglia are destroyed by the antiserum, and conversely dissociated ganglionic neurons can survive in culture only in the presence of NGF.[50]

It has been suggested repeatedly that neuroblastoma cells are able to mature in vivo and that the clinical effects of the tumor correlate with its degree of maturation. The demonstration by Goldstein[51] that neuroblastoma cells will undergo complete maturation if transferred from their host to an in vitro environment strongly indicated that it is a host's condition, rather than intrinsic cellular properties, which supports the persistence or the growth of the neuroblastoma; and it is its fluctuations which are at the base of corresponding fluctuations in the morphology and the clinical manifestations of the tumor. The simplest of such conditions would be a chemical agent, produced by the host and affecting the growth and/or the differentiation of the tumor cells. NGF appears to be a ready-made candidate for such an agent. It affects growth and differentiation in cells which, like the neuroblastoma cells, are neural crest derivatives, can be produced outside the responsive tissue, and, furthermore, can undergo structural changes which affect its biological activity. However, before NGF can be accepted for such a role in the pathology of the tumor, evidence must be obtained that (a) neuroblastoma patients show NGF abnormalities, whether qualitative or quantitative or both; (b) variations of these abnormalities are paralleled by tumoral changes; and (c) the survival, growth, or maturation of the tumor cells are affected by normal or abnormal NGF.[52]

Nerve growth factor and its antibody have profound effects on sympathetic tissue. It seems, therefore, that there might be a number of ways in which these substances could affect neoplastic tissue of sympathetic origin, such as neuroblastoma:

1. Anti-NGF might destroy a neuroblastoma just as it destroys non-neoplastic sympathetic tissue.

2. NGF might cause a neuroblastoma to mature.

In vitro, NGF causes changes in cultured sympathetic cells, including increases in neurite formation and cell size, which could be interpreted as maturation. Thus, it seems possible that the administration of NGF to children with widespread neuroblastoma might accelerate maturation and retard or even stop the growth of the tumor. For this reason, it was decided that three children suffering from widespread neuroblastoma would be treated with intramuscular injections of NGF. But the injections did not seem to influence the course of their tumors.[53]

In another study, examination of sera from 621 normal individuals and 7 children with neuroblastoma failed to provide evidence that children with neuroblastoma had abnormally high levels of NGF activity.[54] Earlier studies[55,56] had suggested that there might be a relationship between presence of the NGF in the serum and regression of neuroblastoma. But subsequent studies did not confirm this hypothesis.

The main object of this study was to explore the possibility of a relationship between the NGF/anti-NGF system, and the factors which initiate and determine the progress of neuroblastoma. Many children's tumors should probably be regarded not merely as groups of disorganized cells but as manifestations of inborn abnormalities involving the whole patient. If a neuroblastoma were initiated by an inborn metabolic error involving NGF, it might be reflected in abnormal NGF activity in the serum. The observation that the NGF activity of the sera of 7 children with neuroblastoma was normal is evidence against a disturbance of NGF metabolism being the cause or the result of these tumors.[54]

So far we have been unable to demonstrate that the NGF/anti-NGF system has any relevance to development or regression of neuroblastoma, but it remains possible that our failure was due to the fact that so little is known about the chemistry and biology of these substances. Evidence is accumulating that NGF is a group of proteins of varying molecular weights with similar biological effects. Assuming that the different preparations owe their activity to a particular structure of one part of a large molecule, much work is being devoted to the discovery of an NGF with a low molecular weight. But it seems that we are being forced to conclude that NGF probably has no role in the treatment of neuroblastoma.[54]

NEUROBLASTOMA IN SITU

In infants dying of non-neoplastic causes, small foci of cells morphologically reminiscent of neuroblasts can sometimes be found in the adrenals of fetuses and newborns up to the age of three months (Figure 10).[57,58] This finding has been called neuroblastoma in situ by

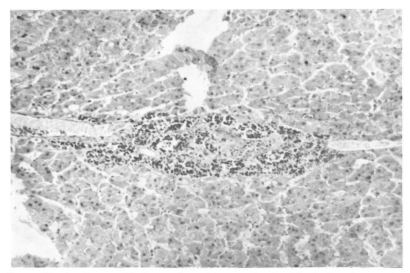

Figure 10. In situ neuroblastoma adjacent to central vein of fetal adrenal cortex in a 20-hour-old premature infant (H and E × 210). (Courtesy of Dr. D. Shanklin and *Biology of the Neonate*[60])

Beckwith and Perrin.[59] In situ neuroblastomas are minute, incidentally encountered adrenal tumors which appear to represent an early stage in the histogenesis of neuroblastomas. These tumors are cytologically identical with typical malignant neuroblastoma, but are rendered distinctive by their microscopic size and by the absence of demonstrable metastases. Neuroblastoma in situ is present in the adrenals of about 1 out of 250 new-born infants (Table 2).[59,60,61,62] Frank neuroblastoma, however, develops in only about 1 in every 10,000 live-born infants. Thus, the frequency of incidental or in situ

Table 2
Incidence of Neuroblastoma In Situ from
Reported Series

Authors	Cases of In Situ Neuroblastoma	Number of Patients Surveyed
Guin, 1969	6	2,596
	4	155
	1	100
Shanklin, 1969	3	471
Beckwith, 1963	7	1,571
Total	21	4,893
Average incidence	1	233

neuroblastomas in children under three months of age exceeds the clinical occurrence of these tumors by a factor of 40.[59,60,62] If indeed neuroblastoma in situ is a primal expression of a neuroblastoma gene, a considerable proportion of such tumors must, with age, disappear, mature, or convert to forms no longer recognizable as neuroblastomas.[63]

Oncogenetic significance of in situ tumors Thus, neuroblastomas in situ have important implications from the standpoint of the natural history of these tumors, particularly in regard to their spontaneous regression (Figure 11). There are several possible interpretations of the significance of in situ neuroblastomas. One is that they do not represent malignant neuroblastomatous foci at all but are residua of normal fetal anlage. Fetal neuroblasts are indistinguishable morphologically from their malignant counterparts postnatally. Another interpretation is that they are early neuroblastomas which would have gone on to become clinically apparent, had their "host" not succumbed to another condition. Morphologic observations support this concept, since their appearance differs in no way from typical malignant neuroblastomas, and there is evidence of both proliferative and invasive activity. However, the frequency with which in situ neuroblastomas are encountered is very much against

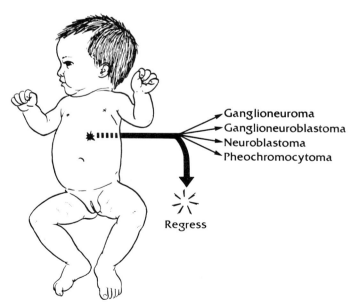

Ganglioneuroma
Ganglioneuroblastoma
Neuroblastoma
Pheochromocytoma

Regress

Figure 11. The possible fates of in situ neuroblastomas. The leading theoretical possibilities are shown.

this concept. If we assume that every potential neuroblastoma is present at the time of birth as recognizable tumor, then the incidence of early neuroblastomas in the adrenal glands of a random population of young infants should not exceed the proportion of liveborn infants who will eventually be found to have primary adrenal neuroblastomas. It is probable that neuroblastomas may take origin beyond the period of infancy, since immature neural crest tissue persists at least until puberty. In this case, the expected incidence of early tumors in infants should be even lower.[59]

In situ neuroblastomas represent a broad spectrum. The earliest lesions are microscopic in situ tumors. A more advanced stage in the development of the neuroblastoma is also observed. The tumor in these cases may replace the medulla and compress the cortical tissue but does not grossly enlarge the adrenal gland. In still other cases the tumor expands the adrenal gland, replaces the medulla, focally destroys the cortex, compresses the remaining cortical tissue, and impinges upon the capsule of the gland. Evidence of necrosis and fibrosis may be present, suggesting beginning resolution. No metastases are present in these cases, and none of the tumors produce clinical symptoms.[62]

The frequent association of in situ neuroblastoma and congenital anomalies is considered to be spurious rather than real.[60] The concordance of these disorders nevertheless provides a fortuitous opportunity to observe the various stages in the natural history of neuroblastoma. The dramatic cutoff point of 3 months of age, beyond which no in situ tumors are found, implies an important time-growth relationship with regard to the natural history of neuroblastoma, recalling its potential for spontaneous resolution.

Investigation of excretion patterns of catecholamines and metabolites in infants may offer a feasible approach to early diagnosis of neuroblastoma.[62,64] With regard to earlier diagnosis the application of the urine spot test or dipstick test* on a widespread public health basis could now become a reality.[64] This has been done successfully in phenylketonuria which has approximately the same incidence as neuroblastoma. One testing would not suffice, of course, but routine tests during well-child visits either on wet diapers or fresh urine could become an integral part of standard care. If this were done three times during the first year, twice during the second year, and annually thereafter to the age of 5, there is reason to believe the survival rates in neuroblastoma would be sharply improved. This is being done in some areas of this country and in Japan.[64] However, the total cost of

*Testrip⁸ is made by Kallestad Laboratories, Inc., Minneapolis, Minnesota.

such a screening program has been thought by some to be prohibitively high.[65] We must weigh this cost against the dismal outcome in older children after costly prolonged and painful therapy, bearing in mind the excellent cure rates in very young children with early lesions. In addition, the reliability of this test has been questioned and further studies in evaluation are needed.[66] This test cannot be easily or simply evaluated. False positive tests may cause undue alarm in the parents and require a considerable amount of the pediatrician's time in explorations. A positive test would be a signal for more thorough laboratory (biochemical) evaluation, not necessarily for prolonged and costly x-ray examinations.

FAMILIAL NEUROBLASTOMA

The occurrence of neuroblastoma in more than one member of a sibship has been reported in a total of only six families.[67] Therefore, neuroblastoma has not been thought to be hereditary in origin.[68] The incidence of familial neuroblastoma is difficult to ascertain because of the extreme variability of the natural course of the tumor. There has been such a poor survival rate that weak penetrance could well be masked. Chatten and Voorhess[69] observed a family of five siblings, four of whom had neuroblastoma. In another family, studies of two siblings with neuroblastoma and one of their parents suggested gene mutation and an autosomal dominant pattern of inheritance.[70]

Neuroblastomas have been thought to be the result of somatic mutation because of the scarcity of familial case aggregates.[71,72] However, it is possible that a tumor of neural crest origin can arise as a result of mutation of those genes that will form the neural crest and be transmitted in an autosomal dominant pattern. This possibility is best exemplified by the mode of inheritance of multiple neurofibromatosis and pheochromocytoma. Neurofibromas, ganglioneuromas, pheochromocytomas, and neuroblastomas (all of which are of neural crest origin) have been shown to co-exist in various combinations within the same individual. Bolande and Towler[63] found ultrastructural similarities among ganglioneuroma, neurofibroma, and neuroblastoma maturing into ganglioneurofibroma and theorized that neurofibromatosis may in some instances be derived from disseminated neuroblastoma or aberrantly migrating neural crest cells. Thus, it is conceivable that neuroblastoma may be transmitted in a dominant manner after mutation of the genes governing neural crest formation. The increased excretion of VMA in the urine of parents and unaffected siblings suggests that there may be some abnormality of neural crest origin (possibly in situ neuroblastomas) in unaffected family members.[63,69,73] In those children who actually develop a clinically manifest neuroblastoma, host factors and modifying genes may play a role in development of the tumor.

The etiology of neuroblastoma remains unknown. Studies of the relatives of children having neuroblastoma and children of survivors of neuroblastoma may delineate the true familial incidence of this tumor, as well as provide clues to host factors or modifying genes which may determine the clinical appearance of the tumor.[70] In one case familial neuroblastoma occurred in association with trisomy 13.[74]

Several genetic mechanisms might explain the distribution of affected members in these families. Autosomal dominant inheritance was suggested and this mechanism is believed to be the cause of most familial tumors. To explain the relatively large number of non-familial cases of neuroblastoma, including three examples of discordant twin pairs, it must be assumed that many sporadic cases arise by mutation and represent lethal genes, or that the dominant gene has variable penetrance or expression. Thus, some families with more than one affected member may not be identified because the tumor is present as an in situ lesion, spontaneously regresses, or matures into a benign tumor. It is also possible that neuroblastoma represents a combination of genes controlling neural-crest development. The café-au-lait spots in the paternal members of one family may represent a second genetic factor contributing to the incidence of tumor in the offspring.[69]

The case of a child affected with three tumors—neuroblastoma, ganglioneuroma, and neurofibromatosis—was reported.[75] Germinal mutation is probably the cause of this coincidence. In view of the dominant inheritance of neuroblastomatosis and of pheochromocytoma, the inference is made that neuroblastoma generally may be attributable to a dominant mutation which in the past has been lethal but which, as a result of therapeutic progress, may be inherited by the offspring of survivors in the future, as has been noted for retinoblastomas.[75,76]

NEUROBLASTOMAS IN ANIMALS

An animal tumor model for neuroblastoma has been sought for many years. There is a mouse tumor, the C-1300 in the A/J mouse, which has many points of similarity with the human neoplasm.[77]

Neuroblastomas seem to be rare in domestic animals; the cases reported are too few to indicate any species prevalence. They have been observed in the dog, pig, ox, horse, cat, rabbit, and chicken. Unlike neuroblastoma in man, incidence generally increases with age. No cases have been reported in very young animals. There is no apparent breed or sex prevalence.[78] These tumors are usually solitary but may be multiple. In all animals they are most commonly found in the adrenal medulla and in the abdominal and pelvic sympathetic chain of ganglia and associated celiac and mesenteric ganglia. They are also found in the cervical and thoracic parts of the sympathetic system and the ganglia within the visceral organs.[78]

Willis referred to the occurrence of adrenal ganglioneuromas in two rats. Ganglioneuromas are not uncommon in whales and in other fish. A six-month-old rabbit with neuroblastoma of the neck and metastases to lungs, liver, and spleen is mentioned.[79] Metastatic neuroblastomas were also described in cows. Neuroblastoma occurred in a 9½-year-old Chihuahua dog. The tumor originated in both adrenal glands and caused venous distension and edema of the hind legs. There was no mention of metastases to the liver or to other organs.[80] A 15-year-old male Irish Setter dog developed a large neuroblastoma in the periadrenal area. There were metastases to liver and lungs.[81] A 2-year-old Boxer dog developed an abdominal neuroblastoma with metastases to liver, heart and skin.[82] Neuroblastomas and ganglioneuromas occur in chickens. In one case there were liver metastases.[83] However, widespread dissemination of neuroblastomas has not been described in fowl.

SUMMARY AND CONCLUSIONS

Neuroblastomas may occur in the fetus. When they do, they may cause stillbirth or, in rare instances, catecholamine-related symptoms in the mother. Neuroblastomas occurring during infancy are unique because of the occurrence of skin "metastases," the high incidence of liver "metastases," and the high rate of spontaneous cure. The high incidence of liver involvement may in part be due to the peculiarities of the fetal circulation causing increased perfusion of the liver by blood from the systemic circulation and bypassing or shunting of blood past the lungs. Newborn infants and young children with neuroblastoma may have widely disseminated disease in the liver, skin, and other soft tissues (stage IV-S). But, paradoxically, they may still respond well to therapy and show a high rate of cure. Nerve growth factor probably plays no significant role in either the development or regression of neuroblastomas.

Neuroblastoma in situ is present in the adrenal glands in about 1 in 250 fetuses and infants who are less than three months of age, whereas clinically manifest neuroblastoma has an incidence of about 1 in 10,000 live births. It is believed that the surplus cases of neuroblastoma in situ regress spontaneously. Familial occurrence of neuroblastoma has been noted in a few cases. Certain other members of these neuroblastoma families show persistent increase in urinary excretion of VMA. Neuroblastomas occur in domestic animals, but they are rare and tend to occur in older age groups rather than during very early life as in humans.

REFERENCES

1. Schneider, K., Becker, J., and Krasna, I.: Neonatal neuroblastoma. *Pediatrics* 36: 359–366, 1965.

2. Becker, J., Schneider, K., and Krasna, I.: Neonatal neuroblastoma. *Progress Clin. Cancer* 4: 382–386, 1970.

3. MacKenzie, D., Ham, J., and Hyslop, R.: Congenital neuroblastoma. *Aus. N.Z. J. Surg.* 34: 173–177, 1968.

4. Rickham, P., and Johnston, J.: *Neonatal Surgery.* London: Butterworths, 1969, pp. 591–595.

5. Olsen, A., and Bennett, S.: Congenital neuroblastoma. *J. Amer. Med. Wom. Ass.* 18: 548–551, 1963.

6. Pepper, W.: A study of congenital sarcoma of the liver and suprarenal; with report of a case. *Amer. J. Med. Sci.* 121: 287–299, 1901.

7. Hutchison, R.: On suprarenal sarcoma in children with metastases in the skull. *Quart. J. Med.* 1: 33–38, 1907.

8. Erp, J.: Cutaneous metastases in neuroblastoma. *Dermatologia* 136: 265–269, 1968.

9. Hornstein, O., and Muckle, G.: Kutan metastasierendes Neuroblastoma sympathicum mit "spontan" regressiven Verlauf. *Dermatologica* 120: 35–52, 1960.

10. Montgomery, H., and O'Leary, P.A.: Multiple ganglioneuromas of the skin. *Arch. Derm. Syph.,* 29: 26–53, 1934.

11. Helson, L., Fleisher, M., Bethune, V., et al.: Urinary Cystathionine, Catecholamine, and Metabolites in Patients with Neuroblastoma. *Clin. Chem.* 18: 613–615, 1972.

12. Helson, L.: Neuroblastoma; early diagnosis a key to successful treatment. (C. Pochedly, ed.) In *Clinical Management of Cancer in Children.* Acton, MA.: Publishing Sciences Group, Inc., 1975.

13. Falkenburg, L.W., and Kay, M.N.: A case of congenital

sympathagonioma (neuroblastoma) of the right adrenal simulating erythroblastosis fetalis. *J. Pediat.* 42: 462–465, 1953.

14. Strauss, L., and Driscoll, S.: Congenital neuroblastoma involving the placenta; report of two cases. *Pediatrics* 34: 23–31, 1964.

15. Anders, D., Kindermann, G., and Pfeifer, U.: Metastasizing fetal neuroblastoma with involvement of the placenta simulating erythroblastosis, report of 2 cases. *J. Pediatr.* 82: 50–53, 1973.

16. Berger, R.: Neonatal malignancy; report of 2 cases. *Amer. Osteopath. Ass. J.* 66: 825–839, 1967.

17. Evans, A., D'Angio, G.J., and Randolph, J.: A proposed staging for children with neuroblastoma. *Cancer* 27: 374–378, 1971.

18. Sutow, W.W.: Prognosis in Neuroblastoma of Childhood. *Amer. J. Dis. Child.* 96: 299, 1958.

19. Rothner, A.D.: Congenital "dumbbell" neuroblastoma with paraplegia. *Clin. Pediat.* 10: 235–236, 1971.

20. Rosedale, R.: Neuroblastoma of nodose ganglion of infant vagus nerve. *Arch. Otolaryng.* 80: 454–459, 1964.

21. Mehta, M., and Bubariwalla, R.: Neuroblastoma in the newborn. *Indian Pediat.* 8: 74–75, 1971.

22. Shuangshoti, S., and Ekarapbanich, S.: Congenital neuroblastoma and hyperplasia of islets of Langerhaus in an infant. *Clin. Pediat.* 11: 241–243, 1972.

23. Shown, T., and Durfee, M.: Blueberry muffin baby; neonatal neuroblastoma with subcutaneous metastases. *J. Urol.* 104: 193–195, 1970.

24. Shapiro, M., Simcha, A., Rosenmann, E., and Shafrir, E.: Hypoglycemia associated with neonatal neuroblastoma and abnormal responses of serum glucose and free fatty acids to epinephrine injection. *Israel J. Med. Sci.* 2: 705–714, 1966.

25. Simpson, T., Lynn, H., and Mills, S.: Congenital neuroblastoma in the scrotum. *Clin. Pediat.* 8: 174–175, 1969.

26. Monch, E., Stefan, H., and Kaser, H.: Neuroblastoma of the Pepper type with homocysteinuria. *Helvet. Pediat. Acta.* 25: 530–541, 1970.

27. Bonamico, M., and Cozzi, F.: Ganglioneuroblastoma of the neck in a newborn. *Minerva Pediat.* 24: 266–260, 1972.

28. Pande, S., and Talwar, G.: Congenital extra-adrenal neuroblastoma. *Indian Pediat.* 3: 339–343, 1966.

29. Evans, A.R.: Congenital neuroblastoma. *J. Clin. Path.* 18: 54–62, 1965.

30. Evans, A.E., and Hummeler, K.: The significance of primitive cells in marrow aspirates to children with neuroblastoma. *Cancer* 32: 906–912, 1973.

31. Rose, J., Berdon, W., Sullivan, T., and Baker, D.: Prolonged jaundice as presenting sign of massive adrenal hemorrhage in newborn. *Radiology* 98: 263–272, 1971.

32. Voute, P., Wadman, S., and Von Patten, W.: Congenital neuroblastoma; symptoms in the mother during pregnancy. *Clin. Pediat.* 9: 206–207, 1970.

33. Birner, W.: Neuroblastoma as a cause of antenatal death. *Amer. J. Obst. Gynec.* 82: 1388–1391, 1961.

34. Muller, M.: Metastatic neuroblastoma with intrauterine stillbirth. *Zbl. allg. Path.* 108: 356–358, 1966.

35. Potter, E., and Parish, J.M.: Neuroblastoma, ganglioneuroma, and fibroneuroma in a stillborn fetus. *Amer. J. Path.* 18: 141–151, 1942.

36. Tachdjian, M., and Matson, D.: Orthopedic aspects of intraspinal tumors in infants and children. *J. Bone Joint Surg.* 47-A: 223–248, 1965.

37. van Eys, J., and Flexner, J.: Transient spontaneous remission in a case of untreated congenital leukemia. *Amer. J. Dis. Child.* 118: 507–514, 1969.

38. D'Angio, G.J., et al.: Special pattern of widespread neuroblastoma with a favorable prognosis. *Lancet* 1: 1046–1049, 1971.

39. Hawthorne, H., Nelson, J., Witzleben, C., and Giangiacomo, J.: Blanching subcutaneous nodules in neonatal neuroblastoma. *J. Pediatr.* 77: 297–300, 1970.

40. Wieberdink, J.: Foetal haemic metastasis; an explanation of the Pepper-type metastasis in adrenal neuroblastoma. *Brit. J. Cancer* 11: 378–383, 1957.

41. Fortner, J., Nicastri, A., and Murphy, M.L.: Neuroblastoma; natural history and results of treating 133 cases. *Ann. Surg.* 167: 132–142, 1968.

42. Lehman, E.P.: Adrenal neuroblastoma in infancy; 15-year survival. *Ann. Surg.* 95: 473, 1932.

43. Swank, R., Fetterman, G.H., Sieber, W., and Kiesewetter, W.: Prognostic factors in neuroblastoma. *Ann. Surg.* 174: 428–435, 1971.

44. Breslow, N., and McCann, B.: Statistical estimation of prognosis for children with neuroblastoma. *Cancer Res.* 31: 2098–2103, 1971.

45. Bolande, R.: Benignity of neonatal tumors and concept of cancer repression in early life. *Amer. J. Dis. Child.* 122: 12–14, 1971.

46. Reilly, D., Nesbit, M.E., and Krivit, W.: Cure of three patients who had skeletal metastases in disseminated neuroblastoma. *Pediatrics* 41: 47, 1968.

47. Pochedly, C.: Neuroblastoma in infancy; study of an oncological paradox. Medikon (Ghent) 2: 357–363, 1973.

48. Tefft, M., D'Angio, G.J., Lysor, K., and Urunoy, G.: Neuroblastoma, stage IV-S, a special entity? *Clin. Bull. Memorial Sloan-Kettering Cancer Center* 1: 61–65, 1971.

49. Helson, L.: Regression of neuroblastomas. *Lancet* 1: 1075–1076, 1971.

50. Varon, S.: Nerve growth factors; a selective review. *J. Pediatr. Surg.* 3: 120–124, 1968.

51. Goldstein, M., Burdman, J., and Journey, L.J.: Long-term tissue culture of neuroblastomas. II. Morphologic evidence for differentiation and maturation. *J. Nat. Cancer Inst.* 32: 165–179, 1964.

52. Varon, S.: Possible involvement of nerve growth factors in neuroblastoma pathology. *J. Pediatr. Surg.* 3: 165–166, 1968.

53. Kumar, S., Steward, J., Waghe, M., et al.: The administration of nerve growth factor to children with widespread neuroblastoma. *J. Pediatr. Surg.* 5: 18–22, 1970.

54. Waghe, M., Kumar, S., and Steward, J.: Nerve growth factor in human sera. *J. Pediatr. Surg.* 5: 14–17, 1970.

55. Burdman, J., and Goldstein, M.: Long-term tissue culture of neuroblastomas. III. In vitro studies of nerve growth factor stimulating factor in sera of children with neuroblastoma. *J. Nat. Cancer Inst.* 33: 123–133, 1964.

56. Bill, A.: A study of nerve growth factor in the serum of neuroblastoma patients. *J. Pediatr. Surg.* 3: 171–177, 1968.

57. Reisman, M., Goldenberg, E., and Gordon, J.: Congenital heart disease and neuroblastoma. *Amer. J. Dis. Child.* 111: 308–310, 1966.

58. Beckwith, J.B. and Martin, R.: Observations on the histopathology of neuroblastoma. *J. Pediatr. Surg.* 3: 106–110, 1968.

59. Beckwith, J.B., and Perrin, E.: In situ neuroblastomas; a contribution to the natural history of neural crest tumors. *Amer. J. Path.* 43: 1089–1104, 1963.

60. Shanklin, D., and Sotelo-Avila, C.: In situ tumors in fetuses, newborns and young infants. *Biol. Neonat.* 14: 286–316, 1969.

61. Tubergen, D., and Heyn, R.: In situ neuroblastoma associated with an adrenal cyst. *J. Pediatr.* 76: 451–453, 1970.

62. Guin, G., Gilbert, E., and Jones, B.: Incidental neuroblastoma in infants. *Amer. J. Clin. Path.* 51: 126–136, 1969.

63. Bolande, R., and Towler, W.: A possible relationship of neuroblastoma to Von Recklinghousen's disease. *Cancer* 26: 162–175, 1970.

64. Leonard, A.S., Roback, S.A., Nesbit, M.E., and Freier, E.: The VMA test strip; A new tool for mass screening, diagnosis and management of catecholamine secreting tumors. *J. Pediatr. Surg.* 7: 528–531, 1972.

65. Hallett, G.W.: Urine VMA screening for neuroblastoma; is it worth the cost? *Pediatrics* 51: 757, 1973.

66. Helson, L., Bethune, V., and Schwartz, M.: Clinical evaluation of the VMA test strip. *Pediatrics* 51: 153, 1973.

67. Wagget, J., Aherne, G., and Aherne, W.: Familial neuroblastoma; report of two sib pairs. *Arch. Dis. Childh.* 48: 63–66, 1973.

68. Miller, R.W., Fraumeni, J.F., and Hill, J.A.: Neuroblastoma; Epidemiologic approach to its origin. *Amer. J. Dis. Child* 115: 253–261, 1968.

69. Chatten, J., and Voorhess, M.: Familial neuroblastoma; report of a kindred with multiple disorders, including neuroblastomas in 4 siblings. *N. Engl. J. Med.* 277: 1230–1236, 1967.

70. Wong, K-Y, Hanenson, I.B., and Lampkin, B.: Familial neuroblastoma. *Amer. J. Dis. Child.* 121: 415–416, 1971.

71. Wilfrido, M.S., and Edmonson, J.H.: The developmental defects associated with neuroblastoma—etiologic implications. *Cancer* 22: 234–238, 1968.

72. Hardy, P., and Nesbit, M.: Familial neuroblastoma; report of a kindred with a high incidence of infantile tumors. *J. Pediatr.* 80: 74–77, 1972.

73. Helson, L., Blasco, P., and Murphy, M.L.: Familial neuroblastoma. *Clin. Res.* 17: 614, 1969.

74. Feingold, M., Gherodi, G., and Simons, C.: Familial neuroblastoma and trisomy 13. *Amer. J. Dis. Child.* 121: 451, 1971.

75. Knudson, A., and Amromin, G.: Neuroblastoma and ganglioneuroma in child with multiple neurofibromatosis; implications for the mutational origin of neuroblastoma. *Cancer* 19: 1032–1037, 1966.

76. Griffin, M., and Bolande, R.: Familial neuroblastoma with regression and maturation to ganglioneurofibroma. *Pediatrics* 43: 377–382, 1969.

77. Furmanski, P., and Lubin, M.: Effects of dimethylsulfoxide on expression of differentiated functions in mouse neuroblastoma. *J. Natl. Cancer Inst.* 48: 1355–1361, 1972.

78. Moulton, J.E.: *Tumors in Domestic Animals.* Los Angeles: University of California Press, 1961, pp. 1217.

79. Willis, R.: *Pathology of Tumours* (4th Ed.) New York: Appleton-Century-Crofts, 1967, p. 883.

80. Frye, F., and Clement, E.: Sympathicoblastoma in a dog. *J.A.V.M.A.* 156: 900–901, 1970.

81. Simon, J., and Albert, L.T.: Two cases of neuroblastoma in dogs. *J.A.V.M.A.* 136: 210–214, 1960.

82. Campbell, J.: *Tumours of the Fowl.* Philadelphia: J.B. Lippincott Company, 1969, pp. 243, 245, 246.

83. Vinik, M., et al.: Congenital malignant tumors. *Cancer* 19: 967–979, 1966.

84. Balinski, B.I.: *An Introduction to Embryology.* Philadelphia: W. B. Saunders Company, 1960, p. 143.

2 Neuroblastoma in the Head and Central Nervous System

Carl Pochedly, M.D.

1. Primary intracranial neuroblastomas
2. Metastases to brain in neuroblastoma
3. Periorbital metastases
   a. Incidence
   b. Clinical picture
   c. Pathology and pathogenesis
   d. Other orbital tumors
4. Olfactory neuroblastomas
5. Cerebellar encephalopathy and neuroblastoma
   a. Therapy
   b. Etiology
6. Spinal cord compression due to neuroblastoma
   Summary and Conclusions

The neurological manifestations of neuroblastoma result from rare primary tumors in the brain and, in rare instances, from metastases to the brain or spinal cord from tumors originating elsewhere in the body. Metastases may produce either early or late neurological signs. In this chapter the clinical manifestations of primary and metastatic neuroblastomas affecting the head and central nervous system are described. The various sites of neurological involvement (Figure 1) and the resultant signs, symptoms and clinical course of children with neuroblastomas in the head and central nervous system will be reviewed.

It should be emphasized that brain metastases of neuroblastoma—that is, deposits in the substance of the brain—are practically unknown. There are many examples of compression of the brain, but even extension of neuroblastoma through the dura into the underlying brain or cord is uncommon.

PRIMARY INTRACRANIAL NEUROBLASTOMAS

Neuroblastomas usually originate in the sympathetic ganglia or in the adrenal medulla and rarely arise in the parenchyma of the brain. Neuroblastoma-like tumors in the cerebellum behave like medulloblastomas and should be so managed. (Indeed, some neuropathologists deny the existence of cerebellar neuroblastomas[1]). Metastases to the brain and spinal cord parenchyma are extremely rare. Neurological manifestations of neuroblastoma are almost always the result of compression from metastatic foci in adjoining structures, notably the calvarium, or from invasive disease. There are only a few case reports of primary neuroblastomas of the central nervous system.

Illustrative cases   A 10-month-old boy presented with seizures, weakness of the left arm, and swelling in the right parietal area. Surgery revealed cystic cavities within a tumor mass extending to the lateral ventricles and basal ganglia. Histological sections of the tumor revealed neuroblastoma, and 31 months after surgery there were no neurologic defects or evidence of systemic disease.[1] An adult man with neuroblastoma presented with a one-year history of progressive left hemiparesis.[2] This was followed by left sensory Jacksonian seizures, papilledema, left hemiplegia, and left hemisensory loss. Angiography revealed a right parietal lobe mass. Surgery was performed and a neuroblastoma was removed. Radiotherapy was given. The

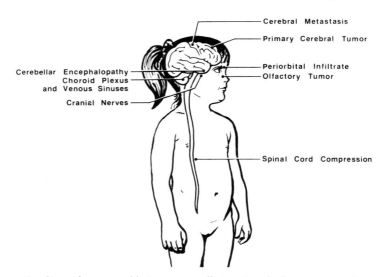

Figure 1.   Sites where neuroblastoma may affect or invade the nervous system.

patient had a 12-year remission before recurrence of symptoms; he died following repeated surgery. At no time was there evidence of metastatic disease elsewhere. In a case of primary so-called neuroblastoma in the posterior fossa there were metastases to bone and elevated VMA excretion.[3] Additional cases of primary cranial neuroblastomas have been reported.[4,5]

METASTASES TO BRAIN IN NEUROBLASTOMA

Metastatic involvement of the brain by compression from adjoining structures occurs fairly often. In a review of 217 cases of neuroblastoma in one series[6] metastatic disease to skull and brain was found in 25 percent of the cases. In contrast, during the neonatal period the reported incidence of intracranial metastases among patients with neuroblastoma was only 6.5 percent.[7]

In 36 cases of neuroblastoma with neurologic manifestations in another series, 22 had pathologic confirmation of the clinical impression of the site of involvement by either post-mortem examination or surgery.[5] Localization, though imprecise, was divided into the following gross areas: cerebral meninges and venous sinuses, 14 cases; spinal cord, 13 cases; spinal nerve roots, 17 cases; cerebrum, 6 cases; and choroid plexus, 3 cases. Many of these patients had multiple areas of involvement.[5]

Neuroblastoma has a definite tendency to infiltrate the meninges and venous sinuses. A somewhat similar tropism is seen in acute lymphoblastic leukemia, but in acute leukemia the meningeal infiltrates commonly involve the pia-arachnoid and result in exfoliation of leukemic cells into the cerebrospinal fluid. On the other hand, the tumor infiltrates in neuroblastoma are confined to bony structures and dura at the base of the brain and behind the orbits. Tumor cells are not commonly found in the CSF.[8] There is frequent involvement of the venous sinuses and the bones of the skull by neuroblastoma. The bony infiltration and resulting involvement of adjacent soft tissues often results in proptosis, periorbital ecchymoses, papilledema, and cranial nerve disturbances.[9,10] Spinal fluid examination may reveal elevated protein; rarely is an increased cell count or presence of tumor cells demonstrated. The common mechanism is when the dural tumor enlarges to act as a space-occupying cerebral lesion by compression, or extends through the dura to invade the brain.[11]

Bone involvement and outgrowth both externally and internally is the key to much of what is seen in the head and face of these

children. Thus, "scalp" nodules are actually subepicranial extensions, proptosis is due to tumor growth from the bone into the
retro-orbital space, etc. Deposits of neuroblastoma involving the calvarium are usually continuous with subperiosteal and extradural
metastases, which may be very bulky. The dura mater seems to act as
a barrier to the deeper penetration by tumor. The brain is rarely, if
ever, involved with neoplasm.

Histologic examination of affected eyes shows the orbital tissue
infiltrated by small, round, undifferentiated cells. Microscopic examination of the globes shows no metastatic intraocular involvement,
however.[12] Occurrence of metastasis from a neuroblastoma or other
solid tumor to the eye of an infant or child has never been reported.
On the other hand, in adults intraocular metastasis from solid tumors
is often described. There is good evidence that neuroblastoma cell
emboli do go to the eye. Such tumor emboli have been seen in the
peripheral blood and even in choroidal vessels. Thus, it appears that
the local environment of the child's eye is unsuitable for support of
metastases of neuroblastoma.[12] These observations support the "infertile soil" hypothesis of cancer metastasis. This is to be distinguished from the Wieberdink hypothesis which relates metastases
to routes of circulation. It seems that the "infertile soil" hypothesis, in
this case, has more to support it in explaining the special pattern of
metastasis of neuroblastoma. (See Chapter 1)

Causes of Increased Intracranial pressure (Table 1)

In some cases there is tumor involvement of the intracranial
venous sinuses. The clinical syndrome includes papilledema, fre-

Table 1
Increased Intracranial Pressure in Neuroblastoma

A. Possible causes
   1. Obstruction of intracranial venous sinuses by metastases in adjoining bones
   2. Compression of the aqueduct of Sylvius by dural infiltrate
   3. Massive ingrowth from calvarial deposits
B. Clinical signs
   1. Engorgement of the scalp veins
   2. Persistent vomiting
   3. Rapid increase in head size
   4. Papilledema
   5. Cranial nerve signs
   6. Widening of the cranial sutures
   7. Increased CSF pressure
   8. Increased CSF protein

quently with marked venous engorgement, increased CSF pressure, and occasionally dilated scalp veins (Figure 2).[5,10] In small children the cranial sutures may be widened (Figure 3), and the head is enlarged as in hydrocephalus. The increased CSF pressure may be due to compression of the aqueduct of Sylvius due to upward pressure of the dural infiltrate at the base of the brain. The result is a form of non-communicating hydrocephalus.

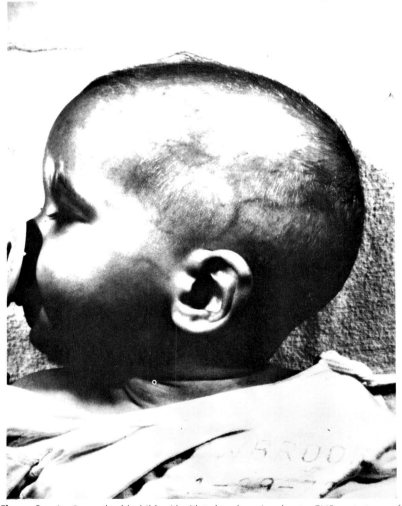

Figure 2. An 8-month-old child with dilated scalp veins due to CNS metastases of neuroblastoma.

Metastases to the venous sinuses can manifest themselves as papilledema as the only neurological sign.[5] The CSF pressure and CSF protein may both be markedly elevated. Intraparenchymal cerebral metastases are rare in neuroblastoma, but when they occur their clinical presentation does not differ from other types of cranial metastatic tumors.[5]

Diagnosis of cranial metastases from neuroblastoma originating elsewhere in the body is usually based on the finding of widened cranial sutures; increased CSF pressure is rarely found even though the head sizes of these patients may increase rapidly. Thus, it appears that widening of the cranial sutures acts chiefly as a mechanism for accommodating bulky extradural metastases.[11] Also, in some cases metastatic neuroblastoma cells may infiltrate the tissues of the cranial sutures and produce marginal bone destruction with resultant widening of the sutures.[11]

At post-mortem examination there may be metastatic infiltrations of the meninges with bulging into the brain substance and extending

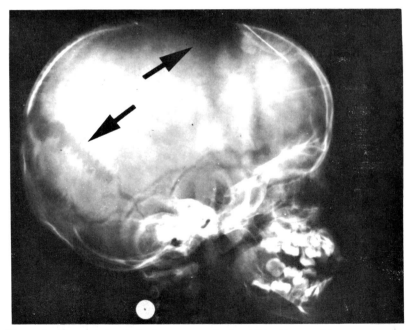

Figure 3. X-ray of the skull of an 18-month-old child with neuroblastoma showing widening of the cranial sutures. The needle shown in the frontoparietal area is inserted into a dilated scalp vein. There was rapid growth of the head and persistent vomiting. (Courtesy of Dr. D. Balsam)

into the orbital cavities.[11] Meningeal infiltration can occur anywhere. The ventricular system may be dilated. The hypothalamus and pituitary may be affected either by downward CSF pressure from the distended third ventricle or by pressure due to infiltration of the meninges at the base of the brain. Rarely, there may be parenchymal metastasis to the frontal and parietal regions of the brain.[5]

Dural metastases without metastases to the calvarium have not been reported.[11] This would support the contention that the initial metastases of neuroblastoma are to bone and that spread to the subperiosteal and extradural spaces occurs later. Partial or complete occlusion of the dural venous sinuses by neuroblastoma has been described only infrequently. On lumbar puncture in such cases increased CSF pressure may be found. It appears that sutural widening in neuroblastoma ordinarily is a mechanism for accommodating large extradural metastases. It is possible that the tumor plaques may interfere with reabsorption of cerebrospinal fluid. Neoplastic infiltration along the sutures and marginal bone destruction may also play a role in sutural diastasis.[11]

The clinical features of Cushing's syndrome in an 11-month-old boy disappeared after removal of neuroblastomas in two ectopic adrenal glands. Brain metastases developed after 5 months with a rapid, fatal course. Although the plasma ACTH level became elevated, none of the clinical manifestations of Cushing's syndrome reappeared.[13] Three other similar cases of Cushing's syndrome in association with adrenal neuroblastoma have been reported.[14,15,16] In suspected cases plasma ACTH assay should be done preoperatively and the tumor should be assayed for biologically active adrenal hormones.

PERIORBITAL METASTASES

Often the first indication of a neuroblastoma is periorbital ecchymosis or proptosis, since the bones of the orbit are frequently the site of metastases (Figure 4). The abducens, oculomotor, optic, and auditory nerves may be involved also. Periorbital metastases may arise from neuroblastomas originating anywhere in the body. Most commonly, however, periorbital metastases are associated with primary abdominal neuroblastomas. These symptoms are caused by metastases in the bones of the skull, which become most readily manifested in the region of the orbit. Thus, the calvarium is usually diffusely involved in these patients when the eye signs become ap-

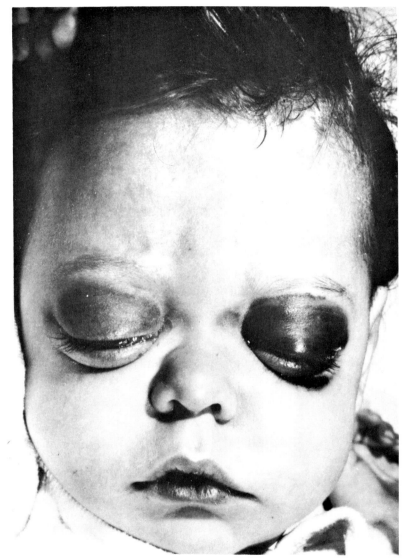

Figure 4. Bilateral proptosis and periorbital ecchymosis in child (same as Fig. 3) with abdominal neuroblastoma. There is swelling over the zygomatic and temporal bones, especially on the right. (Courtesy of Dr. J. Dobbs)

parent. Abdominal neuroblastomas spread preferentially to the orbit and skull on the same side as the abdominal primary tumor.[17] This ipsilateral preponderance of metastases is thought to be suggestive of lymph-borne routes of spread. Cases of neuroblastoma with periorbital metastases are more frequent in children over six months of age.[18]

Incidence

In one series neuroblastomas caused periorbital metastases in 41 out of 108 patients.[12] Thus, more than one-third of the patients with neuroblastoma had periorbital metastases. The sites of the primary tumor in the neuroblastoma patients were the pelvis, abdomen, chest, neck, and multicentric. Periorbital metastases were present in 29 of a total of 64 patients with a primary site in the abdomen. Primary thoracic neuroblastomas resulted in periorbital metastases in only 2 out of 14 cases. In 24 children in whom the primary site could not be definitely determined there were 10 with periorbital metastases. Tumors originated in the neck in 5 children and none developed periorbital metastases. Four of the five patients with cervical neuroblastoma, however, had ptosis resulting from the primary tumor.

Ptosis results from nerve compression.[19] Blockage of impulses to the face along sympathetic nervous system pathways, via cervical or cranial routes, may result in the development of Horner's syndrome, which is characterized by the following signs: meiosis (pupillary constriction), ptosis, anhidrosis (impairment of sweat gland function), flushing of the face due to loss of sympathetic vasoconstrictor control, and enophthalmos (retraction of the eyeball). Ptosis or unequal pupils in a small child are not very obvious signs and do not at once suggest a diagnosis of cervical or mediastinal tumor. In two cases blindness was caused by metastatic neuroblastoma.[20,21] In one case of congenital cervical neuroblastoma, harlequin skin color change was present for several days. A primary neuroblastoma arising from the ciliary ganglion could be confused with an early orbital metastasis. Neuroblastomas arising from the ciliary ganglion, however, have seldom been reported.[12,22]

Clinical Picture

The most common presenting picture of orbital involvement is discoloration of the eyelids or adjacent skin followed in a few weeks by exophthalmos. Ecchymosis and exophthalmos appear simultaneously in some patients; in others, exophthalmos occurs without preceding ecchymoses (Figure 5). Recurrent ecchymoses, limitation of motion of the globe, and localized areas of decreased density in the orbital bone on x-ray examination occur later in some children. With severe proptosis transverse ischemic optic nerve necrosis may occur.[23] Papilledema or optic atrophy may be seen following increased intracranial pressure in patients with skull metastasis.[12]

When the proptosis is first noticed, temporal or cheek swelling is often present. This occurs because there is invariable concomitant bone involvement, and the temporal and zygomatic bones are close to the surface. When metastasis occurs in the frontal process of the zygomatic bone, a temporal swelling is noted and the eye is proptosed down and mediad. When the body of the zygomatic bone is involved, there is cheek swelling and the eye deviates inward.[24] It is usual for the proptosis and the temporal or upper maxillary swelling to appear to be of inflammatory origin. There is marked tendency for the tumor to become necrotic, and, when this occurs in the orbit, it is accompanied by inflammatory signs, ecchymosis, and even hematoma. Unilateral exophthalmos may develop rapidly over a two- or three-week interval, accompanied by swelling of the temporal region or cheek on the side of the proptosis.[24]

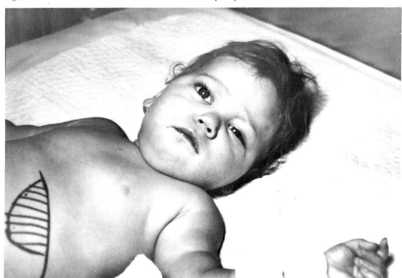

Figure 5. Child with left upper quadrant mass and unilateral proptosis later proven to have a neuroblastoma. Note absence of periorbital ecchymoses.

Thus, the proptosis and swelling sometimes appear to be of inflammatory origin, with edema in the swollen areas, edema of the eyelids, and chemosis of the conjunctiva on the affected side. The swelling of the temporal region or cheek is often necrotic; hence, it may be very soft and associated with ecchymosis of the eyelids on the affected side. Metastases to the xygoma, maxilla, or mandible may cause unilateral swelling resembling that due to an abscessed tooth (Figure 6). At the early stage, x-ray examination of the skull and other bones may be negative, but later both routine skull x-rays and dental x-rays will show bony abnormalities.

In one series of 41 patients, orbital metastases were observed concurrently with the primary in 14 patients, and after the primary in 24. The average time of appearance of orbital metastasis was 3 months following diagnosis of the primary tumor. In one patient orbital metastases occurred 24 months *after* diagnosis of the original neuroblastoma; in another patient orbital metastasis was found 9 months *before* the site of the primary was determined.[12] Orbital metastases were unilateral in 18 patients and bilateral in 23 patients.

Metastasis to the soft tissue of the orbit is due to hematogenous

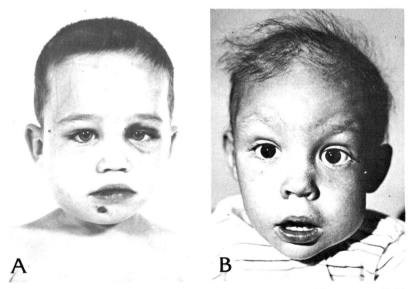

Figure 6. Unilateral facial swelling in two children with neuroblastoma. A: Child with metastasis to the right jaw and left periorbital area from an abdominal neuroblastoma. B: Child with metastasis of the left jaw from an abdominal neuroblastoma. By x-ray examination there were lytic lesions in the mandible and in the tooth follicles. (Courtesy of Dr. Michael Stern and the *Journal of the American Dental Association*[62])

spread, or due to extension from metastatic sites in the orbital bones. Ecchymosis and exophthalmos frequently precede by weeks or months any radiographic evidence of orbital bone involvement. This suggests that metastasis may originate directly in periorbital soft tissues.[12] The pathological picture of orbital metastases is frequently confusing since, when the tumor is incised, it often appears soft, and so vascular as to resemble a hemorrhagic infarct. Often such a tumor entirely collapses, discharging what appear to be masses of clotted blood.[24]

Primary tumors of the cervical or thoracic chain may metastasize to the orbit, but less frequently than do tumors of the abdomen or pelvis. In cervical neuroblastomas heterochromia of the irides may occur, the lighter iris being on the involved side.[19] This finding suggests that the tumor was present in the fetus prior to development of iris pigment.

Other Orbital Tumors

The main malignant tumors of the orbit in children are retinoblastoma, reticulum cell sarcoma, rhabdomyosarcoma, acute leukemic infiltration, and metastatic neuroblastoma. Benign tumors of the orbit include orbital hemangiomas and optic nerve gliomas. Leukemic orbital infiltrations are diagnosed by their characteristic blood and bone marrow findings. Reticulum cell sarcoma and rhabdomyosarcoma have characteristic histopathologic pictures. Usually, the orbit alone is involved in orbital leukemic infiltration, reticulum cell sarcoma, lymphosarcoma, or rhabdomyosarcoma and there is no temporal or upper maxillary swelling. In leukemic orbital infiltration, the proptosis is generally bilateral and the tumor is firm. In orbital reticulum cell sarcoma or lymphosarcoma, the proptosis is usually unilateral and the consistency of the tumor is not so soft as in metastatic orbital neuroblastoma and not so firm as in leukemic infiltration.

OLFACTORY NEUROBLASTOMAS

In very rare cases, primary neuroblastomas may arise in the ciliary, sphenopalatine, otic, or submaxillary ganglia or in the olfactory bulb.[18] Thus, primary extracranial neuroblastomas are found chiefly in the nasopharynx, but may also originate in the orbit and maxilla. Olfactory neuroblastomas are more common in adults and adolescents than in children. They usually present with unilateral nasal obstruction; they grow slowly and tend to remain localized.[25,26]

Olfactory neuroblastoma is seen throughout life with the peak incidence between 10 and 39 years and is slightly more common in males. It is rarely encountered in patients under 10 years of age and, in this respect, is unlike the neuroblastoma of adrenal or sympathetic origin which is seen with greatest frequency below the age of 5 years. When confined to the nasal cavity, the salient clinical features of olfactory neuroblastoma are those of a painless, usually unilateral, polypoid mass causing increasing obstruction and epistaxis. The history of nasal polypectomy or submucous resection for symptomatic relief is, therefore, quite common and understandable. The mass, however, may be small and reside high along the lateral wall of the nasal cavity. Complete anosmia is suggestive of invasion of the cribriform plate. Severe frontal headache may be due to infection of the paranasal sinuses and may not necessarily signify neoplastic invasion of the sinuses or intracranial cavity. Infiltration of the soft tissue of the orbit by tumor may cause diplopia and exophthalmos. Malar swelling may occur due to extension of the neoplasm into the antrum. Distant metastases to the cervical lymph nodes, lung, liver, and other viscera occur.[25,27]

Patients with olfactory neuroblastomas do not show increased urinary excretion of catecholamines.[27] While it is not surprising that tumors of similar histological appearance may have different biological characteristics, the lack of any significant catecholamine excretion may be considered as presumptive evidence that these nasal tumors do not arise from the sympathetic nervous system.[27]

Histologically, olfactory neuroblastomas may be confused with olfactory esthesioneuromas.[28] Olfactory esthesioneuromas are rare tumors of the nasal fossa. They originate from the epithelium and nerves of the olfactory mucosa. From histogenesis and morphology, two types can be distinguished: the olfactory esthesioneuroepithelioma and the olfactory esthesioneurocytoma. Errors in the histological diagnosis occur frequently, particularly in regard to the olfactory esthesioneurocytomas, which are often mistaken for lymphosarcomas or anaplastic carcinomas. The histological recognition of olfactory esthesioneuromas is important because it usually has a benign prognosis. The olfactory esthesioneuroepithelioma appears most likely to give rise to local recurrence and metastasis.

That neuroblastoma-like tumors may arise within the nasal fossa is evident embryologically from the fact that both the epithelial and neural portions of the olfactory mucosa originate from the same neuroectodermal thickening, the olfactory placode. Other possible sites of origin for such tumors which have been suggested are Jacobson's organ and the sphenopalatine ganglion.[29,30] Unlike similar lesions of the adrenal medulla or sympathetic ganglia, most examples of nasal neuroblastoma have pursued a relatively benign clinical course. The fact that the location of these tumors results in early appearance of symptoms, as well as the opportunity for direct visualization and relatively easy extirpation, may have some influence on this difference in behavior.[31]

Neuroblastomas of the olfactory region, or organ of Jacobson, are usually considered to be synonymous with esthesioneuromas. However, the nonmetastatic nature of these tumors does not support the assertion that they are true neuroblastomas. They seem to be histologically and histogenetically related to neuroblastomas, but yet not true neuroblastomas.

Management of localized olfactory neuroblastoma consists of local resection and radiation therapy. However, in addition to regional spread to the paranasal sinuses, or distant metastasis, the tumor shows a strong tendency to invade the cribriform plate and orbitofrontal region of the brain. Intracranial spread of infection from the nasal cavity along pathways created by the invading tumor may result in brain abscess. Awareness of these possible neurological complications as features of the natural history of olfactory neuroblastoma is essential for appropriate neurosurgical evaluation and treatment.[27]

CEREBELLAR ENCEPHALOPATHY AND NEUROBLASTOMA

There have been many reports of children with neuroblastoma who showed signs of acute cerebellar encephalopathy.[32-45,60] The distinctive type of encephalopathy which occurred in these patients has been recognized for many years by neurologists and ophthalmologists. It is referred to variously as opsoclonus, ataxic conjugate movements of the eyes, acute cerebellar ataxia, and myoclonic encephalopathy, though the term acute cerebellar encephalopathy is preferred. In most cases the etiology of this cerebellar syndrome is obscure; its recognition has been important largely to enable clinicians to differentiate it from posterior fossa neoplasms and true infectious types of encephalitis.[36]

In cerebellar encephalopathy there are irregular, hyperkinetic, multidirectional spontaneous eye movements, often accompanied by myoclonic jerks of the face and body and other signs of cerebellar ataxia. The eye movements (opsoclonus) are not always in unison and can be present in sleep with lower amplitude and rate.[32] The chaotic, irregular eye movements offer a sharp contrast to the rhythmicity of nystagmus. In opsoclonus the eye movements are sustained and they are totally irregular, occurring in all planes.[32]

Most cases of cerebellar encephalopathy occur in children with thoracic neuroblastomas.[43] The syndrome may also occur in abdominal and sacral neuroblastomas.[42] Opsoclonus may precede the finding of an occult neuroblastoma by several months.[41,42,45] Normal urinary catecholamine excretion is also common in neuroblastoma with cerebellar encephalopathy.[43]

One child with a neuroblastoma initially showed clinical features resembling myasthenia gravis. The symptoms disappeared after excision of the tumor and the child was living and without evidence of tumor 18 months after treatment by combined surgery, radiotherapy, and chemotherapy.[46] The generalized muscle weakness, with possible associated incoordination, was somewhat suggestive of cerebellar encephalopathy in this case.

Therapy

In most cases the signs of cerebellar encephalopathy improve promptly after therapy of the neuroblastoma with surgery, x-ray therapy, and chemotherapy. Sometimes the neurological improvement is slow or incomplete.[32,36,37,39,41] There may be almost instant and complete cessation of opsoclonus after intravenous injection of diazepam (Valium®). However, a dose of diazepam sufficient to stop a grand-mal seizure, suppressed the opsoclonic activity for only a 5-minute period in one child.[33] In other cases the symptoms of polymyoclonia may be controlled with ACTH.[38]

Although symptomatic control of the ocular symptoms can be achieved by the use of ACTH, it is important to recognize that this unusual ocular symptom may be a manifestation of an occult and potentially curable neuroblastoma. Therefore, one should perform the appropriate diagnostic studies. In view of the known association of cerebellar encephalopathy and neuroblastoma, it would be wise to survey all cases of acute cerebellar encephalopathy with a chest x-ray, an intravenous pyelogram, skeletal survey including spine films, a search of bone marrow aspirate for tumor cells, and an estimation of the urinary excretion of catecholamines.[36]

Etiology

Cerebellar encephalopathy has been linked with postexanthematous types of encephalitis, neurotropic viral encephalitides including that due to poliovirus, and direct involvement of the brain stem or cerebellar hemispheres with primary or metastatic tumor. Opsoclonus has also been seen in such degenerative disorders as multiple sclerosis and Friedreich's ataxia. It should be noted, therefore, that most patients with the distinctive ataxic conjugate eye movement disorders do not harbor malignant tumors.

What is the cause of cerebellar encephalopathy when it occurs in association with neuroblastoma? An etiological factor might be that the neuroblastoma liberates an antigen which stimulates the formation of antibody, and the antigen-antibody complex then damages the nervous system.[36] A second possible etiological mechanism might be the liberation by a neuroblastoma of excessive quantities of some metabolite (catecholamine or cystathionine), which in turn damages the cerebellum by virtue of its toxic chemical properties. The evidence in other cases and among those cited in the literature so far is too inconsistent to support this proposition strongly.[36] Furthermore, the tissue levels of these substances are low in relation to their urinary excretion.[44]

Neuroblastomas do not spread to the brain parenchyma via blood vessels, although they do metastasize to the bones of the skull, causing pressure on the brain. Thus, the cerebellar encephalopathy may be related to local pressure on the brain. Is there an undefined carcinogen that also causes encephalopathy? Are we dealing with a neurotropic oncogenic virus? No specific oncogenic virus has been demonstrated in neuroblastoma. The complete or almost complete absence of pyrexia and the absence of cells in the spinal fluid are partial evidence against existence of a viral infection. Tumor antigens may result in antibody formation, and such an antigen-antibody complex may be injurious to nerve tissue. Since the cerebellum has often been described as a particularly vulnerable part of the nervous system, the cerebellar damage may be either specific or nonspecific.[44]

It is possible that some "silent" neuroblastomas, which involute spontaneously in infants and are never recognized clinically, may produce acute cerebellar encephalopathy. This circumstance seems possible since most of the reported cases of acute cerebellar ataxia never have another specific diagnosis established.[36] But, as mentioned earlier, primary intracerebral neuroblastomas are very rare, making this possible cause of cerebellar encephalopathy an unlikely occurrence.

SPINAL CORD COMPRESSION DUE TO NEUROBLASTOMA

Since neuroblastomas commonly arise from paraspinal sympathetic ganglia, the tumor may have an intraspinal as well as an extraspinal component. It is obvious that the intraspinal portion can produce cord symptoms. The two portions of these "dumbbell" tumors may not grow at the same rate. The cord symptoms may occur prior to, concurrent with, or subsequent to other symptoms. Motor weakness is usually the earliest sign of the cord pressure involvement. The mother's observation that the baby no longer crawls or sits up as well as formerly may occasionally lead to an early diagnosis of a cord tumor. There may be muscle spasm, and in early cases hyperreflexia, followed by hyporeflexia and areflexia.[5,47] Pain in the back and legs is difficult to ascertain in the young child, but it is an important finding in older children. Paraplegia due to neuroblastoma may occur at any age, even in the newborn.[48] "Regressive" bladder and bowel habits may be signs of compression of the lumbo-sacral cord by tumor.

The occurrence of paralysis, due to extradural extension of tumor, as an initial symptom is not uncommon. In one series nearly 20 percent of children with thoracic neuroblastomas had partial or complete paralysis of the lower extremities.[49] Tumors originating in the paravertebral gutter may penetrate through a vertebral foramen, follow the course of a sympathetic nerve fiber, then give rise to a second tumor within the spinal canal[50] (Figure 7). The gross morphology of these tumors suggests the name of "dumbbell" or "hour glass" tumor (Figure 8). The pressure due to growth of the intraspinal portion of the tumor frequently causes paraplegia. Other symptoms that these tumors may cause include radicular pain, and motor weakness or limp.[51] Tumors located at the apex of the lung or lower cervical region may cause Horner's syndrome.

Neuroblastomas in the neck may also be of the "dumbbell" type; they may invade the spinal canal and cause cord symptoms. Pressure on blood vessels and lymphatics may cause swelling of the arm, and pressure on nerve trunks may cause radicular pain.

There have been many reports of spinal cord dysfunction manifested generally as cord compression secondary to extradural neuroblastoma. Spinal cord involvement may occur by invasion of the spinal canal through the intervertebral foramina or by metastases. Out of 30 cases of spinal cord neoplasm in children in one series, 6 were extradural neuroblastomas.[6] In other similar reported series of spinal cord tumors comprising a total of 326 cases, 16 were neuroblastoma.[5] The cases described were all in children. There are also reports of intraspinal extradural neuroblastomas occurring in the neonatal period.[7,52]

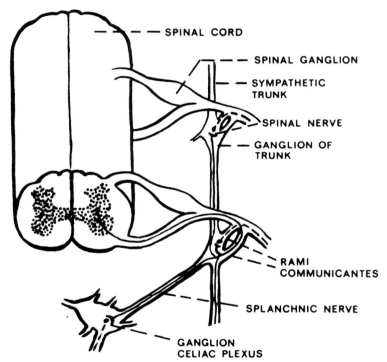

Figure 7. Diagram of a short section of the sympathetic nervous system. Preganglionic fibers (represented by the single solid line) are shown leaving the spinal cord by way of the ventral root of a nerve, entering the sympathetic trunk through the white ramus communicans, and thereafter taking various courses, including leaving the trunk by way of a splanchnic nerve to make connection with a more peripherally placed ganglion. Postganglionic fibers are shown as broken lines. A neuroblastoma originating in a paravertebral sympathetic ganglion may follow the course of its preganglionic fiber, penetrate the vertebral foramen and give rise to a second tumor within the spinal canal. (Adapted from Dr. W. Hollinshead[63])

Neuroblastomas originating in the cervical sympathetic chain may occur at any level.[53,54] Horner's syndrome is common in cervical tumors. In the chest, primary neuroblastomas occur nearly always in the superior and posterior mediastinum. If the tumor is the "dumbbell" type, symptoms of cord compression may be the initial finding. Thoracotomy must be performed as a diagnostic aid, unless a metastatic site yields neuroblastoma. If the cord compression is not promptly relieved, spastic diplegia[55] or permanent paralysis[48] may ensue.

Intraspinal invasion by a pelvic neuroblastoma may cause weakness of the legs, limp, sensory deficit, or radicular pain. Abnormalities of gait and posture, leg weakness, sensory deficit, and abnormal reflexes are the most common complaints and neurologic findings in tumors of the spinal cord in children.

Laboratory Diagnosis

On x-ray examination of the spine widening of the cervical interpediculate distance, increased antero-posterior diameter of the spinal canal, and pedicle erosion suggest an intraspinal lesion. When

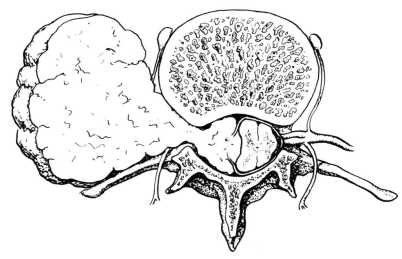

Figure 8. Diagrammatic cross-section of the spine. A dumbbell-shaped neuroblastoma originating from a paraspinal sympathetic ganglion is shown invading the spinal canal through a vertebral foramen and compressing the cord.

there is also an enlarged neural foramen, the findings suggest a "dumbbell" lesion. The tumor may have both an intradural extramedullary component and an extradural component.[56,57] Confirmation by myelography of extradural impingement upon the cord is shown by deviation or blockage of flow of radiopaque fluid in the subarachnoid space.[24,58,59,61]

Neuroblastomas of sympathetic ganglia commonly grow in dumbbell fashion. Most tumors of this type are found in the neck and thorax. Hence, any child with a primary neuroblastoma arising above the diaphragm should be suspected of having an intraspinal component. Plain frontal, lateral, and both oblique views of the spine appropriately centered should be obtained in all such patients. Any of the findings described above virtually establish the presence of an intraspinal tumor.

While preparations are being made for prompt surgery, there should be (1) repeated careful motor, reflex, and sensory examination and evaluation of sphincter function; (2) examination of cerebrospinal fluid dynamics and protein content by lumbar puncture; and (3) myelography whenever any abnormality in the foregoing studies is detected.[59] Indeed, some authorities advocate routine myelography in all children with paraspinal primary neuroblastomas. Surprisingly large intraspinal tumors can be present without detectable neurological findings and with only equivocal changes on plain x-ray films.

SUMMARY AND CONCLUSIONS

The neurological manifestations of neuroblastoma most often are due to metastases to the structures near the CNS. They are rarely caused by tumors originating in the brain or metastasizing there. Periorbital ecchymoses and proptosis are due to metastases to the bones of the orbit, which cause local reaction, inflammation, and hemorrhage. In rare cases primary neuroblastomas may also arise in the ciliary, sphenopalatine, otic, submaxillary, or olfactory ganglia. Opsoclonus (cerebellar encephalopathy) is observed in many cases of neuroblastoma. The mechanism by which neuroblastomas give rise to this syndrome is not known. Since neuroblastomas commonly arise from paraspinal sympathetic ganglia, the tumor may have an intraspinal as well as an extraspinal component. The intraspinal portion of this "dumbell" tumor may produce symptoms due to compression of the spinal cord in the neck, thorax, abdomen, or pelvis.

REFERENCES

1. Miller, A.A., and Ramsden, F.: A Cerebral Neuroblastoma with Unusual Fibrous Tissue Reaction. *J. Neuropath. Exp. Neurol.* 25: 328–340, 1966.

2. Liss, L.: Neuroblastoma (Malignant Gangliocytoma) of the Parietal Lobe. *J. Neurosurg.* 17: 529–536, 1960.

3. Gyepes, M.T., and D'Angio, G.J.: Extracranial Metastases from Central Nervous System Tumors in Children and Adolescents. *Radiology* 87: 55–63, 1966.

4. Durity, F.A., Dolman, C.L., and Moyes, P.D.: Ganglioneuroblastoma of the cerebellum. *J. Neurosurg.* 28: 270–273, 1968.

5. Alpert, J., and Mones, R.: Neurologic manifestations of neuroblastoma. *J. Mt. Sinai Hospital* (New York) 36: 37–47, 1969.

6. Gross, R.E., Farber, S., and Martin, L.W.: Neuroblastoma Sympatheticum; A Study and Report of 217 Cases. *Pediatrics* 23: 1179, 1959.

7. Schneider, K.M., Becker, J.M., and Krasna, I. I.: Neonatal Neuroblastoma. *Pediatrics* 36: 359, 1965.

8. Farr, G.H., and Hajdu, S.: Exfoliative cytology of metastatic neuroblastoma. *Acta Cytol.* (Baltimore) 16: 203–206, 1972.

9. Alfano, J.: Ophthalmological aspects of neuroblastomatosis; a study of 53 verified cases. *Trans. Amer. Acad. Ophthal. Otolaryng.* 72: 830–848, 1968.

10. Mones, R.J.: Increased Intracranial Pressure due to Metastatic Disease of Venous Sinuses. *Neurology* 15: 1000–1007, 1965.

11. Carter, T., Gabrielson, T., and Abell, M.: Mechanism of split cranial sutures in metastatic neuroblastoma. *Radiology* 91: 467–475, 1968.

12. Albert, D., Rubenstein, R., and Scheie, H.: Tumor metastases to the eye. II. Clinical study in infants and children. *Amer. J. Ophthal.* 63: 727–732, 1967.

13. Normann, T., Havnen, J., and Mjolnerod, O.: Cushing's syndrome in an infant associated with neuroblastoma in two ectopic adrenal glands. *J. Pediatr. Surg.* 6: 169–175, 1971.

14. Kaplan, L.I.: Sympathicoblastoma with metastases, associated with the clinical picture of Cushing's syndrome; Report of a case. *Arch. Neurol. Psychiat.* 62: 696, 1949.

15. Kogut, M.D., and Donnel, G.N.: Cushing's syndrome in association with renal ganglioneuroblastoma. *Pediatrics* 28: 566, 1961.

16. Kenny, F.M., Stavrides, A., Voorhess, M.L., and Klein, R.: Cushing's syndrome associated with an adrenal neuroblastoma. *Amer. J. Dis. Child.* 11: 3611, 1967.

17. Oniugbo, W.: Cephalic spread of neuroblastomas in children. *Arch. Dis. Childh.* 36: 526–529, 1961.

18. Dargeon, H.W.: Neuroblastoma. *J. Pediatr.* 61: 456–463, 1962.

19. Apple, D.: Metastatic orbital neuroblastoma originating in the cervical sympathetic ganglionic chain. *Amer. J. Ophthal.* 68: 1093–1095, 1969.

20. Shubert, E.E., Oliver, G.L., and Jaco, N.: Blindness due to neuroblastoma. *Canad. J. Ophthal.* 4: 100, 1969.

21. Bond, J.V.: Unusual presenting symptoms of neuroblastoma. *Brit. Med. J.* 2: 237–238, 1972.

22. Levy, W.J.: Neuroblastoma. *Brit. J. Ophthal.* 41: 48, 1957.

23. Manschat, M.: Transverse ischemic optic nerve necrosis in neuroblastoma. *Arch. Ophthal.* 81: 707–709, 1969.

24. Mortada, A.: Clinical characteristics of early orbital metastatic neuroblastoma. *Amer. J. Ophthal.* 6: 1787–1793, 1967.

25. Hope-Stone, H.: Extra-adrenal neuroblastoma. *Brit. J. Surg.* 48: 424–429, 1961.

26. Fitz-Hugh, L.S., et al: Olfactory neuroblastoma. *Arch. Otolaryng.* 81: 161, 1965.

27. Robinson, F., and Solitaire, G.: Olfactory neuroblastoma; neurosurgical implications of an intranasal tumor. *J. Neurosurg.* 25: 133–139, 1966.

28. Gerard-Marchant, R., and Micheau, C.: Microscopical diagnosis of olfactory esthesioneuromas; General review and report of 5 cases. *J. Nat. Cancer Inst.* 35: 75–82, 1965.

29. Schall, L., and Lineback, M.: Primary intranasal neuroblastoma; report of 3 cases. *Ann. Otol. Rhinol. Laryng.* 60: 221–229, 1951.

30. Fisher, E.R.: Neuroblastomas of the nasal fossa. *Arch. Pathol.* 60: 435–439, 1955.

31. McCormack, L., and Harris, H.E.: Neurogenic tumors of the nasal fossa. *J.A.M.A.* 157: 318–321, 1955.

32. Solomon, G., and Chutorian, A.: Opsoclonus and occult neuroblastoma. *New Engl. J. Med.* 279: 475–477, 1968.

33. Davidson, M., Tolentino, Y., and Sapir, S.: Opsoclonus and neuroblastoma. *New Engl. J. Med.* 279: 948, 1968.

34. Dyken, P., and Kolar, O.: Dancing eyes, dancing feet; infantile polymyoclonia. *Brain* 91: 305–320, 1968.

35. Lemerle, J., Lemerle, M., Aicardi, J., et al.: Three cases of neuroblastoma associated with an oculo-cerebello-myoclonia syndrome. *Arch. Franc. Ped.* 26: 547–558, 1969.

36. Bray, P., Ziter, F.A., Lahey, M.E., and Myers, G.: The coincidence of neuroblastoma and acute cerebellar encephalopathy. *J. Pediat.* 75: 983–990, 1969.

37. Brissaud, H., and Beauvais, P.: Opsoclonus and neuroblastoma. *New Engl. J. Med.* 280: 1242, 1969.

38. Moe, P., and Nellhaus, G.: Infantile polymyoclonia-opsoclonus syndrome and neural crest tumors. *Neurology* 20: 756–764, 1970.

39. Forster, C., and Weinmann, H.: Symptomatic infantile polymyoclonus. *Z. Kinderheilk.* 111: 240–246, 1971.

40. Martin, E., and Griffith, J.F.: Myoclonic encephalopathy and neuroblastoma; report of a case with apparent recovery. *Amer. J. Dis. Child.* 122: 257–258, 1971.

41. Sandok, B., and Kranz, H.: Opsoclonus as the initial manifestation of occult neuroblastoma. *Arch. Ophthal.* 86: 235–236, 1971.

42. Korobkin, M., Clark, R., and Palubinskas, A.: Occult neuroblastoma and acute cerebellar ataxia in childhood. *Radiology* 102: 151–152, 1972.

43. Leonidas, J., et al.: Neuroblastoma presenting with myoclonic encephalopathy. *Radiology* 102: 87–88, 1972.

44. Malmstrom-Groth, A.: Cerebellar encephalopathy and neuroblastoma. *Europ. Neurol.* 7: 95–100, 1972.

45. Williams, T., House, R., Burgert, E.O., and Lynn, H.: Unusual manifestations of neuroblastoma; chronic diarrhea, polymyoclonia-opsoclonus and erythrocyte abnormalities. *Cancer* 29: 475–480, 1972.

46. Robinson, J., and Howard, N.: Neuroblastoma presenting as myasthenia gravis in a child aged 3 years. *Pediatrics* 43: 111–113, 1969.

47. Bodian, M.: Neuroblastoma. *Pediatr. Clin. N. Amer.* 6: 449–472, 1959.

48. Rothner, D.: Congential "dumbbell" neuroblastoma with paraplegia. *Clin. Pediat.* 10: 235–236, 1971.

49. Ware, G.: Thoracic neuroblastoma. *J. Pediatr.* 49: 765–773, 1956.

50. Lepintre, J., Schweisguth, O., and LaBrune, M.: Neuroblastoma with spinal cord compression; study of 22 cases. *Arch. Franc. Ped.* 26: 829–847, 1969.

51. Bulmer, J.H.: Scoliosis complicating ganglion cell tumours. *Brit. J. Surg.* 53: 619–624, 1966.

52. Elefant, E., Vojta, V., and Benes, V.: Intraspinal neuroblastoma in a newborn baby. *Arch. Dis. Childh.* 33: 212, 1958.

53. Pulliam, R.: Ganglioneuroblastoma; a case involving the superior cervical ganglion. *Arch. Otolaryng.* 74: 40–44, 1961.

54. Adams, L.: Neuroblastoma; review of the literature and report of 18 cases. *North Carolina Med. J.* 27: 113–125, 1966.

55. Citipitioglu, B.: Spastic diplegia following mediastinal neuroblastoma. *Turk. J. Pediat.* 12: 98–105, 1970.

56. Prakash, B.: Neuroblastoma and ganglioneuroblastoma causing spinal cord compression. *J. Oslo City Hospital* 19: 200–210, 1969.

57. Binet, E., Lustgarten, M., and Markarian, B.: Enlarged neural foramen in a child. *New York State J. Med.* 71: 449–452, 1971.

58. Haft, H., Ransohoff, J., and Carter, S.: Spinal cord tumors in children. *Pediatrics* 23: 1152–1159, 1959.

59. Tachdjian, M., and Matson, D.: Orthopedic aspects of intraspinal tumors in infants and children. *J. Bone Joint Surg.* 47-A: 223–248, 1965.

60. Senelick, R., Bray, P., Lahey, M.E., et al.: Neuroblastoma and myoclonic encephalopathy: two cases and a review of the literature. *J. Pediatr. Surg.* 8: 623–632, 1973.

61. Fagan, C., and Swischuk, L.: Dumbbell neuroblastoma or ganglioneuroma of the spinal canal. *Amer. J. Roentgenol.* 120: 453–460, 1974.

62. Stern, M., Turner, J., and Coburn, T.: Oral involvement in neuroblastoma. *J.A.D.A.* 88: 346–351, 1974.

63. Hollinshead, W.H.: *Textbook of Anatomy.* New York: Hoeber Medical Books, 1967, p. 57.

3 Neuroblastoma in the Neck, Chest, Abdomen, and Pelvis

Carl Pochedly, M.D.

1. Neck
   a. Primary tumors
      (1) Clinical features and x-ray findings
   b. Metastases
      (2) Route
2. Chest
   a. Clinical features
   b. Radiographic findings
      (1) Paravertebral widening
   c. Distinguishing between primary and metastatic chest tumors
3. Abdomen
   a. Clinical features
   b. Radiographic findings
   c. Functionally active neurogenic tumors
4. Pelvis
   a. Clinical features and x-ray findings

Neuroblastomas may arise from any site where one would normally find elements of the sympathetic nervous system. Thus, the adrenal medulla and any segment of the sympathetic chain of the neck, thorax, abdomen or pelvis, including the carotid ganglia, aortic bodies, and bodies of Zuckerkandl, may be sites of origin. Neuroblastomas have also been reported as arising in intestine, mesentery, uterus, coccygeal body, skin, subcutaneous tissue, carotid body and in an ovarian teratoma.[1,2] However, two-thirds of neuroblastomas originate in the upper abdomen, arising from either the adrenal medulla or from nearby lumbar sympathetic ganglia (Figure 1).

Although there are many general and nonlocalizing symptoms (Figure 2), [3-15] neuroblastomas may also show symptoms peculiar to the location of the primary tumor. Thus, symptoms and signs of neuroblastoma vary from local to regional to systemic. The clinical

59

findings of extra-adrenal neuroblastoma depend upon its specific site of origin in the sympathetic nervous system: cervical sympathetic, thoracic sympathetic, lumbar sympathetic, or sacral sympathetic.

NECK

In the neck there may be confusion of neuroblastoma with lymphadenitis, lymphoma, branchial cysts, teratomas, lipomas, and intramuscular hemorrhage from trauma.[16] Primary tumors may be high or low in the neck, depending not only on the sympathetic ganglion of origin, but also on the extent of the growth (Figure 3). Tumors at the level of the mandibular ramus may arise from the submaxillary ganglion. Others occur in the supraclavicular fossa. The covering sternocleidomastoid muscle may initially conceal the tumor

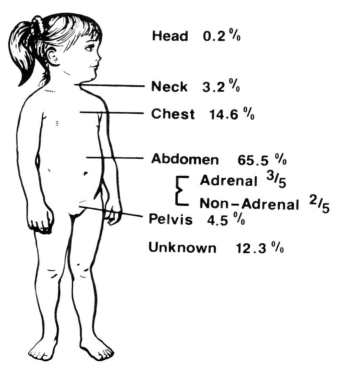

Head   0.2 %

Neck   3.2 %

Chest   14.6 %

Abdomen   65.5 %
$$\begin{cases} \text{Adrenal } 3/5 \\ \text{Non-Adrenal } 2/5 \end{cases}$$
Pelvis   4.5 %

Unknown   12.3 %

Figure 1.   Diagram showing primary sites of neuroblastomas in 1,303 cases accumulated from recently reported series.[3-15]

and make recognition difficult. X-ray examination may show a soft-tissue mass and possibly some tracheal deviation. Neuroblastomas in this region may also be of the "dumbbell" type; they may invade the spinal canal and cause cord symptoms. Pressure on blood vessels and lymphatics may cause swelling of the arm, and pressure on nerve trunks may cause radicular pain.

Tumors in the neck often give rise to ptosis resulting from nerve compression.[17] Cervical neuroblastomas, like those originating in other sites, may also metastasize to the orbit.[18] Heterochromia of the irides may occur, with the lighter iris being on the involved side. This finding suggests that the tumor was present in the fetus prior to development of iris pigment.[17] Neuroblastoma of the lower jaw may originate from the submandibular ganglion.[19] Thus, neuroblastomas originating in the cervical sympathetic chain may occur at any level. Horner's syndrome (ptosis, enophthalmos, and contracted pupil) (Figure 4), tracheal deviation, and edema of the arm from compression of blood vessels and lymphatics are common in cervical tumors.[20]

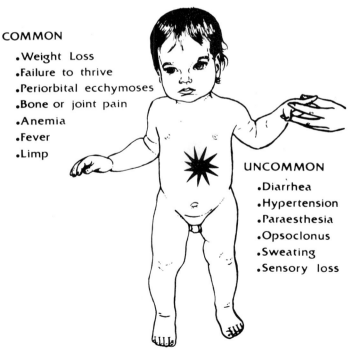

COMMON

- Weight Loss
- Failure to thrive
- Periorbital ecchymoses
- Bone or joint pain
- Anemia
- Fever
- Limp

UNCOMMON

- Diarrhea
- Hypertension
- Paraesthesia
- Opsoclonus
- Sweating
- Sensory loss

Figure 2. Nonspecific and nonlocalized symptoms and signs that may be observed in a child with neuroblastoma.

In the cervical area a relatively small mass may cause displacement and distortion of the laryngopharynx, often with resulting stridor.[21] Stippled calcifications within the mass increase the chances of its being a neuroblastoma. The mass may cause displacement or distortion of the hypopharynx, trachea, or esophagus as seen on x-ray examination. On examination of the cervical spine there may be widening of the cervical interpediculate distance, enlarged neural foramena of the cervical spinal canal, and pedicle erosion suggesting an intradural lesion.[22]

In *metastatic* neuroblastomas, enlargement of the cervical lymph nodes, beginning with the left supraclavicular or Virchow's node, may be the first indication that the child is ill (Figure 5). A persistent cervical mass in a child should be especially suspect. A child who presents with painless swelling of a left supraclavicular lymph node, even if small, should have an x-ray examination of the chest and an intravenous pyelogram to exclude the possibility of metastasis from an abdominal neuroblastoma. Lymphadenopathy may be an early

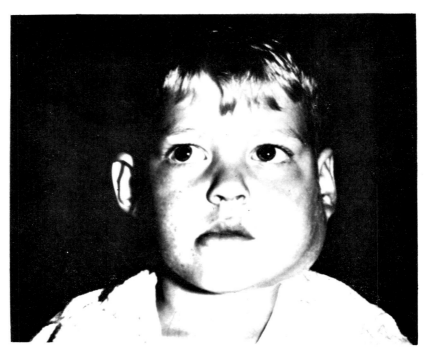

Figure 3. A child with a primary neuroblastoma of the neck. (Courtesy of Dr. G. Fendrick)

sign of tumors arising in the thorax or cervical region. In these cases biopsy of an enlarged cervical or supraclavicular node may lead to an early diagnosis.

Metastases frequently involve the mandible or maxilla, but not as often as they do the skull and tubular bones. These are often painless lesions with a variable amount of underlying bone destruction. Neuroblastomas originating in the nasopharynx and orbit have been reported but are rare.[8] Primary cervical neuroblastomas have less tendency to metastasize, possibly because they come to the attention of the physician earlier than do tumors in the other sites.[8] Priebe and Clatworthy reported 92 consecutive cases of neuroblastoma. Three of these were in the neck, all were in the favorable age group of one year or under, and all three were cured by a combination of surgical excision and postoperative x-ray therapy.[10]

Fourteen cases of metastatic neuroblastoma of the mandible were reviewed.[23-34] One case was a 21-month-old white girl who had a reddish, tender, friable, and easily bleeding exophytic tumor that involved the body and ascending ramus of the left side of the mandible. The primary tumor was found to be arising from the right adrenal

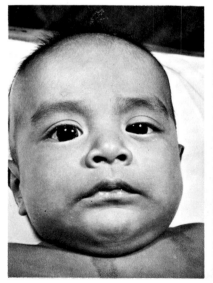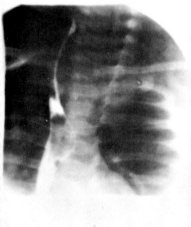

Figure 4. **Left:** three-month-old girl with left-sided Horner's syndrome due to neuroblastoma in the left lower cervical area. The tumor was treated with excision only. Horner's syndrome cleared. **Right:** preoperative barium swallow showing compression of the esophagus by a left-sided tumor mass in the lower neck and upper mediastinum. (Courtesy of Dr. Howard Wechsler)

gland. In spite of chemotherapy the patient died 2½ months after diagnosis.[33] Metastatic neuroblastoma to the mandible may present with the appearance of "floating teeth" on x-ray examination.[35] With careful searching, it is not uncommon to find jaw metastases in neuroblastoma.[36]

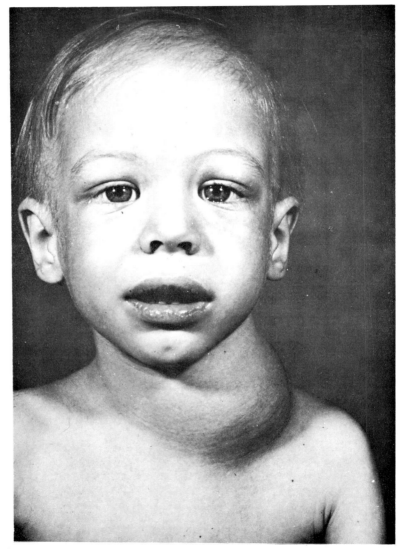

Figure 5. A child with massive metastasis to the left supraclavicular lymph nodes from a left adrenal primary neuroblastoma. (Courtesy of Dr. F. Ordonez)

With metastases of neuroblastoma from adrenal to mandible, there is a peculiar and unexplained lack of pulmonary involvement. According to the classical theory of blood-borne tumor metastasis, tumor-cell emboli from an abdominal neuroblastoma should enter the venous system, travel to the lungs, and then to the mandible and other bones. In one series of 12 cases the lung was involved in only one instance, but even in this case, the pulmonary involvement did not seem to be caused by a blood-borne metastasis, but rather to be a direct extension from the primary tumor located in the posterior mediastinum. Thus, the classical theory of blood-borne tumor metastasis fails to explain adequately the occurrence of mandibular metastases.[33]

It is possible that mandibular involvement in metastatic neuroblastoma is related to the mechanism of blood-borne tumor metastasis advanced by Batson. According to this concept, the tumor-cell emboli from an abdominal or thoracic neuroblastoma enter the vertebral venous system and are carried directly to the mandible, bypassing the lung entirely. This route is facilitated further in the instance of neuroblastoma by the usual finding of increased intra-abdominal pressure that is responsible for the diversion of blood flow from the caval system to the vertebral veins.[33] On the other hand, pulmonary metastases are rare in any patient with neuroblastoma, despite the fact that the long bones, ribs, pelvis, and multiple other bony sites commonly are involved. It would seem that the lung, for reasons that are only speculative, does not provide a suitable soil for neuroblastoma cells. This latter explanation seems more plausible in explaining the occurrence of mandibular metastases in the absence of lung metastases.

CHEST

Because of the adaptability of the mediastinal contents and the lungs to slowly growing tumors, the diagnosis of either primary or metastatic neuroblastoma in this region is only rarely made before considerable growth of the tumor has occurred (Figure 6). Primary neuroblastomas occur nearly always in the superior and posterior mediastinum. Symptoms of cough and tracheal compression are rare, but if fever and pulmonary symptoms predominate, mediastinal neuroblastoma may be misdiagnosed as an inflammatory lung lesion.[37] One neonate had a mediastinal neuroblastoma of such great size that she was initially diagnosed as respiratory distress syndrome.[38] Swelling of the neck and face are present when the superior vena cava

66

and other upper mediastinal vessels become compressed. Physical examination of the thorax is not usually revealing until massive metastases produce tracheal, pulmonary, or cardiac signs. If the tumor is of the "dumbbell" type, symptoms of cord compression may be the initial finding.

Intrathoracic neurogenic tumors which commonly occur in infants and children include neuroblastomas, ganglioneuromas, and ganglioneuroblastomas. In children under 5 years of age, the most common tumor is the neuroblastoma.[39] Tumors composed in various proportions of benign ganglioneuroma and malignant neuroblastoma, called ganglioneuroblastomas, are not uncommon. The degree of malignancy of these tumors is probably the same as for pure neuroblastomas.[40] In some cases, histological maturity in the tumor may favor a better prognosis but degree of maturity of the tumor cannot be used as a guide to treatment.[14] The finding of an increase in catecholamines in the urine is strong evidence for the diagnosis, but biopsy for histopathology is necessary to establish the diagnosis.

Of 13 cases in one series with primary intrathoracic origin of

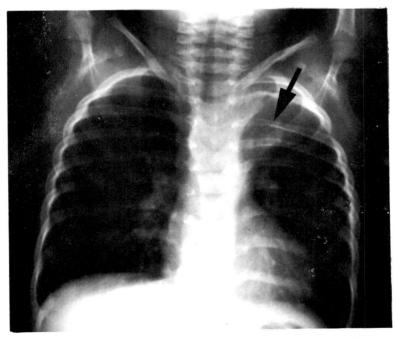

Figure 6. X-ray of the chest showing tumor mass in left superior mediastinum, causing bony erosion of ribs (arrow).

neuroblastoma, the time interval from onset of symptoms to diagnosis was usually just a few weeks.[41] Only three of these cases were symptomatic for more than a month before diagnosis. Most of this group manifested a symptom complex that pointed to the intrathoracic location of the patient's disease. Dyspnea, cough, tachypnea, wheezing, stridor, pain, and cyanosis were the prominent symptoms and signs. However, two of this group manifested only leg weakness because the tumor in both of these cases was small, paravertebral, and infiltrating into the neural foramina. One patient in this group was totally asymptomatic when a large intrathoracic tumor was clinically detected during a routine physical examination.[41]

A pleural tumor may occur, but pleural effusion is uncommon. In one case of primary mediastinal neuroblastoma, the patient presented with pleural effusion and respiratory distress secondary to tracheal compression.[8,19] Another case of pleural effusion occurred in a child with metastases to pleura from an adrenal primary.[42] In a one-year-old girl infarction of a mediastinal neuroblastoma resulted in rupture into the right pleural cavity. The tumor had undergone nearly complete necrosis and had ruptured into the pleural cavity, producing hemorrhage with pleural effusion as the presenting sign.[43] With mediastinal neuroblastoma and pleural effusion, neuroblastoma cells may be identified in the pleural fluid (Figure 7).[44,45]

There are only rare reports of neuroblastomas arising in the anterior mediastinum. A 10-month-old boy with neuroblastoma of the anterior mediastinum remained well 8 months after surgery.[46] The site of origin of the neoplasm in this report can only be surmised. It might possibly have arisen in ganglionic tissue overlying the heart. Another possibility is that it originated in a cervical sympathetic ganglion with downward extension into the anterior mediastinum.[46] The rarity of neuroblastomas originating in the anterior mediastinum is undoubtedly related to the paucity of ganglionic tissue in this area.[47,48]

Neuroblastomas seldom metastasize to the lungs; when present, pulmonary metastases usually occur in far-advanced disseminated disease. This is a helpful point in differentiating neuroblastomas from Wilms' tumor, with which they are often confused. When neuroblastomas metastasize to the chest there may be mediastinal lymphadenopathy, pulmonary atelectasis, involvement of the lung parenchyma, and occasionally signs of mediastinal obstruction.

The occurrence of paralysis as an initial symptom due to extradural extension of neuroblastomas originating in the chest is not uncommon. In one series nearly 20 percent of children with thoracic neuroblastomas had partial or complete paralysis of the lower extremities.[48] Tumors originating in the paravertebral gutter may penetrate through a vertebral foramen, following the course of a sympathetic nerve fiber, then give rise to a second tumor within the spinal canal.[49] The gross morphology of these tumors suggests the name of "dumbbell" or "hour-glass" tumor. The pressure due to growth of the intraspinal portion of the tumor frequently causes paraplegia. Other symptoms that these tumors may cause include radicular pain, and motor weakness or limp.[39] Tumors located at the apex of the lung may cause Horner's syndrome.

Severe scoliosis may develop in children with neuroblastoma, ganglioneuroblastoma, or ganglioneuroma, especially when the primary tumor is in the mediastinum. Such a tumor arises from the sympathetic chain or from adrenal medulla close to the spinal column. Scoliosis may be present initially or may develop as long as four years after treatment of the original tumor.[50] Scoliosis in these cases is

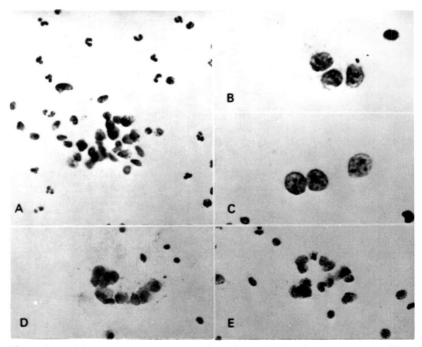

Figure 7. Exfoliated tumor cells in pleural fluid of a child with metastatic neuroblastoma. B and C (×900) show cells with scanty cytoplasma and distinct nucleoli. Note pleomorphic nuclei of cells in D and E (×350). Papaniculaou stain is used. (Courtesy of Dr. G. Farr and *Acta Cytologica*[44])

commonly concave toward the side of the mass. Removal of the tumor may result in correction of the scoliosis.[50]

Radiographic Findings

X-ray examination may show mediastinal adenopathy and parenchymal involvement, possibly producing some mediastinal shift, or pulmonary atelectasis. Compression of the superior vena cava may be seen on suitable contrast studies. A large neuroblastoma in the posterior-superior mediastinum can cause displacement of the trachea, esophagus, heart, and great vessels (Figure 8). Calcifications may be present in the tumor. Skeletal involvement of vertebrae or ribs is common and can be detected as asymmetrical loss of vertebral height, pedicle blurring, widening of neural foramina, thinning of ribs and intercostal widening.[8,14,50,51] These findings are often associated with intraspinal protrusion of the mass. Myelography is indicated in such cases, even in the absence of neurological signs. Confirmation by myelography of extradural impingement upon the cord is shown by blockage of flow of radiopaque dye in the thoracic subarachnoid space.[14]

Calcification, which is commonly present in abdominal (retroperitoneal) neuroblastomas, is rarely found in intrathoracic tumors, and is best seen in overpenetrated films.[8] Calcification is rarely if ever seen in metastases. Hence, the presence of calcification indicates that the tumor is probably primary. The finding of stippled or amorphous calcification in a thoracic, abdominal, pelvic, or cervical mass should alert the diagnostic radiologist to the possibility of a neuroblastoma.

Paravertebral widening on x-ray Retroperitoneal (Figure 9) or mediastinal (Figure 10) paravertebral widening is often seen in children with neuroblastoma. It is almost always seen in children with neuroblastomas originating in the mediastinum. Paravertebral widening is due both to direct contiguous extension of the tumor and also to foci of retroperitoneal metastases. This paravertebral widening is not seen in children with Wilms' tumor. Although it is not a pathognomonic sign of neuroblastoma, it is of critical diagnostic importance in the evaluation of the child with a thoracic or abdominal mass.[41]

Widening of the retroperitoneal paravertebral region in patients with neuroblastoma has a unique radiographic appearance. In this situation, the antero-posterior view of the lower thoracic or upper lumbar region demonstrates a segmental bulge, or a lateral convexity, of variable degree, which corresponds in length to the height of one to several vertebral bodies. The presence of this finding in patients known to have or suspected to have neuroblastoma usually signifies that the tumor has spread by contiguity to the paravertebral tissue or has metastasized to the retroperitoneal lymph nodes. Paravertebral

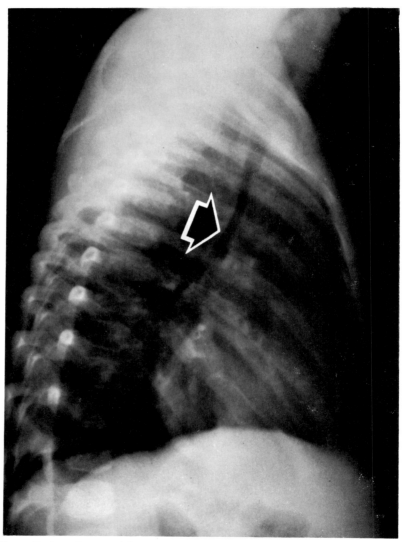

Figure 8. Lateral x-ray of the chest of a 22-month-old child showing indentation on the posterior wall of the trachea by neuroblastoma.

widening in retroperitoneal primary tumors is a bad prognostic sign, especially if it is contralateral, because it means that lymph node metastasis has occurred. It is, therefore, a potentially valuable sign in that it aids in the preoperative staging of the tumor and, also, signifies the need for additional therapy when it develops in the postoperative patient. When paravertebral widening is seen in a patient with an undiagnosed abdominal mass, it is quite likely that neuroblastoma is present.[41]

The child with neuroblastoma in the thorax has a better chance for prolonged survival than one with an abdominal tumor.[7] Review of large series of neuroblastomas originating in the thorax indicates that tumors arising in this location show increased likelihood to re-

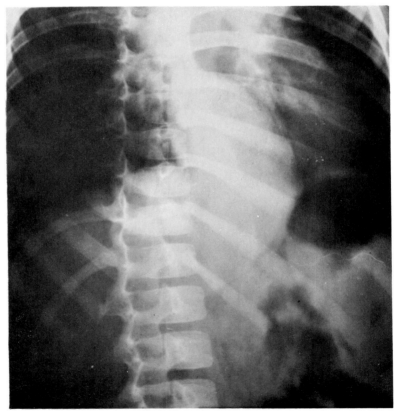

Figure 9. Abdominal x-ray showing a large, ovoid retroperitoneal neuroblastoma, with thinning of adjacent posterior ribs.

spond well to therapy.[14,39,53,54] The relation of prognosis to site of the primary tumor is discussed in Chapter 13. A neuroblastoma that arises in the mediastinum usually can be successfully treated even if

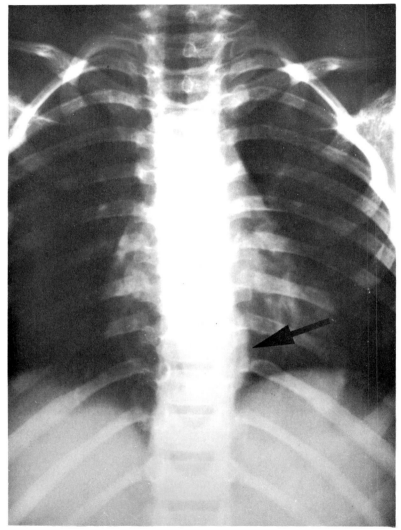

Figure 10. Chest x-ray showing a paraspinal mass in the left lower mediastinum (arrow). This represented direct extension of a left adrenal neuroblastoma.

the tumor has spread to produce clinical signs that ordinarily indicate a poor prognosis in a patient with cancer. The primary tumor should be excised as completely as possible, even in the presence of distant metastases.[55]

Distinguishing Between Primary and Metastatic Chest Tumors

The diagnosis of primary intrathoracic neuroblastoma is made by exclusion. If there is a mediastinal neuroblastoma but examination of the abdomen does not show an adrenal mass and if there is no calcification, displacement, or distortion of the superior pole of the kidney on intravenous pyelography, one assumes that the mediastinal tumor is of thoracic origin.

The symptoms and signs of a mediastinal neuroblastoma often lead the clinician to suspect an intrathoracic origin during the initial examination of such a patient. It is pertinent to stress, however, that occasionally this is misleading in that the intrathoracic mass is not the primary lesion but represents a metastasis. X-ray examination of the abdomen in these instances indicates the suprarenal, retroperitoneal origin by demonstrating renal displacement and suprarenal calcification. If the primary tumor arises in a sympathetic ganglion, signs of a paravertebral mass with or without intraspinal extension will then be found. Lymph node metastases are common in either situation, and commonly are present bilaterally. Palpable masses can then be identified, and appropriate radiographic studies will reveal displacement of retroperitoneal and intra-abdominal structures.

The importance of searching for these signs of intra-abdominal neuroblastoma in the child presenting with a mediastinal mass is stressed because, if it is documented that transdiaphragmatic metastases have occurred, radiation therapy along or in combination with chemotherapy is the treatment of choice rather than thoracotomy and attempted excision of a metastasis.[41] Although neuroblastoma has the highest rate of spontaneous regression among malignant neoplasms, it is commonly lethal, especially when adrenal in origin and locally advanced or metastatic. In contrast, extra-adrenal neuroblastoma, even with advanced local involvement, has a very high rate of prolonged survival. Therefore, careful study is necessary to accurately distinguish between primary mediastinal (extra-adrenal) neuroblastoma and mediastinal metastasis from a hidden primary lesion in the adrenal gland.[14]

ABDOMEN

There is much confusion with regard to the so-called Pepper and Hutchison syndromes in abdominal neuroblastoma. In 1901 Pepper reported some remarkable similarities in six cases.[56] The initial symptoms of each patient appeared by the age of 5 weeks; each patient was dead by the age of 16 weeks; each had extensive metastasis to the liver; and the primary tumor of each was in the right adrenal gland. The clinical picture was that of abdominal distention due to enlargement of the liver and abdominal lymph nodes. Hutchison, in 1907, described 10 cases of "sarcoma of the suprarenal gland" with metastases to the orbit and the skull.[57] In four of these patients the primary tumor was in the right adrenal gland and in six it was in the left adrenal gland. The striking clinical features were swelling about the skull, proptosis, and discoloration of the eyelids.

Nothing indicates that either Pepper or Hutchison intended to identify a syndrome, whether clinical or anatomical. It was Frew, in 1911, who introduced the concept of the Pepper and Hutchison syndromes.[58] He ascribed the clinical picture of abdominal swelling and enlargement of the liver to metastases from neuroblastomas of the right adrenal. This he called the "Pepper syndrome." The clinical picture of swelling about the skull and orbital and skeletal metastasis he believed due to primary tumors of the left adrenal, and he termed this the "Hutchison syndrome." Frew's theory has been repeatedly proven incorrect. There is no difference in the routes of metastases between neuroblastomas arising in the right or in the left adrenal glands. Although the contributions of Pepper and Hutchison to the early literature on neuroblastoma were of considerable importance, the concept of the Pepper and Hutchison syndromes as described by Frew had best be laid to rest.

It is truly the retroperitoneal space, including the adrenal gland and other structures of chromaffin origin rather than the abdomen, that is the most common site of origin for neuroblastomas. As with thoracic tumors, extensive growth may occur before any symptoms or signs are noted. In large upper abdominal neuroblastomas, it is difficult to decide whether the tumor originated in an adrenal gland or in a lumbar sympathetic ganglion.[13] The mass, when palpable, is generally in the flank or subcostal region. Its margins are usually not well defined. It is firm but, because of the insulating effect of the bowel and abdominal wall, may feel softer than it actually is. It may often be confused with an enlarged spleen, kidney, or cyst. If on the right side, it may push the liver downward, adding further difficulty in palpation. Tumor cells may be present in bone marrow smears. Soft tissue metastases are more common in the younger age group[59] (Figure 11).

The differential diagnosis of flank masses in small children includes the following:

1. Enlarged spleen
2. Renal cystic lesions
3. Hydronephrosis
4. Wilms' tumor and other renal neoplasmas
5. Neuroblastoma
6. Perinephric abscess
7. Adrenal cyst
8. Adrenal abscess[60]
9. Adrenocortical neoplasm
10. Pheochromocytoma
11. Retroperitoneal sarcoma
12. Hepatic neoplasm and hamartoma
13. Abnormal hepatic lobe
14. Mesenteric cyst
15. Choledochal cyst
16. Pancreatic cyst
17. Enteric duplication

Radiographic Findings

Abdominal neuroblastomas may be confused on palpation with enlarged viscera but may be accurately differentiated only by x-ray examination. The presence of calcification in the mass favors a diagnosis of neuroblastoma. On the intravenous pyelogram, the collecting system of the kidneys may appear normal, but one kidney is often considerably displaced by a neuroblastoma. The kidney is usually not directly invaded, but rather it is displaced downward and laterally. This creates the "drooping lily" deformity of the calyces[61] (Figure 12). Obliteration of the psoas shadow is sometimes observed, and occasionally hydronephrosis due to ureteral compression may be present.

In the intravenous pyelogram, neuroblastomas rarely produce a significant degree of hydronephrosis in the adjacent kidney, and deformities of renal calyces or nonfunction are uncommon in this disease. Usually the kidney outline is maintained in the presence of neuroblastoma which helps to differentiate it from Wilms' tumor. The deformity which may exist from neuroblastoma is an extrinsic one rather than the intrinsic one, such as is found with Wilms' tumor. Excretory pyelograms will often show the kidney displaced downward and outward. If there is upward or medial displacement the condition is more likely to be a renal tumor. Lateral x-ray films are helpful to show anterior displacement of the kidney especially in relation to the calcific areas in the tumor.[58,62] The urinary system can be involved in neuroblastoma by direct extension of the tumor or metastasis. In one study of 62 patients with neuroblastoma, 27 showed involvement of the urinary system. Alterations also occurred chiefly from direct pressure effects by the tumor. Evidence of tumor invasion of the kidney on I.V.P. in neuroblastoma is an unfavorable prognostic sign.[63]

Other radiographic studies which are a mandatory part of the work-up of the child suspected to have a neuroblastoma are x-ray films of the chest and of the skeleton. Pulmonary metastases are rare in neuroblastoma. They have no characteristic radiographic pattern when present.

One of the characteristic roentgenographic findings in neuroblastoma is calcification in the soft-tissue tumor. Intra-tumor calcifications

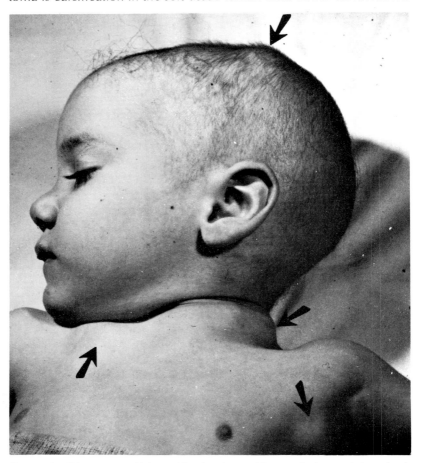

Figure 11. This 2½-year-old boy with adrenal neuroblastoma had several sites of soft tissue metastases (arrows).

visible by x-ray occur in about half the primary abdominal neuroblas-tomas[64] (Figure 13). Calcium present in a neuroblastoma is usually finely scattered within the tumor causing a mottled or stippled appearance. Hemangioendotheliomas and hepatomas may also contain calcifications. Calcified metastases in the retroperitoneal lymph nodes are occasionally seen, but they are rare in hepatic metastases.[65] The liver is involved either by direct spread or by metastases in one-third of the patients when they are first seen.

Centrally located, fine stippled calcification is found in neuro-blastomas about five times as often as it is seen in any other type of tumor in this area, and it rarely occurs in Wilms' tumor. Whenever plaque-like or linear calcifications are seen near the periphery of a flank tumor, calcification within a subcapsular hemorrhage in a Wilms' tumor or within hematoma due to trauma should be con-

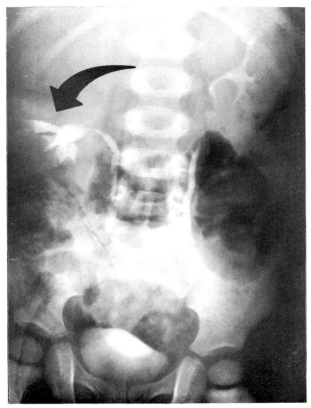

Figure 12. I.V.P. showing marked downward and lateral displacement of the right kidney, the "drooping lily" deformity (arrow).

sidered. If such calcification is found in association with flocculent calcifications centrally, then the diagnosis of neuroblastoma is virtually assured. Thus, a stippled calcific shadow in the adrenal region with separate calcifications in the liver or paravertebral region is highly suggestive of neuroblastoma.[64] Liver metastases from neuroblastoma that calcify are very rare. But calcification of the adrenal from neonatal trauma and calcification in the liver associated with hemangioma, though rare, is probably seen with equal frequency.

Tumoral calcification in neuroblastoma is dystrophic in type—in other words, it is the result of a change in the chemical structure of the intercellular substances. The mechanism by which this occurs is complex and imperfectly understood. Why calcification occurs in some necrotic tumors and not in others is unknown. Since it is more common in embryonic tumors in children than in adult carcinomas, it might be considered more likely to appear in rapidly growing, large tumors which outstrip their blood supply, with consequent necrosis and calcification. The prognosis in calcified malignant tumors has not

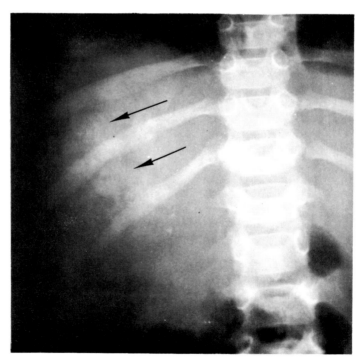

Figure 13. X-ray of abdomen showing mottled calcifications in a large neuroblastoma of the right adrenal area (arrows).

been shown to differ, however. from that in noncalcified tumors when the patients are of similar age. Calcification in abdominal neuroblastomas is less common in infants than in older children, and, since neuroblastoma in infancy has a better outlook than at a later age, the overall prognosis in calcified neuroblastomas is not quite so good as when the tumor is not calcified. The size of the calcified primary tumor and the occurrence of metastases is not greater than that of uncalcified ones.[58,64,65]

Functionally active intrathoracic or abdominal neuroblastomas Under certain circumstances so far undefined, neuroblastomas and ganglioneuromas may be associated with secretion of pressor amines in sufficient amounts to cause clinical symptoms. The signs and symptoms associated with functioning neurogenic tumors are presumably caused by excessive production of norepinephrine and epinephrine. Hypertension, diarrhea, excessive sweating, flushing or pallor, rash, polyuria, and polydypsia are the characteristic findings associated with excess urinary excretion of catecholamines or VMA. Considerable variation exists in the symptomatology of patients showing these manifestations, possibly because of variability in the predominant metabolite of the catecholamine secreted by the tumor.

Hawfield and Daisley[66] recorded for the first time in 1952 the association of diarrhea with neurogenic tumors. Since then 18 such cases have been described. In many of these the tumor was an incidental finding, either as a space-occupying lesion seen in the chest x-ray, as a palpable abdominal mass, or as calcifications in the abdomen. The relationship to diarrhea was only attributed to the tumor when diarrhea ceased abruptly after surgical removal of the tumor.[67] The site of the tumor is usually in the mediastinum or in the abdomen, but it may also be in the pelvis.

Ganglioneuroblastomas, neuroblastomas, and ganglioneuromas may secrete epinephrine and other adrenergic metabolites which can cause episodes of hypertension and flushing. However, the mechanism by which these tumors cause diarrhea is not understood. The association between sympathetic tumors and diarrhea was firmly established in 1959 when Green and co-workers.[68] as well as Greenberg and Gardner,[69] presented several instances of neuroblastoma in association with chronic diarrhea. Diarrhea ceased after complete removal of the tumor in each patient.

Mason reported an infant with an adrenaline-secreting intrathoracic neuroblastoma which was successfully removed.[70] The preoperative symptoms (sweating, pallor, tachycardia, and hypertension) were completely relieved by extirpation of the tumor. A similar case was reported by Smith.[71] Preoperatively, a 3½-year-old girl behaved clinically as though she had a pheochromocytoma. She had increased sweating, tachycardia, hypertension, and irritability during the two years before a thoracic neuroblastoma was diagnosed. Chronic diarrhea was not present. Urinary catecholamines were markedly elevated. All these abnormalities disappeared following surgical removal of the tumor.

In a review of 28 patients with adrenergic symptoms or with increased secretion of catecholamines or both, 14 had neuroblastoma, 8 had ganglioneuroblastoma, and 6 had ganglioneuroma.[72] Hypertension was present in 15 patients, diarrhea in 12, profuse sweating in 8, palpitation in 5, pallor in 4, a rash in 3, paroxysmal attacks in 3, polyuria and polydipsia in 3, flushing in 2, and 3 patients were asymptomatic despite increased excretion of catecholamines. Diarrhea and hypertension were both present in 3 patients. Hypertension, diarrhea, other adrenergic symptoms, and increased secretion of catecholamines or VMA occurred in association with the different types of tumor. Hypertension was found in 10 patients with neuroblastoma, 3 with ganglioneuroblastoma, and in 1 with ganglioneuroma. Diarrhea was present in 6 patients with ganglioneuroma, 4 with ganglioneuroblastoma, and in 2 with neuroblastoma.[72]

The occurrence of Cushing's syndrome has been found in association with increased secretion of catecholamines in a few patients. An 18-month-old girl with Cushing's syndrome and virilization was found to have bilateral suprarenal masses which, at surgical removal, proved to be an adrenal ganglioneuroblastoma and an adrenal adenoma. One year after surgery the patient was without evidence of recurrent disease.[73] Cushing's syndrome has been seen in association with ganglioneuroblastoma and adrenal neuroblastoma.[74,75,76] It is likely that these neuroblastomas were asymptomatic. Thus, these are examples of the detection of a malignant tumor (neuroblastoma) only because of the symptoms of a probably benign tumor (adrenocortical adenoma).

A few cases have been reported in which there was the occurrence of chronic diarrhea with abdominal distention and wasting (celiac-like syndrome) as the presenting symptoms in patients who had either a ganglioneuroma or a ganglioneuroblastoma. The diarrhea could not be attributed to other known causes.[68,77,78] Preoperatively there was elevated excretion of catecholamines. Following removal of the tumor, the diarrhea subsided and the children began to gain weight.[67] Improvement in the child's appetite and general behavior was dramatic. Excessive sweating and abdominal distention also diminished strikingly.

It appears that this clinical picture is not rare and that neuroblastoma should be kept in mind when a child presents with the "celiac triad": diarrhea, weight loss, and enlargement of the abdomen.[79] The radiographic findings are of special interest since alteration of colonic motility may be of particular importance in the pathogenesis of the symptoms in these unusual cases. Follow-up studies would show that the urinary excretion of catecholamines returns to normal and barium enema should show return of the colon to normal caliber. Fourteen months after operation one such child was completely well.[79] Other similar cases have been reported.[68,78,80-82]

The mechanism of production of diarrhea is as yet unknown, but it is suggested that these tumors secrete a substance which either stimulates peristalsis or alters absorption or excretion of water and/or electrolytes in the gut. Neuroblastomas, which secrete epinephrine and related neurohumors at a constant or intermittent rate, may cause diarrhea by producing recurrent periods of hypermotility in the intestinal wall; this hypermotility may be related to the refractoriness of the neuroeffector junctions to these adrenergic mediators. Another theory presented by Hamilton suggests that abnormal catecholamine secretion from these tumors may cause diarrhea by adversely affecting blood flow to the intestinal absorptive mucosa.[83] However, not all patients with catecholamine-secreting neurogenic tumors have diarrhea, and patients with pheochromocytomas do not usually have diarrhea as a prominent symptom.[80] It is not known whether a certain combination of catecholamines or their metabolites is necessary to produce the diarrhea, or whether the symptom is caused by the release of a noncatechol agent from these neoplasms. The latter theory is favored in those patients with tumor and diarrhea in whom levels of VMA and catecholamine excretion are within normal limits.[82,84]

PELVIS

Neuroblastomas originating from sacral sympathetic ganglia comprised only 4.5 percent of 1,303 cases compiled from recently reported series (Figure 1). Sacral neuroblastomas often respond well to therapy, even when they are very large and cannot be completely resected.[14,19]

In the sacral sympathetic area, a neuroblastoma may originate either from the sacral plexus or from the para-aortic bodies of Zuckerkandl. When a neuroblastoma originates in the pelvis, symptoms are usually related to bowel or bladder dysfunction. The tumor may be felt on rectal examination in a child who had disturbed bowel function. Compression of the bladder (Figure 14) or compression of the rectum (Figure 15) may cause symptoms of partial or complete obstruction.[85] There may be hydroureter or hydronephrosis. Pressure on blood vessels and lymphatic vessels may produce edema, dimin-

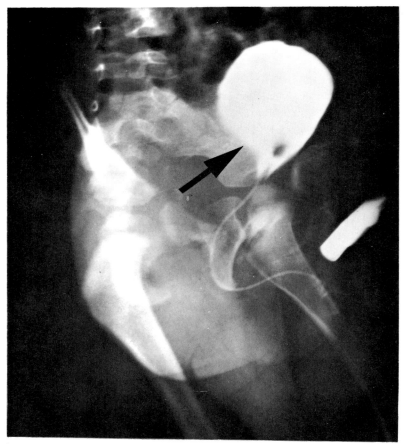

Figure 14. Cystogram showing anterior displacement of the bladder (arrow) due to pelvic neuroblastoma.

ished warmth, or cyanosis of the legs (Figure 16). Extension of the tumor through the sacrosciatic notch may result in swelling of the buttock.[86] Downward extension of tumor may cause swelling of the scrotum.[87] Intraspinal invasion by the tumor may cause weakness of the legs, limp, sensory deficit, or radicular pain. Involvement of the sacral plexus may produce a neurogenic bladder.[19,88,89] A child who is toilet trained may show loss of sphincter control due to involvement of the lumbar and sacral nerve roots by the tumor. Opsoclonus may also occur in children with neuroblastomas originating in the pelvis. Even incomplete removal of a sacral neuroblastoma followed by x-ray therapy and chemotherapy may cure the patient.

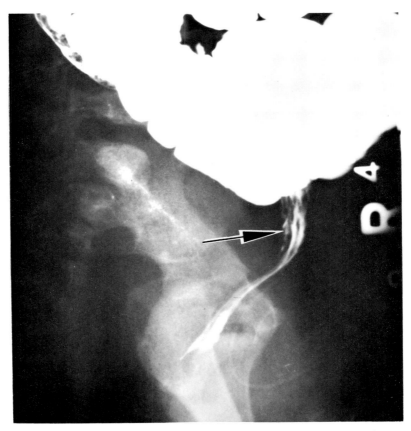

Figure 15. Barium enema showing narrowing and anterior displacement of the rectum by an extrinsic mass which proved to be a pre-sacral neuroblastoma.

84

SUMMARY

Neuroblastomas may arise from any site where one would normally find elements of the sympathetic nervous system—this includes the adrenal medulla and the sympathetic chain on either side of the neck, thorax, abdomen and pelvis. Neuroblastomas present with a wide range of clinical manifestations which may be systemic (Figure 2) or dependent upon the local site of origin or site of metastasis (Table 1).

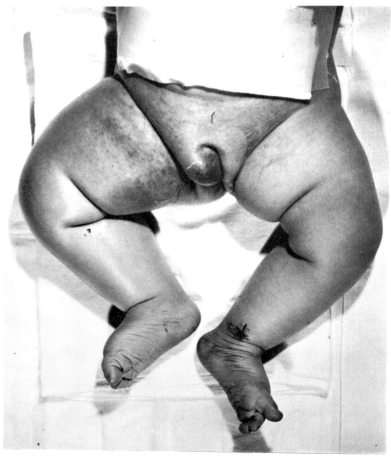

Figure 16. A six-month-old girl with large presacral neuroblastoma causing venous engorgement and edema of the right leg and vulva.

Table 1
Clinical Manifestations of Neuroblastomas Occurring in Various Parts of the Body

Site of Primary Neuroblastoma	Clinical Manifestations	
	Symptoms	Commonest Physical or X-Ray Findings
Head	Cranial nerve palsy Nasal obstruction Proptosis	Edema of face Horner's syndrome Heterochromia of irides
Neck	Mass in neck Radicular pain	Horner's syndrome Heterochromia of irides Lymphadenopathy Tracheal deviation
Chest	Leg weakness or limp Cough or dyspnea Arm weakness Chest pain Dysphagia	Posterior mediastinal mass Erosion of rib Scoliosis Superior vena cava syndrome Block on myelogram
Abdomen	Enlarged abdomen Abdominal pain Leg weakness	Abdominal mass Hepatomegaly Displaced kidney on I.V.P. Calcifications
Pelvis	Limp Loss of bowel or bladder control Constipation Radicular pain	Mass in pelvis Mass in rectum or buttock Compression of bladder Hydronephrosis Poor sphincter tone Edema or cyanosis of legs

REFERENCES

1. Hutchinson, J.E., Nash, A., and McCord, C.: Neuroblastoma of the anterior mediastinum in an adult. *J. Thorac. Cardiovasc. Surg.* 56: 147–152, 1968.

2. McCollough, C.D., and Hardart, F.: Neuroblastomatous Transformation in a Benign Cystic Teratoma. *Obst. & Gynec.* 21: 259–261, 1963.

3. Bodian, M.: Neuroblastoma. *Pediat. Clin. N. Amer.* 6: 449–472, 1959.

4. Gross, R.E., Farber, S., and Martin, L.W.: Neuroblastoma Sympatheticum; A study and report of 217 cases. *Pediatrics* 23: 1179, 1959.

5. Chapman, K., and Sheridan, A.: Neuroblastoma; 10 year experience. *Surgery* 48: 1101–1106, 1960.

6. King, R.L., Storasli, J.P., and Bolande, R.P.: Neuroblastoma: Review of twenty-eight cases and presentation of two cases with metastases and long survival. *Amer. J. Roentgenol.* 85: 733–747, 1961.

7. Koop, C., and Hernandez, J.: Neuroblastoma; experience with 100 cases in children. *Surgery* 56: 726–733, 1964.

8. Adams, L.: Neuroblastoma; review of the literature and report of 18 cases. *North Carolina Med. J.* 27: 113–125, 1966.

9. Lingley, J.F., Sagerman, R.H., Santulli, T.V., and Wolff, J.A.: Neuroblastoma; Management and Survival. *New Engl. J. Med.* 277: 1227, 1967.

10. Priebe, C., and Clatworthy, W.: Neuroblastoma; evaluation of the treatment of 90 children. *Arch. Surg.* 95: 538–545, 1967.

11. Fortner, J., Nicastri, A., and Murphy, M.L.: Neuroblastoma: Natural History and Results of Treating 133 Cases. *Ann. Surg.* 167: 132, 1968.

12. deLorimier, A., Bragg, K., and Linden, G.: Neuroblastoma in childhood. *Amer. J. Dis. Child.* 118: 441–450, 1969.

13. Stella, J., Schweisguth, O., and Schlienger, M.: Neuroblastoma; a study of 144 cases. *Amer. J. Roentgenol.* 108: 324–332, 1970.

14. Young, L., Rubin, P., and Hanson, R.: The extra-adrenal neuroblastoma; high radiocurability and diagnostic accuracy. *Amer. J. Roentgenol.* 108: 75–91, 1970.

15. Swank, R., Fetterman, G.H., Sieber, W., and Kiesewetter, W.: Prognostic factors in neuroblastoma. *Ann. Surg.* 174: 428–435, 1971.

16. Rosenfeld, L., Graves, H., and Lawrence, R.: Primary neurogenic tumors of the lateral neck. *Ann. Surg.* 167: 847–855, 1968.

17. Albert, D., Rubenstein, R., and Scheie, H.: Tumor metastasis to the eye. II. Clinical study in infants and children. *Amer. J. Ophthol.* 63: 727–732, 1967.

18. Apple, D.: Metastatic orbital neuroblastoma originating in the cervical sympathetic ganglionic chain. *Amer. J. Ophthal.* 68: 1093–1095, 1969.

19. Hope-Stone, H.: Extra-adrenal neuroblastoma. *Brit. J. Surg.* 48: 424–429, 1961.

20. Pulliam, R.: Ganglioneuroblastoma; a case involving the superior cervical ganglion. *Arch. Otolaryng.* 74: 40–44, 1961.

21. Dawson, D.: Nerve cell tumors of the neck and their secretory activity. *J. Laryngol.* 84: 203–216, 1970.

22. Heitzman, E.R., and Markarian, B.: Enlarged neural foramena in a child with cervical neuroblastoma. *N.Y. State J. Med.* 71: 449–452, 1971.

23. Rosendal, T.: Two cases of sympathicoblastoma of the suprarenal gland with metastasis to the cranium and the tubular bones. *Acta Radiol.* 23: 462, 1942.

24. Burford, W.N.: Symposium on 18 cases of benign and malignant lesions of the oral cavity from the Ellis Fischel State Cancer Hospital, Columbia, Mo. *Amer. J. Orthodont.* 33: 1, 1947.

25. Burch, R.J.: Metastasis of neuroblastoma of the mandible; report of a case. *J. Oral Surg.* 10: 160, 1952.

26. Blum, T.: Instructive clinical case reports. *Oral Surg.* 10: 1239, 1957.

27. Levine, M.: Neuroblastoma of adrenal gland with metastasis to mandible. *Dalhousie Dent. J.* 1: 161, 1961.

28. Pedler, J.A.: Secondary neuroblastoma of the mandible. *Oral Surg.* 1: 989, 1961.

29. Montana, R.A.: Metastatic neuroblastoma of the mandible, recurrent. *J. Clin. Stomat. Conf.* (Columbia Univ.) 6: 30, 1965.

30. Hoffman, S., and Green, G.H.: Neuroblastoma with metastasis to the mandible; report of a case. *J. Oral Surg.* 24: 75–81, 1966.

31. Bradley, P.F., and Rowe, N.L.: Mandibular metastasis of a neuroblastoma; report of case. *J. Oral Surg.* 28: 781–784, 1970.

32. DeLeon, E.L., et al.: Neuroblastoma with metastasis to maxilla and mandible; review of literature and report of case. *J. Oral Surg.* 28: 773–780, 1970.

33. Angelopoulos, A., Tilson, J., and Stewart, R.W.: Metastatic neuroblastoma of the mandible; review of literature and report of a case. *J. Oral Surg.* 30: 93–106, 1972.

34. Dehner, L.P.: Tumors of the mandible and maxilla in children. II. A study of 14 primary and secondary malignant tumors. *Cancer* 32: 112–120, 1973.

35. Keusch, K., Poole, C., and King, D.: The significance of "floating teeth" in children. *Radiology* 86: 215–219, 1966.

36. Stern, M., Turner, J., and Coburn, T.P.: Oral involvement in neuroblastoma. *J.A.D.A.* 88: 346–351, 1974.

37. Mullaney, P.J., Mullaney, J., and Coffey, V.: Primary thoracic neuroblastoma; report of two cases. *Irish J. Med. Sci.* 410: 81–86, 1960.

38. Delaitre, R., Testard, R., Migner, C., et al.: Neonatal res-

piratory distress due to thoracic neuroblastoma. *Arch. Franc. de Pediat.* 29: 557, 1972.

39. Schweisguth, O., Mathey, J., Renault, P., and Binet, J.: Intrathoracic neurogenic tumors in infants and children; a study of forty cases. *Ann. Surg.* 150: 29–41, 1959.

40. Saenger, E., and Dorst, J.: Radiation therapy. (Shirkey, H., ed.) In *Pediatric Therapy*. St. Louis: C.V. Mosby Company, 1968. Pp. 975–977.

41. Eklof, O., and Gooding, C.: Intrathoracic neuroblastoma. *Amer. J. Roentgenol.* 100: 202–207, 1967.

42. Ghosh, P.: Pleural effusion due to neuroblastoma. *Brit. J. Dis. Chest.* 62: 219–220, 1968.

43. Rath, R., and Touloukian, R.: Infarction of a mediastinal neuroblastoma with hemorrhage and pleural effusion. *Ann. Thorac. Surg.* 10: 552–555, 1970.

44. Farr, G., and Hajdu, S.: Exfoliative cytology of metastatic neuroblastoma. *Acta Cytol.* (Baltimore) 16: 203–206, 1972.

45. Sutton, J., Parker, E., and Pratt-Thomas, H.R.: Nonepithelial malignant tumors of the lung and mediastinum. *American Surg.* 34: 605–610, 1968.

46. Oberman, H.: Sympathicoblastoma of the anterior mediastinum. *Dis. Chest* 43: 314–317, 1963.

47. Buthker, W., Feltkamp-Broom, T., Goren, A.S., and Wieberdink, J.: Sympathicoblastoma in the anterior mediastinum. *Dis. Chest* 46: 531–536, 1964.

48. Filler, R., Traggis, D., Jaffe, N., and Vawter, G.: Favorable outlook for children with mediastinal neuroblastoma. *J. Pediat. Surg.* 7: 136–143, 1972.

49. Ware, G.: Thoracic neuroblastoma. *J. Pediatr.* 49: 765–773, 1956.

50. Bulmer, J.: Scoliosis complicating ganglion cell tumors. *Brit. J. Surg.* 53: 619–624, 1966.

51. Smith, R., Whitehead, T., Morris, L., and Williams, H.: Functionally active intrathoracic neuroblastoma. *Arch. Dis. Childh.* 36: 82–89, 1961.

52. Griff, L., and Griff, R.: Neuroblastoma; emphasis on the mediastinal neuroblastoma. *Amer. J. Roentgenol.* 103: 19–24, 1968.

53. Alexander, L.L.: Primary mediastinal neuroblastoma in an infant; a 21 year survival following radiation therapy. *J. Nat. Med. Ass.* 53: 36–38, 1961.

54. Wieberdink, J.: Foetal haemic metastasis; an exploration of the Pepper-type metastasis in adrenal neuroblastoma. *Brit. J. Cancer* 11: 378–383, 1957.

55. Mayo, P.: Intrathoracic neuroblastoma in a newborn infant. *J. Thorac. Cardiov. Surg.*, 45: 720–724, 1963.

56. Pepper, W.: A study of congenital sarcoma of the liver and suprarenal; with report of a case. *Amer. J. Med. Sci.* 121: 287–299, 1901.

57. Hutchison, R.: On suprarenal sarcoma in children with metastases in the skull. *Quart. J. Med.* 1: 338–38, 1907.

58. Frew, R.S.: On carcinoma originating in the suprarenal medulla in children. *Quart. J. Med.* 4: 123–140, 1911.

59. Benson, C., Mastard, W., Ravitch, M., et al. (eds.): *Pediatric Surgery*. (Vol. II). Chicago: Year Book Medical Publishers, 1962, pp. 874–885.

60. Favara, B., Akers, D.R., and Franciosi, R.: Adrenal abscess in a neonate. *J. Pediatr.* 77: 682–685, 1970.

61. Berdon, W., and Baker, D.: Radiographic findings in adrenal disease in infants and children. *New York State J. Med.* 69: 2773–2778, 1969.

62. Ecklof, O., and Lundin, E.: Renal pelvis appearances in nephro- and neuroblastomas; diagnostic value of true lateral projections. *Acta Radiol. Diagnosis* 8: 209–220, 1969.

63. Varkarakis, M., Bhanalaph, T., and Murphy, G.: Kidney involvement in neuroblastoma. *New York State J. Med.* 72: 2753–2756, 1972.

64. Ross, P.: Calcification in liver metastasis from neuroblastoma. *Radiology* 85: 1074–1079, 1965.

65. Hope, J., Borns, P., and Koop, C.: Diagnosis and Treatment of Neuroblastoma and Embryoma of the Kidney. *Radiol. Clin. North America* 1: 593–620, 1963.

66. Hawfield, H.H., and Daisley, G.: A report of a case of a functional adrenal ganglioneuroma. *Clin. Proc. Child. Hosp.* (Washington, D.C.) 8: 98–102, 1952.

67. Sindhu, S., and Anderson, C.: Ganglioneuroma as a cause of diarrhea and failure to thrive. *Aust. Paediatr. J.* 1: 56–60, 1965.

68. Green, M., Cooke, R., and Lattanzi, W.: Occurrence of chronic diarrhea in three patients with ganglioneuromas. *Pediatrics* 23: 951–955, 1959.

69. Greenberg, R.E., and Gardner, L.I.: New diagnostic test for neural tumors of infancy; increased urinary excretion of 3-methoxy-4-hydroxymandelic acid and norepinephrine in ganglioneuroma with chronic diarrhea. *Pediatrics* 24: 683, 1959.

70. Mason, G., Hart-Nercer, J., Miller, E.J., et al.: Adrenaline-secreting neuroblastoma in an infant. *Lancet* 2: 322–325, 1957.

71. Smith, R.A., Whitehead, T., Morris, L., and Williams, H.P.:

Functionally active intrathoracic neuroblastoma. *Arch. Dis. Childh.* 36: 82–89, 1961.

72. Kogut, M., and Kaplan, S.A.: Systemic manifestations of neurogenic tumors. *J. Pediatr.* 60: 694–704, 1962.

73. Dahms, W.T., Gray, G., Vrana, M., and New, M.: Adrenocortical adenoma and ganglioneuroblastoma in a child; a case presenting as Cushing syndrome with virilization. *Amer. J. Dis. Child.* 125: 608–611, 1973.

74. Kogut, M., and Donnell, G.: Cushing's syndrome in association with renal ganglioneuroblastoma. *Pediatrics* 28: 566–577, 1961.

75. Normann, T., Havnen, J., and Mjolnerod, O.: Cushing's syndrome in an infant associated with neuroblastoma in two ectopic adrenal glands. *J. Pediatr. Surg.* 6: 169–175, 1971.

76. Omenn, G.S.: Ectopic hormone syndromes associated with tumors in childhood. *Pediatrics* 47: 613–622, 1971.

77. Fregonese, B., Cottafova, F., Vignola, G., et al.: Tumors of the neural crest with chronic diarrhea. *Minerva Pediatr.* 21: 1699–1704, 1969.

78. Rosenstein, B.J., and Engelman, K.: Diarrhea in a child with catecholamine-secreting ganglioneuroma. *J. Pediatr.* 63: 217–221, 1963.

79. McCrea, W.: Neuroblastoma and the coeliac triad. *Scot. Med. J.* 10: 65–69, 1965.

80. Stickler, G.B., Hallenbeck, G.A., Flock, E.F. and Resevear, J.W.: Catecholamines and diarrhea in ganglioneuroblastoma. *Amer. J. Dis. Child.* 104: 598–602, 1962.

81. Cameron, D., Warner, H., and Szabo, A.: Chronic diarrhea in an adult with hypokalemic nephropathy and osteomalocia due to a functioning ganglioneuroblastoma. *Amer. J. Med. Sci.* 253: 417–424, 1967.

82. Peterson, H.D., and Collins, O.D.: Chronic diarrhea and failure to thrive secondary to ganglioneuroma. *Arch. Surg.* 95: 934, 1967.

83. Hamilton, R.J., Radde, I.C. and Johnson, G.: Diarrhea associated with adrenal ganglioneuroma. *Amer. J. Med.* 44: 453, 1968.

84. Galbert, M.: Chronic diarrhea with ganglioneuroblastoma. *Clin. Pediatr.* 10: 476–479, 1971.

85. Hepler, A.: Presacral sympathicoblastoma in an infant causing urinary obstruction. *J. Urol.* 49: 777–782, 1943.

86. Dargeon, H.: Neuroblastoma. *J. Pediatr.* 61: 456–462, 1962.

87. Simpson, T., Lynn, H., and Milla, S.: Congenital neuroblastoma in the scrotum. *Clin. Pediatr.* 8: 174–175, 1969.

88. Pochedly, C., Sarrafi, G., and Kenigsberg, K.: Removal of sacral neuroblastoma by posterior route with prolonged survival. *J.A.M.A.* 224: 1186–1187, 1973.

89. Mann, C., Leape, L., and Holder, T.M.: Neonatal urinary ascites; a report of two cases of unusual etiology and a review of the literature. *J. Urol.* III: 124–128, 1974.

4 Neuroblastoma in the Skeletal System

Carl Pochedly, M.D.
Dvorah Balsam, M.D.

1. Factors influencing location of bone metastases in neuroblastoma
2. Bone marrow demonstration of metastases in neuroblastoma
3. Incidence and locations of bone lesions
4. X-ray appearance of metastases in neuroblastoma
5. Differential diagnosis of x-ray findings suggesting neuroblastoma metastases
   a. Local bone diseases
   b. Systemic diseases
6. Detecting occult bony metastases by scanning techniques
   Summary

Skeletal lesions are a common feature of metastatic neuroblastoma. Metastases to bone have a broad spectrum of clinical signs and symptoms. The distribution of bone involvement can be determined only by a thorough radiographic evaluation and by post-mortem examination.

FACTORS INFLUENCING LOCATION

Skeletal metastases most frequently localize in the spine, pelvic bones, femur, skull, ribs, and humerus. In those bones commonly involved by metastasis, the medullary cavity contains red bone marrow. Because of atrophy of bone marrow in the peripheral skeleton which progresses with age, the bones of the forearm and foreleg have a low incidence of metastases.[1] In general, factors

93

influencing the location of metastases include: (1) the mode of extension; (2) filtering barriers encountered by the cancer; (3) the status of the capillary bed receiving the tumor deposit; and (4) variations in the growth potential of tumors that metastasize to bone.[1]

Malignant tumors may spread by the blood stream into the bone marrow. This deduction is based on the following observations: (1) metastases to bone occur in the medullary cavity; (2) subperiosteal invasion often begins in the region of large foramina which serve as a point of egress for the veins; and (3) individual cancer cells in the bone marrow lie within definite channels which are arranged in a manner similar to that of the veins present in the marrow.[1]

It is uncertain whether there are lymphatics within bone structure. Tumors may, however, extend to the bone structure by direct invasion from the periosteum previously involved through lymphatic extension. Where such extension occurs, bones near the primary growth have a higher incidence of involvement—for example, in carcinoma of the breast the upper humerus, scapula, clavicle, and ribs are commonly involved.[1]

The vertebral vein system forms a valveless plexus; it is a separate pool for blood forced from the veins of the thoracoabdominal system by any act of coughing, sneezing, lifting, or straining. This venous system includes the epidural venous plexus, which communicates with the venous dural sinuses and drains the spinal cord and vertebral column. It communicates with various segmental veins of the body at the various intervertebral foramina. Metastases, therefore, may be distributed anywhere along the vertebral system without involving the portal, the pulmonary, or the caval systems of veins. The latter venous systems drain into barriers which filter the tumor cells and may prevent widespread peripheral vascular metastases.

Cancer cells have been found floating in the regional venous systems of various parts of the body of patients with known primary sites of cancer. Yet there is little evidence, in many cases, that metastatic foci are present. The particular circumstances of the tumor-host relationship in each case determine the development and character of metastases and the route of dissemination. Secondary deposits from certain tumors are more capable of survival and growth in distant regions than are those of other neoplasms—for example, extension to bone occurs more often in patients with mammary, renal, prostatic, and bronchogenic carcinoma. In general, there is a relationship between the type of cancer and its mode and extent of spread.[1]

When metastases are present, the elements constituting the normal bone marrow eventually are completely replaced by tumor tissue. Microscopic examination reveals a relentless and continuous spread of tumor through the haversian systems, invading and destroying the surrounding bone of the cortex. Reactive bone will often form about such areas of invading tumor in an attempt to contain the metastatic area by new osteoid tissue. Depending on the degree of success of reactive bone activity, radiography of skeletal lesions shows either predominant osteolytic or osteoblastic bone changes.[1]

BONE MARROW DEMONSTRATION OF METASTASES

The finding of distinctive tumor cells in smears of aspirates from bone marrow of neuroblastoma patients was reported in 1938 by Kato and Wachter.[2] The value of this method in the diagnosis of neuroblastoma is well established.[3-6] The morphologic characteristics of neuroblastoma cells as they appear in smears of bone marrow are distinctive. The recognition of neuroblastoma cells in smears of marrow may in many instances be of considerable clinical importance.[6] Neuroblastoma cells are readily distinguished from normal marrow cells. The typical pattern of neuroblastoma is the arrangement of tumor cells in ball-like clumps or mosaics. This appearance reflects the tendency of neuroblastoma cells to grow in ball-like agglomerations. The clumps of cells in bone marrow smears present a mosaic pattern with indistinct cell boundaries (Figure 1). There is often a suggestion of pseudorosette formation.[6]

Neuroblastoma cells are usually larger than myeloblasts. Nuclei tend to be round in cells that appear singly but they appear polygonal in cells arranged in clumps. The nuclei are large with an immature chromatin pattern. Staining of the fine network of chromatin is usually deep purple-blue, but somewhat paler in partially degenerated or aging cells. Nucleoli can often be identified. Mitotic figures are rare. Cytoplasm is scant and faintly basophilic, without granules. Cytoplasmic vacuoles are rarely observed.[6] In an instance in which the neuroblastoma cells are not present in clumps but tend to be scattered singly, it becomes difficult to distinguish them from cells of reticulum cell sarcoma, lymphosarcoma, or acute leukemia.[6]

Observers differ as to the degree of reliability of bone marrow smears in the diagnosis of neuroblastoma. Positive bone marrow smears provide a strong presumptive diagnosis of neuroblastoma in patients who also have increased VMA or catecholamines in the urine. The tendency of cells of metastatic carcinoma in general to form clumps in smears of aspirates from bone marrow is well known. It is impossible to differentiate with certainty clumps of metastatic cells from various forms of carcinoma and those of neuroblastoma. But in attempting to classify tumor cells found in smears of bone marrow from infants and children, the clinician is strongly influenced by the knowledge that neuroblastoma is by far the leading cause of bone marrow metastases in this age group. The most common error in the interpretation of metastatic neuroblastoma cells in smears of bone marrow is to regard them as representative of acute leukemia. Where the characteristic mosaic aggregates (clumps) of neuroblastoma cells are present, such confusion should not occur.[6]

Bone marrow metastases of neuroblastoma may also be demonstrated histologically, in sections of biopsied bone marrow, in children with negative smears of aspirated marrow. The histology of the bone marrow as seen on 40 biopsies from 31 children with neuroblastoma was studied. Marrow invasion was seen in 20 samples. Tumor invasion of the marrow may be partial, with presence of

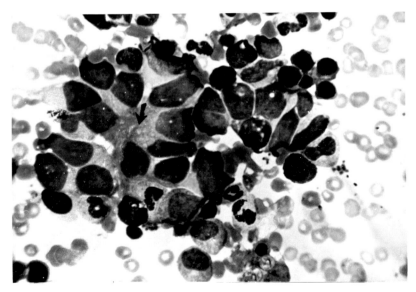

Figure 1. Photomicrograph of bone marrow smear showing a clump of neuroblastoma cells (arrow). A few normal granulocytes and erythroid precursors are also present.

small tumor nodules and without any marked cellular reaction by the bone marrow. On the other hand, there may be total invasion with areas of tumor necrosis and associated myelosclerosis.[7] The reticulin network may be abnormally developed and hemorrhagic areas may be seen both in the invaded and in the normal marrow. A comparative study of the result of marrow biopsy, smears of aspirated bone marrow, the peripheral blood, and the x-ray of the skeleton have shown the biopsy to be a useful adjunct to define the extent of the disease and the cause of anemia in neuroblastoma.[7]

The presence of neuroblastoma cells in bone marrow need not be accompanied by the presence of skeletal lesions visible on x-ray examination. The early bone metastases involve marrow spaces and hematopoietic tissue rather than osseous tissues proper. In addition, the involvement of marrow in neuroblastoma is often diffuse rather than focal.[6] It should be noted, however, that, in young children with stage IV-S neuroblastoma, bone marrow involvement as demonstrated by presence of tumor cells in bone marrow smears is of far less grave significance than when bone changes are demonstrated by x-ray examination (see Chapter 10).

INCIDENCE AND LOCATIONS OF BONE LESIONS

Metastatic neuroblastoma has a special predilection for the skeleton. Survey roentgenograms of the skull, spinal column, pelvis, and long bones should be done when the diagnosis of neuroblastoma is suspected or is histologically proven. Skeletal metastases have a significant relationship to the age of the patient, occurring more frequently in the older age group than among patients two years of age or younger. Neuroblastoma patients with radiographically demonstrable skeletal metastases (rather than a positive marrow examination) have an almost uniformly fatal outcome. Therefore, a careful search for these lesions at the time of initial presentation is mandatory.

Metastases from neuroblastoma are actually most frequent in the retroperitoneal lymph nodes, but by x-ray examination metastases are most easily recognized in the skeleton. Hepatic and lymph node metastases are not radiographically obvious unless calcified, or unless there is noticeable hepatomegaly. There is a very high incidence of skeletal metastases at the time of initial diagnosis in children with neuroblastoma. In one series, 37 out of 50 patients with neuroblastoma (74 percent) showed one or more areas of bone metastasis. In

26 out of 37 (70 percent) there was evidence that more than one bone was involved. A solitary bone lesion was the presenting finding in several cases.[8] In another series of 73 proved neuroblastomas reviewed as to the results of x-ray therapy, there were only 26 patients (35 percent) with bone metastases on admission.[9] The same percentage was seen by Benson.[10] No skeletal region is immune from involvement. However, as the lesions generally follow the distribution of the red bone marrow, the lesions are statistically commonest proximal to the elbows and knees.[8] Figure 2 lists the common and uncommon sites of bone invasion by neuroblastoma.

X-RAY APPEARANCE OF BONE METASTASES

Since the earliest changes in neuroblastoma may be very slight and subtle, the best possible roentgenograms are needed. The diagnosis of early bone involvement requires films of exceptional quality taken with the object of demonstrating individual trabeculae. A fine focal spot is helpful, and the absence of any motion is essential.

Skeletal metastases from neuroblastoma are predominantly osteolytic in type. Fine, patchy areas of bone loss with indistinct margins are characteristic, but larger ovoid or irregular lytic defects or long fusiform areas of involvement may also be seen. In the long bones, the metastases, which tend to be in the metaphyses, are often strikingly symmetrical, even in the absence of widespread skeletal involvement. Two common sites should be scrutinized for early metastases: the medial aspect of the distal metaphysis of the femur, and a similar position on the proximal metaphysis of the humerus.[10]

Another important feature of the skeletal lesions is the frequency of cortical destruction. This is most commonly seen in the long bones, less often in the flat bones. When cortical destruction is present, the tumor mass may be seen in some instances to extend into the adjacent soft tissues (Figure 3). This occurred in one case in which there was extensive metastatic destruction of a portion of the clavicle.[11]

Periosteal reaction is a common finding in the involved bones, especially in the long bones and skull. Kincaid found periosteal reaction associated with 60 percent of the long bone lesions in his series. This is related to tumor infiltration under the periosteum and is most commonly of the parallel type showing either one layer or multilayer "onion-skin" lamination (Figure 4). Less commonly, it is of the "sunburst" or perpendicular type (Figure 5). Periosteal reaction may be seen at a time when the underlying bone appears normal or virtually normal, and has the same significance as does a lytic defect of bone. Occasionally, the periosteal reaction extends almost the entire length of the shaft of a long bone.

Pathologic fractures (Figure 6) sometimes occur in the long

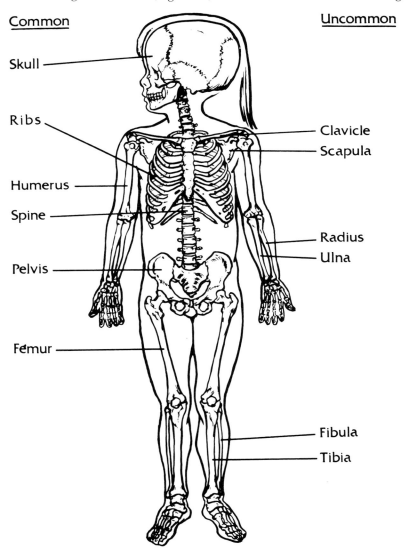

Common

Skull

Ribs

Humerus

Spine

Pelvis

Femur

Uncommon

Clavicle

Scapula

Radius

Ulna

Fibula

Tibia

Figure 2. Sites of bone metastases in metastatic neuroblastoma.

100

bones and in the spine, generally at the site of massively destructive lesions. Such fractures were present in two patients in one series, one in the surgical neck of the humerus and one in a thoracic vertebra.[11]

Metastases are often generalized and in all bones proximal to the elbow and knee joints; they are not rare even below these joints. Spread to metacarpal and metatarsal bones, such as is seen in leukemia, is relatively unusual in neuroblastoma, as is involvement of

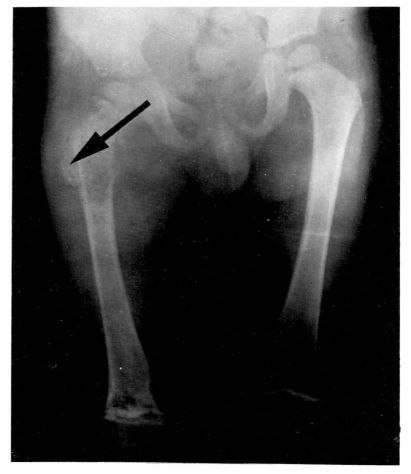

Figure 3. Osteolytic lesions in the femur of a child with neuroblastoma originating in the left adrenal gland. There was a pathological fracture on the right. In the right hip (arrow) there appeared to be extension of the metastatic bone lesion into the adjacent soft tissues. Also note that the lower femoral lesions are bilateral.

epiphyseal ossification centers.[12,13,14] Transverse bands of decreased density at the metaphyses, formerly thought to be pathognomonic of leukemia, have been seen in generalized neuroblastoma as well as in a variety of other conditions.

When generalized, destructive metastases may also take the form

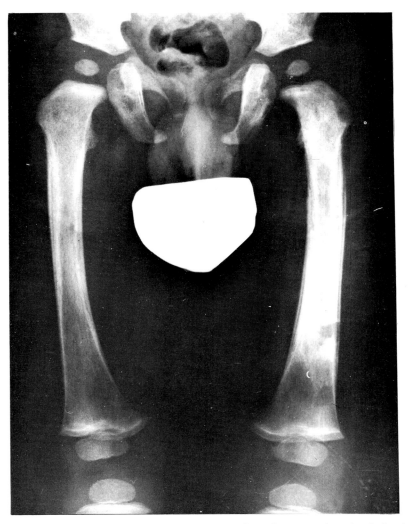

Figure 4. Multilayer "onion-skin" periosteal new bone formation along the shafts of both femurs in a child with neuroblastoma. There are also small, ill-defined areas of bone destruction.

of a diffuse loss of calcium in the skeleton, resembling osteoporosis, similar to that seen in leukemia[1] (Figure 7). Erosion of contiguous bones, enlargement of intervertebral foramina, and separation of ribs on the affected side may indicate extension into the spinal canal.

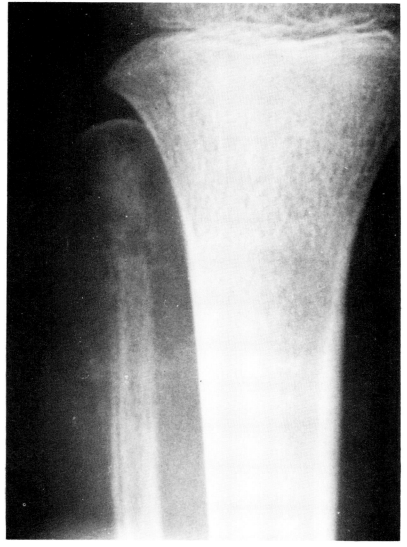

Figure 5. Periosteal new bone formation along the fibula in this patient was of the "sunburst" type as well as the parallel type. (Courtesy of Drs. D. Baker and W. Berdon)

Metastatic spread to the calvarium is more common than spread to the base of the skull. Although occasionally only one or more rather discrete lesions develop in the skull, usually large areas are involved. Metastases to the meninges or brain, with or without evidence of increased intracranial pressure, are often associated with skull metastasis. Roentgenologic evidence of suture separation is often seen, suggesting meningeal involvement (see Figure 3, Chapter 2). This is due either to spreading apart of the cranial bones, or to destruction of the bones at their edges, at the dural attachments. When combined with moth-eaten osteolytic lesions in the skull, and a perpendicular or "sunburst" type of periosteal reaction, such a picture is highly characteristic of neuroblastoma (Figure 8). These findings may develop within a few weeks.

Metastasis to the orbit is a common feature of neuroblastoma and is considered a result of direct extension from metastatic lesions in the skull and meninges. X-ray views of the skull and orbits show increased soft tissue density over the involved orbit, with or without areas of destruction in the bony orbital walls. In one case only the mandible was involved and the tumor mass caused extrusion of a tooth.[11]

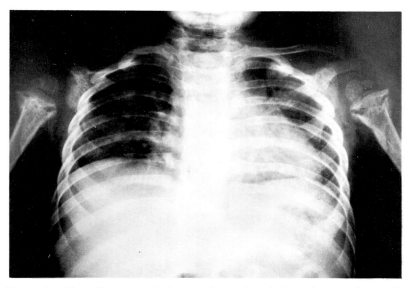

Figure 6. Bilaterally symmetrical upper humeral pathologic fractures in an 18-month-old girl with widespread metastatic neuroblastoma. The patient had been receiving vincristine and cyclophosphamide therapy for some time, and there is evidence of healing.

Course of Bone Lesions

The progression of metastatic involvement may be strikingly rapid. Some insight into the rapidity of development of the bone changes was furnished by five cases in which serial x-ray examinations were done. Two patients presented normal appearing bones at the first examination, but within 23 days in one and within two months in the other fairly pronounced involvement was visible. Several additional patients showed an increase of two to three times in the size of bone destruction within a period of two months.

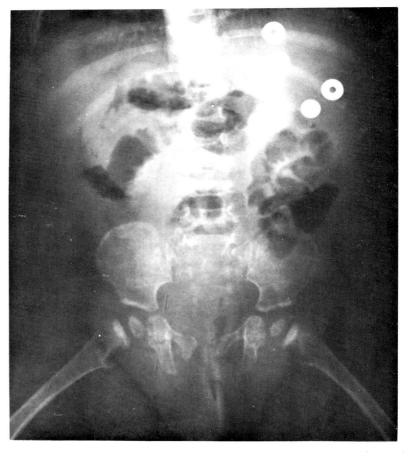

Figure 7. The skeleton in this girl with metastatic neuroblastoma shows widespread demineralization, with uniform loss of vertebral height. Pathologic fractures are evident in both femoral necks.

Repair of bone lesions following treatment was studied in a few patients. In one, an area several inches in length returned to normal within three months after x-ray therapy. Most cases show some degree of recalcification and a decrease in size of the lesion after radiotherapy.[8]

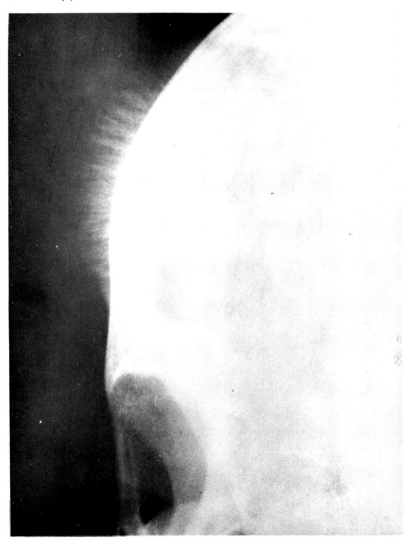

Figure 8. Perpendicular "sunburst" periosteal new bone in a calvarial metastasis. A lump on the head was this three-year-old girl's presenting sign. (Courtesy of Dr. D. Baker and W. Berdon)

In summary, the x-ray findings in skeletal neuroblastoma include:

1. A predominance of fine patchy osteolytic lesions
2. A marked tendency to bilaterally symmetrical distribution of the lesions
3. Frequent finding of cortical destruction and periosteal reaction
4. Occasional extension of the tumor process into the adjacent soft tissues
5. Occasional presence of pathologic fractures
6. Presence of destructive skull lesions, suture separation, and sunburst periosteal reaction
7. Rapid progression of the lesions
8. Response to radiotherapy and chemotherapy.

DIFFERENTIAL DIAGNOSIS OF X-RAY FINDINGS SUGGESTING NEUROBLASTOMA

On x-ray examination, neuroblastomas must be differentiated from leukemia, lymphosarcoma and Hodgkin's disease, primary bone neoplasms (such as Ewing's tumor and osteogenic sarcoma), retinoblastoma, osteomyelitis, tuberculosis, reticuloendotheliosis, Wilms' tumor, and hydronephrosis. A few other conditions under special circumstances may cause confusion (Table 1).[8,15]

The skeletal metastases alone, despite the characteristic ap-

Table 1
Diseases That May Mimic the Radiographic Picture of Metastatic Neuroblastoma

1. Ewing's sarcoma
2. Osteogenic sarcoma
3. Acute leukemia
4. Lymphosarcoma
5. Reticulum cell sarcoma
6. Hodgkin's disease
7. Reticuloendotheliosis
8. Wilms' tumor
9. Retinoblastoma
10. Osteomyelitis
11. Tuberculosis of bone

pearances discussed in the previous section, often cannot be identified with absolute certainty as lesions of neuroblastoma. The radiologist must correlate the chest and abdominal films, and the urographic findings, with the skeletal manifestations.

Since neuroblastomas present often as abdominal masses, the problem of differentiation from Wilms' tumor arises. In excretory urograms, a neuroblastoma is extrinsic to the kidney and therefore tends to push the kidney away from its normal axis and position, producing more displacement than distortion. Since this tumor lies outside the kidney, renal invasion is a relatively late phenomenon. Wilms' tumor, in contrast, is an intrinsic renal tumor. Calcification, while it may occur in Wilms' tumor, is infrequent and, if present, is generally smaller and less confluent than in neuroblastoma. It lacks the specific sand-like appearance of neuroblastoma calcifications. A greater incidence of associated hydronephrosis, ureteral abnormality, and confinement of the disease to the abdomen are additional points favoring a Wilms' tumor. Rarely, a neuroblastoma may directly invade the kidney, and, if there are no other distinguishing features, the roentgenologist may not be able to tell whether the growth is a Wilms' tumor or a neuroblastoma.[16] The frequency of lung metastases in Wilms' tumor and the infrequency of bone metastases would prove helpful in such instances, since lung metastases are rare in neuroblastoma.

Other malignant abdominal tumors of children, such as retroperitoneal rhabdomyosarcoma and other soft tissue sarcomas, can also occasionally cause a differential diagnostic dilemma. Such tumors may metastasize to bone, with resultant destructive bone lesions. But most of them, unlike neuroblastoma, often give rise to early pulmonary metastases.

The conditions which have to be excluded in a case of suspected skeletal neuroblastoma fall into two groups: (1) localized bone disease which may have systemic manifestations; and (2) systemic disease with localized manifestations in bone. Although the list of theoretical possibilities is long, the conditions which, in practice, have to be differentiated are few.[17,18]

Local Bone Diseases

In the occasional case in which neuroblastoma first presents as a single bone lesion, careful search must be made for other foci of the disease. These will usually be found in other bones, in the abdomen, or in the chest. If not, the differential diagnosis must include primary bone tumors and infections.

Most *Ewing's tumors* occur in a somewhat higher age range than neuroblastomas; Ewing's tumors are rare in children under 5 years of age, the age group in which neuroblastoma is most common. Many show a somewhat different x-ray appearance from the rare "solitary" neuroblastomas in bone. Ewing's tumor is usually symmetrically located in bone, of a fusiform shape and in the midshaft; it shows fine patchy destruction and a parallel type of periosteal reaction. Ewing's tumor begins and remains as a single bone lesion for a longer time than neuroblastoma before additional areas of disease develop either in the lung, liver, or other bones; these additional areas tend to be few and localized.

Osteogenic sarcoma tends to have a characteristic x-ray appearance, but it can be mimicked by a solitary metastasis. Constitutional disturbances in bone sarcoma, when present, are not as marked as in neuroblastoma. Most important, metastases to the lungs are frequent, while multiple bone deposits are rare.

Osteomyelitis causes reactive proliferation of bone and periosteal reaction, combined with foci of destruction which may simulate the changes of neuroblastoma. The symmetrical involvement of multiple bones in metastatic neuroblastoma will usually serve to differentiate the two conditions, but a solitary metastasis may pose a problem. The most common difficulty arises when inadequate treatment with antibiotics has been given, with some apparent improvement. The association of a lowered hemoglobin level with a raised sedimentation rate should lead to intensive investigation, including open biopsy, rather than a clinical trial with a different antibiotic.

The early stages of *bone tuberculosis,* before the radiographic changes are marked, may be difficult to distinguish from neuroblastoma. If the diagnosis is still in doubt after full investigation, biopsy should be preferred to a clinical trial with antituberculous drugs.

The lesions of *reticuloendotheliosis* in the skull and long bones tend to be more sharply punched out than the ill-defined lesions of neuroblastoma. Periosteal reaction is, however, seen in both conditions.

In metastatic retinoblastoma the radiographic characteristics of the skeletal lesions are identical to those of neuroblastoma. Only the discovery of the primary tumor can differentiate the two conditions.

Systemic Diseases

Neuroblastoma may closely simulate the joint pains of *rheumatic fever* or *rheumatoid arthritis,* without radiographic changes in the early stages. A persistent raised sedimentation rate, despite symptomatic improvement, may be the only early sign of neuroblastoma.

Neuroblastoma involving the skeleton is probably more often confused with *leukemia* than with any other condition. An investigation was made of the x-ray appearance of bone changes in leukemia, based on 72 proved cases.[8] The bone abnormalities observed were demineralization, fine patchy bone destruction, periosteal reaction, transverse lines of diminished density at the metaphyses and, very infrequently, slight productive changes. These were usually bilateral and symmetrical. Of the above, only transverse lucent bands at the metaphyses are uncommon in neuroblastoma. The difficulty in differentiating this constellation of findings from neuroblastoma in the skeleton is obvious, particularly in aleukemic leukemia. At times only the IVP, chest film, bone marrow examination, and urinary catecholamine determination can resolve the question.

DETECTING OCCULT METASTASES OF NEUROBLASTOMA BY SCANNING TECHNIQUES

Neuroblastoma is well recognized to be a functioning tumor. Increased secretions of catecholamines and cystathionine are found in the urine of patients with this neoplasm. Identification of all the compounds of catecholamine metabolism in the urine of children harboring the tumor is a valuable diagnostic tool and aids in evaluating the success of therapy. Elevation of the urinary content of cystathionine is also useful.

An attempt was made to exploit for diagnostic purposes the ability of neuroblastoma cells to synthesize cystathionine. Selenium-75 methionine was given to four patients with known metastatic neuroblastoma. Localization within the tumor was confirmed on scans obtained three to six hours after the injection of the radionuclide in three of the patients. Two of the patients showed incorporation of radioisotope into the tumor specimen obtained at surgery.[19]

Bone metastasis indicates poor prognosis in neuroblastoma patients; yet, by the time it can be recognized on routine x-ray examination, extensive demineralization has already occurred and the disease is often widespread. It had previously been shown that metastases to bone in adult cancer patients could be detected by strontium-85, fluorine-18,[20] or technetium[99m] polyphosphate scans before their roentgenographic appearance.

The mechanism of Tc^{99m} polyphosphate deposition in bone is thought to be adsorption onto the hydroxyapatite crystal. Technetium, with a half-life of six hours, causes minimal radiation dosage, when compared with Ca^{47} and Sr^{85}. Technetium also produces high count rates with good scanning resolution, permitting rapid total body scanning two to four hours after injection.[21] It is also easily available to any nuclear medicine department, since the necessary tin-polyphosphate complex is commercially available in kit form, and has largely replaced F^{18}, whose short half-life required rapid transportation from a nearby nuclear reactor or cyclotron.

If, during the initial evaluation of the patient, bone metastases are suspected but are not borne out by standard roentgenographic procedures, total body bone scans are indicated.

False negative bone scans have been seen in patients with small metaphyseal metastatic lesions detectable by x-ray. This is most likely due to the normal uptake of isotope at the growing epiphysis and adjacent bone. The additional uptake by the lesion at this site—that is, at the growing epiphysis and adjacent bone—could not be detected.[22]

Colloidal gold-198 is clinically useful for imaging the marrow reticuloendothelial system (RES) in the detection of metastatic carcinoma. This technique has been used for detection of metastatic disease in adult patients by RES marrow scans. In some cases, marrow involvement has been detected when the routine radiographs were negative.[23] In three children with neuroblastomas, a tumor which commonly invades the bone marrow, reticuloendothelial activity as viewed by scan was found to be markedly decreased. Only one of the three had an abnormality in the liver scan.[23] Decrease of RES activity in bones is interpreted as indicating probable sites of metastasis of neuroblastoma.

A total RES scan (liver, spleen, and RES marrow) was performed in pediatric patients using a minor modification of the method described for adults, using the Anger gamma camera. A dose of 6.0 mCi of Tc^{99m} sulfur colloid per 1.7 m^2 was used for patients in the pediatric age group. With this dose, the RES marrow image was made by accumulating counts for a pre-set time of six minutes. Liver and spleen views were recorded in the standard fashion by accumulating 350,000 counts. The images were comparable to those obtained with the larger doses used in adults.[23] It was found that the RES marrow scan procedure is safe, simple, and not traumatic to the child. The procedure may prove to be a very useful adjunct in the initial evaluation and subsequent management of childhood neoplasms.[23]

SUMMARY

Metastatic neuroblastomas have a special tendency to invade the skeletal system. The tumor cells tend to accumulate in the bone marrow in sites of active hematopoiesis. Accordingly, the metastases of neuroblastoma are most commonly found in the axial skeleton and in the proximal portions of the arms and legs. Neuroblastoma cells can be distinguished morphologically from normal hematopoietic cells in bone marrow smears, but they cannot be distinguished with certainty from other solid tumors. Tumor cells can be present in the bone marrow without the finding of bone abnormalities on x-ray examination. Bone abnormalities are commonly found on x-ray examination in children with neuroblastoma, especially in those over two years of age. This finding is a very bad prognostic sign. The radiographic changes seen in the bones of children with neuroblastoma may be mimicked by those changes caused by primary bone sarcomas, acute leukemia, lymphosarcoma, and osteomyelitis. Bone metastases not visible by x-ray examination may be demonstrated by special radioisotopic scanning techniques.

REFERENCES

1. Copeland, M.: Metastases to bone from primary tumors in other sites. *Proc. Nat. Cancer Conf.* 6: 743–756, 1970.

2. Kato, K., and Wachter, H.E.: Adrenal neuroblastoma in children, with special reference to biopsy of sternal marrow and of mestastatic nodule in the skull. *J. Pediatr.* 12: 149–162, 1938.

3. Luhby, A.L., and Diamond, I.K.: Neuroblastoma metastases: diagnosis by bone marrow aspiration with note on therapy with radioactive phosphorus and nitrogen mustard. *Proc. Amer. Fed. Clin. Res.* 3: 52–53, 1947.

4. Piney, A., Mallarme, J., and Ross, M.S.: The bone marrow in Hutchison's syndrome. *J. Clin. Path.* 3: 230–238, 1950.

5. Koss, I.G., and Ginsberg, V.: The value of bone marrow studies in neuroblastoma: report of case. *Arch. Pediatr.* 69: 21–32, 1952.

6. Gaffney, P., Hansman, C., and Fetterman, G.: Experience

with smears of aspirates from bone marrow in the diagnosis of neuroblastoma. *Amer. J. Clin. Path.* 31: 213–221, 1959.

7. Tchernia, G., Gerard-Marchant, R., View, F., et al.: Histological study of bone marrow of 31 children with neuroblastoma. *Rev. Eur. Etud. Clin. Biol.* 17: 471–482, 1972.

8. Sherman, R., and Leaming, R.: The roentgen findings in neuroblastoma. *Radiology* 6: 837–849, 1953.

9. Wittenborg, M.H.: Roentgentherapy in neuroblastoma; A review of 73 cases. *Radiology* 54: 679–688, 1950.

10. Benson, C. Mastard, W., Ravitch, M., et al. (Eds.): *Pediatric Surgery.* (Vol. II). Chicago: Year Book Medical Publishers, 1962, pp. 874–885.

11. Kincaid, O., Hodgson, J., and Dockerty, M.: Neuroblastoma; a roentgenologic and pathologic study. *Amer. J. Roentgenol.* 78: 420–436, 1957.

12. Wyatt, G., and Farber, S.: Neuroblastoma sympathicum; roentgenological appearances and radiation treatment. *Amer. J. Roentgenol.* 46: 485–496, 1941.

13. Ackerman, L., and del Regato, J.: *Cancer; Diagnosis, Treatment, and Prognosis.* St. Louis: C.V. Mosby Company, 1962, pp. 911–921.

14. Dargeon, H.: Neuroblastoma. *J. Pediatr.* 61: 456–462, 1962.

15. Pochedly, C.: The broad clinical spectrum of neuroblastoma. *Postgrad. Med.* 51: 79–85, (April) 1972.

16. Caffey, J.: *Pediatric X-Ray Diagnosis* (Vol. 2). Chicago: Year Book Medical Publishers, 1972, pp. 808–812.

17. Hansman, C., and Girdany, B.: The roentgenographic findings associated with neuroblastoma. *J. Pediatr.* 51: 621–633, 1957.

18. Busfield, P.: Neuroblastoma in orthopedic practice. *J. Bone Joint Surg.* 40-B: 47–57, 1958.

19. D'Angio, G.J., Loker, M., and Nesbit, M.: Radionuclear (Se[75]) identification of tumor in children with neuroblastoma. *Radiology* 93: 615–617, 1969.

20. Helson, L., Watson, R., Benua, R., and Murphy, M.L.: F[18] radioisotope scanning of metastatic bone lesions in children with neuroblastoma. *Amer. J. Roentgenol.* 115: 191–199, 1972.

21. Charkes, N.D., Valentine, G., and Cravetz, B.: Interpretation of the normal Tc[99m] polyphosphate bone scan. *Radiology* 107: 563–570, 1973.

22. Berdon, W.: Personal communication, 1974.

23. Judisch, J., and McIntyre, P.: Recognition of metastatic neuroblastoma by scanning the reticuloendothelial system (RES). *Johns Hopkins Med. J.* 130: 83–86, 1972.

5 Catecholamine Metabolism in Neuroblastoma

Stanley E. Gitlow, M.D.*
Laura Bertani Dziedzic, Ph.D.
Stanley W. Dziedzic, Ph.D.

1. Catecholamine metabolism
2. Screening tests
3. Specific procedures for assay of catecholamine metabolites
4. Effect of drugs and diet upon biochemical testing
5. Normal values
6. Biochemical diagnosis
7. Relationship of therapy to catecholamine metabolism
8. Relationship of catecholamine metabolism to prognosis of neuroblastoma
9. Catecholamine metabolism within neuroblastoma tissue

Neuroblastoma, one of the most common solid malignancies of childhood, shares with ganglioneuroma and pheochromocytoma a common cytogenetic origin—the neural crest. The difference in the clinical symptomatology associated with pheochromocytoma in contrast to neuroblastoma may have delayed recognition of their basic biochemical similarity—namely, the excessive synthesis of the catecholamines. The observation between 1957 and 1959 of children presenting with the combination of an abdominal or thoracic tumor with elevated blood pressure led to the appreciation of neuroblastoma as a tumor capable of synthesizing catecholamines.[1,2]

Since neither blood pressure nor norepinephrine excretion in the majority of patients with neuroblastoma achieved those levels ob-

* Supported by Grant GM-19443 from the National Institutes of Health and by Grant C1-59F from the American Cancer Society.

115

served in association with pheochromocytoma, it was perhaps fortuitous that the period between 1957 and 1959 witnessed a rapid growth in our knowledge of the biochemical pathways of catecholamine metabolism. Thus, it was in 1959 that Greenberg and Gardner noted the association of a ganglioneuroma with increased vanillylmandelic acid (VMA) excretion,[3] and Stickler, Hallenbeck, and Flock[4] described a patient with a ganglioneuroblastoma with a similar elevation of the excretion of this newly discovered by-product of catecholamine metabolism.[5] Within the next two years, excessive dopamine (DA)[6] as well as 3,4-dihydroxyphenylalanine (DOPA)[7] excretion was noted in association with these malignant neural crest lesions.

This common childhood malignancy, possessing the highest rate of spontaneous regression of any human cancer,[8] failed to demonstrate a significant improvement in its prognosis despite advances in chemotherapy since 1956.[9,10] It has been suggested that this tragic fact may be due, at least in part, to the difficulties inherent in early diagnosis[11,12] and clinical management of this illness.[13] Not only has neuroblastoma been confused with lymphoma, carcinoma, sarcoma, Wilms' tumor, retinoblastoma, Ewing's sarcoma, Burkitt's lymphoma, leukemia, or such non-neoplastic diseases as Still's disease, osteomyelitis, rheumatic fever, tuberculosis, or certain of the reticuloendothelioses,[14-17] but cytologists continue to have occasional difficulties in establishing a definitive diagnosis from either bone marrow aspirates or surgical pathology specimens.[18] Such difficulties with clinical diagnosis[11,12,16] could be significantly alleviated by the availability of chemical assays which could detect abnormalities specifically associated with these tumors. Similarly, the medical management of patients with neuroblastoma might be simplified by possession of techniques for evaluating the status of the malignancy in a more subtle and precise manner than that permitted by the assessment of fever, anemia, pain, or tumor size.

Today it is well established that neuroblastoma almost universally produces one or more of the catecholamines and their metabolites in excessive quantities. However, the enormous variability in both the quantitative and qualitative spectra of these compounds makes it difficult to describe which metabolite should be selected for diagnostic, prognostic, or investigative studies.[19] Despite the fact that the catecholamine metabolites, VMA and homovanillic acid (HVA), are relatively simple to measure and among the most frequently elevated in neuroblastoma,[13] there are cases of "non-secreting" tumors,[20] in which circumstance other less commonly assayed metabolites might be helpful in establishing a diagnosis or assessing the progress of the disease. It is therefore apparent that diagnosis and medical management of the neural crest lesions require a detailed understanding of the synthesis, storage, and metabolism of the catecholamines, their precursors, and their by-products.

CATECHOLAMINE METABOLISM

Following the discovery of dopa decarboxylase (DDC) by Holtz in 1938,[21] and the realization that N-methylation would interfere with the function of this enzyme, Blaschko proposed a scheme for the synthesis of epinephrine (E). This scheme involved the hydroxylation of phenylalanine (PA) via tyrosine (TYR) to DOPA, its decarboxylation to dopamine (DA), and the β-carbon oxidation to form the then unobserved precursor of epinephrine, norepinephrine (NE).[22] The validity of this theory was demonstrated during the ensuing years with the discovery of the specific enzymes for each of the biochemical steps proposed by Blaschko, and the observation of norepinephrine as the primary adrenergic neurotransmitter.

All of the enzymes necessary for the biosynthesis of norepinephrine (NE) from phenylalanine are present in the post-ganglionic sympathetic nerve fibers and in chromaffin cells. The initial steps of ring-oxidation to form tyrosine and DOPA are catalyzed by tyrosine hydroxylase (TH), a soluble enzyme requiring a reduced pteridine co-factor and believed to be present in the axoplasm of the adrenergic neuron.[23,24] As the rate-limiting step in the synthesis of the catecholamines, it appears to be largely controlled by the process of end-product inhibition.[25] Dopamine decarboxylase is broadly distributed but is also localized in the cytoplasm of adrenergic tissue;[26,27] with its pyridoxal co-factor, it catalyzes the conversion of DOPA to dopamine (DA). At this juncture in this biosynthetic pathway, the neurotransmitter storage vesicle assumes prime importance.

The copper-containing enzyme, dopamine-beta-hydroxylase (DBH), is associated with the storage vesicle, possibly reacting with dopamine at the granule membrane and ultimately resulting in the formation and storage of norepinephrine within this entity.[28-31] The granules containing approximately 7 percent catecholamines are transported to the nerve ending at which point neurohumoral transmission results in the release of their contents by the process of exocytosis.[32] Measurable levels of dopamine-beta-hydroxylase are thereby attained in the serum.[33] The primitive catecholamine cell system in the ganglia[34] as well as certain other tissues failing to synthesize norepinephrine do not contain dopamine-beta-hydroxylase.[35] Such tissues would obviously result in the formation and storage of dopamine rather than norepinephrine or epinephrine. On the other hand, the presence of phenylethanolamine-N-methyltransferase (PNMT) and S-adenosylmethionine (SAM) in the cytoplasm of the adrenal medullary cells permits the formation from norepinephrine and storage of epinephrine. This biosynthetic step can apparently be inhibited by high concentrations of dopamine and requires high concentrations of glucocorticoids for its optimal function.[34]

Since the catabolic enzymes for catecholamine destruction are present within adrenergic and chromaffin tissue, the storage vesicles appear essential for protection of the intact neurotransmitters. Their absence would logically result in rapid enzymatic degradation of the catecholamines into their less physiologically active products. Not only are these vesicles capable of storing those catecholamines synthesized within their own sub-cellular or cellular borders, but they are also able to store distantly synthesized catecholamines as well. This mechanism represents one means by which the body can discontinue the physiological response to those catecholamines previously released. The other mechanism is that of enzymatic degradation by catechol-O-methylation and amine oxidation. Catechol-O-methyltransferase (COMT) is a ubiquitous cytoplasmic enzyme found in especially high concentrations in the soluble portions of liver and kidney; for maximal activity it requires a divalent cation and SAM as a methyl donor.[36,37,38] The product, normetanephrine (NM), of the rapid conversion of norepinephrine by this enzyme is non-pressor. Circulating catecholamines are largely catabolized by this mechanism.

Within the biosynthetic tissue, however, amine oxidation assumes relatively greater importance as a catabolic step. Monoamine oxidase (MAO) is apparently concentrated in the insoluble component of the outer layer of the mitochondria.[39,40] It is quite non-specific in its choice of substrate but requires flavin adenine dinucleotide (FAD) for full activity.[39,40] In the case of catecholamines, it results in the formation of an unstable aldehyde congener which, under the influence of aldehyde dehydrogenase (ADH) or reductase, ultimately forms an acid or alcohol (glycol) derivative of the original catecholamine (Figure 1).

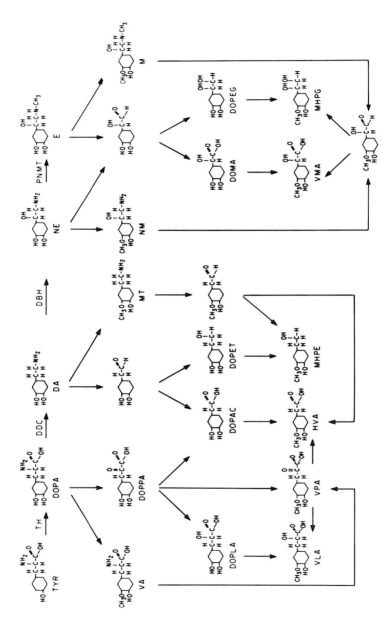

Figure 1. Major Metabolic pathways of the catecholamines. (For abbreviations see Appendix A.)

SCREENING TESTS

The complexity of the quantitative, specific assay procedures gave impetus to the formulation of screening tests which could be rapidly, easily, and broadly applied to biological specimens from patients suspected of having a neuroblastoma. A screening test was developed by Gitlow and coworkers in 1960 for use in patients with pheochromocytoma.[41] This screening test was utilized by Bell and Steward[42,43] and slightly modified by Young and his coworkers[44] for detection of excess catecholamine catabolites in urine specimens from patients with neuroblastoma. Young et al. eliminated one extraction, carried internal standards of VMA throughout the procedure, and restricted intake of foods containing caffeine, bananas, vanilla, and citrus fruits. Although the 13 children with neuroblastoma all showed positive results with this screening test, several false positives were obtained. These were later found to be normal by quantitative chromatographic methods.[44] Bell reported that this screening test was positive in 70 percent of patients with neuroblastoma.[43]

In 1968, a urinary spot test was described by LaBrosse for the detection of neuroblastoma.[45] A drop of urine was placed on filter paper and sprayed with a freshly prepared solution of diazotized paranitroaniline. A rapidly appearing purple color suggested an abnormal elevation of urinary VMA. Seventy-five percent of neuroblastomas gave positive screening values by this method. This technique was evaluated by Evans et al. and found to be helpful in both diagnosis and follow-up of some children with neuroblastoma.[46]

In 1970, Gitlow and his coworkers developed a rapid, bedside screening test for the diagnosis of neuroblastoma which was positive in 92 percent of patients with untreated neuroblastoma.[13] By June 1973, this test yielded positive results in 102 of 109 patients with untreated neuroblastoma followed at this laboratory. A schematic representation of this method is presented in Figure 2. This test was negative in urine specimens from all normal children as well as from those who had diseases of other than neural crest origin.

The VMA "test strip" represents the most recent screening method for neuroblastoma.[47] The obvious advantages of a simple paper dip test, not requiring special glassware or refrigeration of reagents, were somewhat compromised by the instability of the strips during storage. The authors reported a false positive incidence of 1:400. Although they described 24 cases in which patients with neuroblastomas resulted in positive strip test findings, they gave no data regarding their incidence of false negative observations. Using *fresh* test strips, the majority of those specimens yielding a positive result by the technique noted in Figure 2, gave rise to positive strips.

SPECIFIC PROCEDURES FOR ASSAY OF CATECHOLAMINE METABOLITES

Although screening tests may be useful in detecting patients with neural crest lesions, their lack of absolute reliability demands confirmation by quantitative and specific assay procedures. In addition, the small percentage of patients with neuroblastoma who fail to yield a positive screening test, but in whom the index of suspicion is high, require further quantitative testing as well.

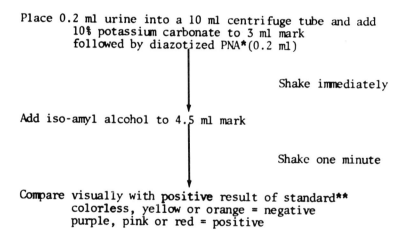

SCREENING TEST FOR NEUROBLASTOMA

Place 0.2 ml urine into a 10 ml centrifuge tube and add 10% potassium carbonate to 3 ml mark followed by diazotized PNA*(0.2 ml)

Shake immediately

Add iso-amyl alcohol to 4.5 ml mark

Shake one minute

Compare visually with positive result of standard** colorless, yellow or orange = negative purple, pink or red = positive

*Diazotized PNA: A solution of 0.5 g para-nitroaniline in 10 ml concentrated hydrochloric acid and 490 ml water is mixed with 0.2% sodium nitrite (1:1 by vol.) immediately before use. All reagents must be refrigerated.

** Standard: normal urine + 5 μg VMA carried throughout the procedure.

Figure 2. Schematic representation of the rapid biochemical screening test for neuroblastoma.

Although it is accepted that the more metabolites that are studied, the greater the possibilities for diagnostic accuracy, routine clinical laboratories are equipped to perform only the relatively simple assays. The most commonly assayed metabolites of catecholamines in urine are VMA and HVA. These compounds may be simultaneously determined by the bi-directional paper chromatographic technique of Armstrong et al.[5] (Figure 3) or the high voltage electrophoretic method of von Studnitz.[48] Colorimetric methods for the determination of VMA have generally failed to prove specific enough to satisfy criteria for a truly quantitative assay procedure.[44,49,50] Similarly, the early gas-liquid chromatographic procedure developed by Williams and Greer for VMA and HVA proved to be too insensitive to permit evaluation of subtle variations from the norm.[51] Sensitive and specific gas-liquid chromatographic methods for the assay of VMA[52] and HVA[53] were thereafter developed, but these required considerable experience with gas-liquid chromatographic methodology, a circumstance unlikely to be found in a routine clinical laboratory. Other less commonly utilized methods for the measurement of VMA included uni-directional paper chromatography[54] and thin-layer chromatography.[55] Fluorimetric methods have been more broadly used for measurement of HVA[56,57,58] than colorimetric methods.[59]

In 1959, 3-methoxy-4-hydroxyphenylethyleneglycol (MHPG) was isolated and characterized by Axelrod et al.[60] Although paper chromatography was employed for the determination of MHPG,[61] it was not until the development of the gas-liquid chromatographic technique of Wilk et al. that a suitably sensitive analytical procedure was available for the quantitative measurement of this metabolite.[62]

In 1962, Pisano et al.[63] developed a photometric assay for measurement of total metanephrines in urine. Minor modifications of this procedure led to its use in the clinical testing of patients suspected of having a pheochromocytoma.[64,65] Gas-liquid chromatography,[66] thin-layer chromatography[67] as well as fluorimetric methods[68] were employed for measurement of the metanephrines. The gas-liquid chromatographic technique of Bertani et al.[66] also permitted quantitation of the dopamine product, 3-methoxytyramine (MT).

Several minor metabolites of the catecholamines including 3,4-dihydroxyphenylacetic acid (DOPAC),[69,70] tyramine,[71] 3-methoxy-4-hydroxyphenylethanol (MHPE),[72,73] vanilpyruvic acid (VPA),[74] 3-methoxy-4-hydroxyphenyllactic acid (VLA),[75] N-acetyltyramine,[76] N-acetyldopamine,[77] and N-acetylnorepinephrine[78] have been identified in urine. A review of the methodology employed for the deter-

A urine volume equivalent to ¼ mg creatinine (all chromatograms done in duplicate)

↓

Make up to 2 ml with water and acidify to pH <1 with hydrochloric acid

↓

Extract 3 times with ethyl acetate (4,2,2 ml); discard aqueous layer

↓

Remove ethyl acetate, extract with capillary pipette; avoid water drops

↓

Blow ethyl acetate extract to dryness by gentle air stream (do not exceed 50°C)

↓

Add 1 ml of absolute ethanol, washing sides of tubes and re-evaporate

↓

Add 3 drops (2X) of ethyl acetate for chromatogram spotting on 1 foot square Whatman No. 1 paper

↓

Standards* are spotted for comparison with unknown

↓

Chromatograms are put in covered cylindrical tanks containing 50 ml mixture of isopropanol:ammonium hydroxide:water (40:9:1) for at least 10 hours

↓

After drying they are run in perpendicular direction for 6 hours in tanks containing a mixture of benzene:propionic acid:water (20:15:1)

↓

After air drying they are placed in 250°C oven for 2 minutes and sprayed with a mixture of para-nitroaniline, sodium nitrite and potassium carbonate (1:1:2) in that order (Para-nitroaniline prepared as in Figure 2, 0.2 percent sodium nitrite and 10 percent potassium carbonate)

↓

For quantitation the VMA and HVA spots are compared visually with the reference standards at their respective rf values. A factor of 4 permits expression as μg/mg creatinine.

---

* Standards: VMA—0.25, 0.50, 0.75, 1.0 μg
             HVA—0.50, 1.00, 1.50, 2.0 μg

Figure 3. Bi-directional paper chromatographic technique for VMA and HVA.

mination of the known minor metabolites of the catecholamines can be found in an article by Gjessing.[79]

Although DOPA and its biosynthetic products dopamine, norepinephrine, and epinephrine may be measured in human urine, the procedures have generally proven less satisfactory than those in which their degradation products were assayed.[7,69,80-88]

EFFECT OF DRUGS AND DIET UPON BIOCHEMICAL TESTING

Apparent elevation of the excretion of the catecholamines or their metabolites may result from the use of non-specific assay procedures in the face of ingestion of a foodstuff or drug. Modifications in the excretion of the catecholamines may also result from drugs capable of inhibiting those enzymes responsible for their biosynthesis or degradation. Moreover, administration of catecholamines or substances capable of releasing endogenous catecholamines may result in measurements of catecholamines in the urine, which may be misleading from a diagnostic standpoint.[89,90,91] Thus, administration of DOPA may result in marked elevation of dopamine and HVA excretion and modest elevation of other catecholamine metabolites. Likewise, the use of sympathomimetic nosedrops or sprays may yield increased levels of epinephrine and norepinephrine in urine. Alpha-methyldopa administration results in spurious elevation of the urinary catecholamines[92] but fails to significantly interfere with the specific assay procedures for their metabolites.

The number of drugs capable of interfering with fluorimetric assay procedures for catecholamine measurements are too numerous to be mentioned,[41] but rarely do routine medications (sedatives, antibiotics, antihypertensives, analgesics) interfere with the measurement of VMA, total metanephrines (TM), HVA, and MHPG. Drugs which reduce monoamine oxidase (MAO) activity (such as pargyline) or aldehyde dehydrogenase activity (such as disulfiram) as well as those which may reduce effective dehydrogenase activity by competitive inhibition (ethanol) may result in bizarre patterns of catecholamine metabolism, elevating certain metabolites and decreasing others.[93,94] Trihexiphenidyl, methocarbamol, pyridium and certain commercially available cough syrups may result in apparent elevations in VMA, MHPG, or total metanephrines excretion, but these variabilities appear primarily related to the lack of specificity of the commonly used assay procedures. Foodstuffs, on the other hand, appear capable of modifying the results of non-specific quantitative (e.g., colorimetric VMA assays) or screening procedures only. Restriction of coffee, fruits, and vanilla-containing products in the diet is unnecessary for assay of VMA and HVA by bi-directional paper chromatography.[5] These restrictions are also unnecessary for assay of total metanephrines by column chromatography[63,65] and MHPG by gas-liquid chromatography.[62]

NORMAL VALUES

By 1959, it had become apparent in this laboratory that the values for catecholamine metabolite excretion by normal adults differed significantly from those values found in children.[95] Studies designed to determine whether excretion of these substances could best be expressed as a function of body weight, age, surface area, urine volume or in relation to the excretion of other substances (creatinine, creatine plus creatinine, etc.) resulted in the use of two major techniques by the majority of investigators: one involving a 24-hour urine collection and resulting in the expression of the total 24-hour metabolite excretion and the other requiring only a random collection and expressing metabolite excretion in terms of urinary creatinine content. Voorhess in 1967 demonstrated that the daily excretion of dopamine, norepinephrine, epinephrine, and VMA increased progressively with age; she also showed that variability in the expression of such excretion was less in terms of metabolite per kilogram or per square meter of body surface than when expressed on the basis of time alone.[96]

Since total 24-hour urine collections are notoriously difficult to obtain reliably and accurately at any age level, Gitlow et al. evaluated the variability inherent in the expression of catabolite excretion per milligram of urinary creatinine. They ascertained that the diurnal variation in the excretion of these substances (when so expressed) was no greater than the daily variation in one child or the variation among children of the same age, sex, weight, and surface area.[97] Since in the final analysis the method adopted for expression of metabolite excretion should be that which would reduce variability to a minimum while maintaining the usefulness and reliability of the assay for diagnostic purposes, these workers chose to avoid the difficulty inherent in 24-hour urine collections and expressed all catabolite excretion as a function of creatinine content and age.

Unfortunately, many of the early studies could not be compared with one another since they used not only differing collection techniques but assayed for different metabolites; all too often the biochemical procedures used were inadequate in specificity.[44,50] Moreover, the majority of early investigators failed to appreciate the need for large sample sizes at various age levels.[44,98,99,100,101] For this reason, evaluation of any specific compound for diagnostic useful-ness could not be accomplished with any certainty. Bi-directional paper chromatographic assay not only offered such specificity, but permitted simultaneous determination of HVA as well as VMA. Both Gjessing[102] and Gitlow et al.[97] used this procedure in assaying these catecholamine catabolites in urine samples from large numbers of normal children. Such studies have allowed the formulation of pat-terns for the normal excretion of these substances as they vary with age (Figures 4 and 5).

Only Voorhess,[96] Barontini et al.[103] and McKendrick and Ed-wards[50] evaluated comparable groups of normal children for com-

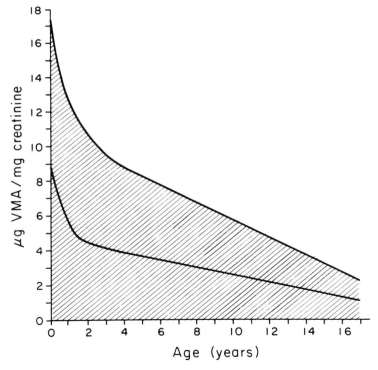

Figure 4. Line of regression for VMA (μg/mg creatinine) as a function of age. Shaded area represents 3 sigma upper normal limit.

parison, but the latter two groups assayed VMA by a non-specific colorimetric method.[49] Both MHPG and total metanephrine excretion were also evaluated in a large number of normal children (Figures 6 and 7). Study of norepinephrine, epinephrine, and dopamine excretion in a normal sample of adequate size was carried out by Voorhess (Figures 8, 9, 10), Barontini et al.,[103] and Sourkes et al.[69] The less common catecholamine metabolites have thus far been determined in too few normal children to permit adequate statistical evaluation of the data.[69-79] Therefore, assay of these substances cannot be readily utilized in the detection, diagnosis and treatment of a child with a neuroblastoma.

The emphasis upon 24-hour urine collections by Voorhess and

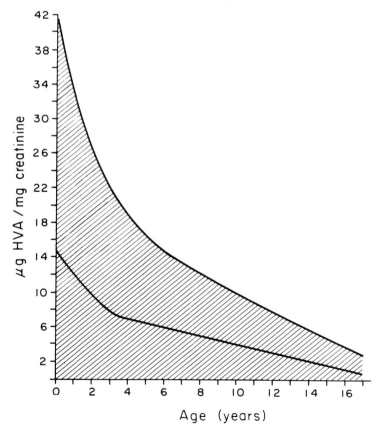

Figure 5. Line of regression for HVA (μg/mg creatinine) as a function of age. Shaded area represents 3 sigma upper normal limit.

Kirkland[104] might well be related to the specific substances (norepinephrine, epinephrine, and dopamine) which these workers studied. The immense variability in the excretion of these catecholamines from moment to moment was well documented during the years in which the unchanged amines represented the only substances which could be measured in the urine samples of patients

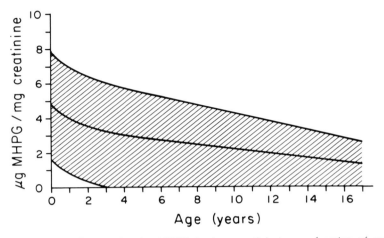

Figure 6. Line of regression for MHPG (μg/mg creatinine) as a function of age. Shaded area represents 3 sigma upper normal limit.

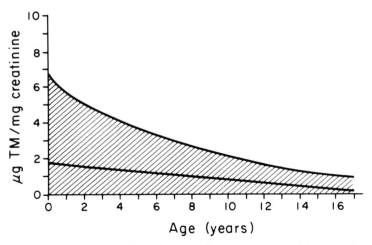

Figure 7. Line of regression for total metanephrines (μg/mg creatinine) as a function of age. Shaded area represents 3 sigma upper normal limit.

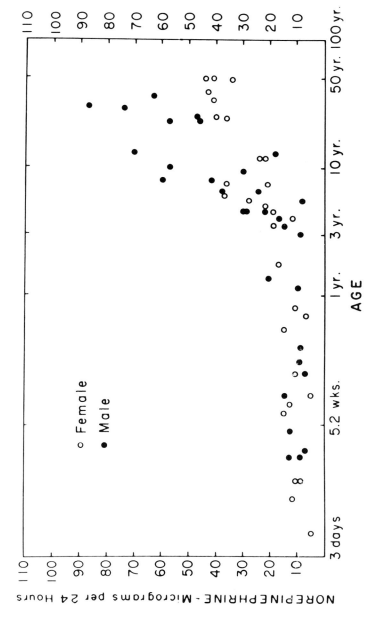

Figure 8. The excretion of norepinephrine as a function of age in normal children. (Courtesy of Dr. M. Voorhess and *Pediatrics*[96])

130

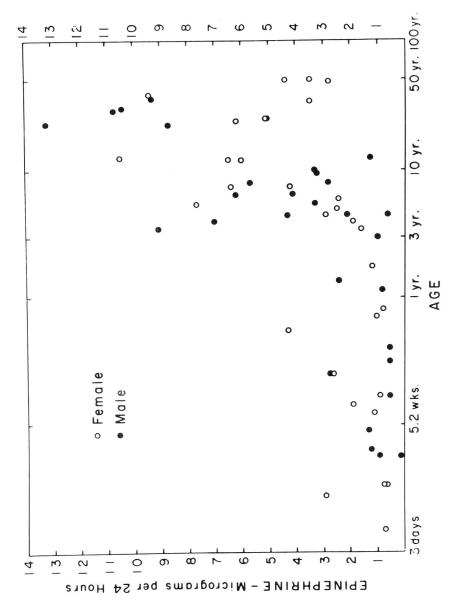

Figure 9. The excretion of epinephrine as a function of age in normal children. (Courtesy of Dr. M. Voorhess and *Pediatrics*[96])

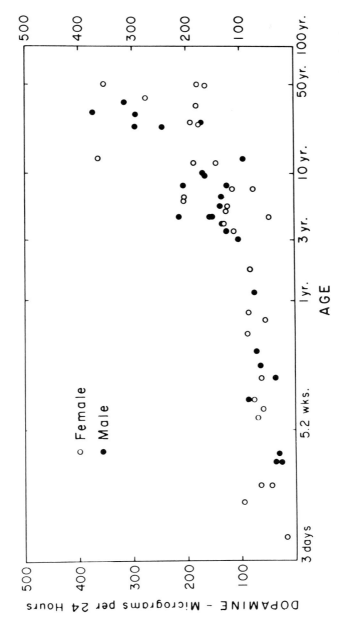

Figure 10. The excretion of dopamine as a function of age in normal children. (Courtesy of Dr. M. Voorhess and *Pediatrics*[96])

suspected of having pheochromocytomas. Indeed, such measurements have fallen into almost total disuse for the detection of these tumors by those groups with extensive experience in this field. Innumerable instances of normal catecholamine excretion in the presence of elevated catecholamine catabolite excretion and a functioning pheochromocytoma have been noted. It is, therefore, not surprising that investigators depending largely upon catecholamine assays deem it necessary to make 24-hour urine collections, whereas those studying the major metabolites of the catecholamines have long recognized the superiority of random urine collections with catabolite excretion expressed in terms of urinary creatinine.[97,102]

A potential difficulty with assay of the unchanged catecholamines lay in the tendency for these substances to become readily elevated in the urine samples of patients undergoing the severe stress of life-threatening illness other than that stemming from a neural crest lesion. Fortunately the excretion of deaminated catecholamine catabolites has been almost uniformly normal in association with illnesses most commonly confused with neuroblastoma. Despite sporadic reports to the contrary[105] the present authors believe that the observation of an abnormally elevated excretion of the deaminated catecholamine catabolites demands the diagnosis of a neural crest neoplasm. The singular exception to this appears to exist in those rare instances in which a patient with a melanoma may excrete minimally elevated quantities of VMA and HVA.[106] Fortunately, these would be unlikely to represent a diagnostic problem.

Since 1971, sensitive and specific assay procedures have been available for determination of dopamine-beta-hydroxylase in human serum. Freedman et al.[33] observed extremely low levels of serum DBH during the first year of life, with the enzyme gradually achieving adult normal concentrations by 16 years of age. Assay of this enzyme in human serum has been used to reflect the degree of catecholamine release by exocytosis.

In view of the strikingly high incidence of neuroblastoma rests (neuroblastoma in situ) in routine post-mortem studies of infants who had apparently died from diseases other than those of the neural crest,[107,108,109] the present authors became interested in their observation of an increased range of excretion of the catecholamine metabolites in the younger age groups. Did this signify the presence of two populations? The distribution of excretion values of HVA and VMA could be expressed as two normal curves.[110] Further statistical evaluation of these data by cluster analysis recently confirmed the existence of a sub-group population of infants excreting quantities of VMA and

HVA in excess of normal, despite the absence of any apparent pathology in these children. One can only speculate upon the relationship of this observation to the incidence of familial neuroblastoma,[111] the obvious association of both the incidence and prognosis of this tumor to age,[10] and the frequency with which neuroblastoma rests have been observed in routine post-mortem studies of infants.[107] The gradual disappearance of elevated catecholamine metabolite excretion as well as neuroblastoma rests with age suggests that normal infants possess a mechanism for eradicating these catecholamine synthesizing cells.

BIOCHEMICAL DIAGNOSIS OF NEUROBLASTOMA

Of 113 patients with untreated neuroblastoma proven by surgical biopsy or necropsy, 97 percent excreted MHPG in excess of 3 sigma confidence limit levels of normal subjects of the same age. This figure fell to 96 percent for VMA, 93 percent for HVA, and 86 percent for total metanephrines.[13,112] The factors by which the patients' catecholamine metabolite excretions exceeded the normal age-related 3 sigma confidence limits were greatest for MHPG and least for HVA. Ninety-seven percent of patients with proven neuroblastoma excreted abnormally elevated quantities of at least three of these four catabolites, whereas less than 2 percent failed to excrete abnormal quantities of at least one of these substances. Such diagnostic precision and reliability demanded quantitative laboratory procedures possessing a high degree of specificity as well as measurement of the excretion patterns of a large enough group of normal children to permit accurate statistical evaluation of the patient. Although assay of MHPG, VMA, HVA, and total metanephrines permitted a high degree of diagnostic reliability, it is possible that determination of other urinary substances such as norepinephrine and dopamine might have replaced such measurements with equal diagnostic reliability.[113] Likewise, if norepinephrine and dopamine were added to the previous laboratory determinations, they might have resulted in a modest improvement in the figures for diagnostic accuracy noted above.[103]

On the other hand, assay of the urinary excretion of the unmetabolized catecholamines might, because of their intrinsic variability, require 24-hour urine collections. Since Voorhess used a VMA assay procedure possessing adequate specificity, her failure to note elevations in the excretion of this catabolite in 20 percent[114] to 40 percent[115] of patients with neuroblastoma could have resulted only from the methods by which she collected her samples. These defects in methodology could have altered the results and obscured differences between her normal and pathological groups. In the final analysis, the clinical value of any assay procedure must rest upon its ability to differentiate pathological from normal. It is obvious that the expression of the excretion of phenolic acids on the basis of 24-hour urine collections fails to yield the diagnostic reliability attainable with their expression as a function of creatinine excretion. Thus, Barontini et al., using a spectrophotometric assay for VMA content of 24-hour urine specimens, failed to differentiate 13 percent of their patients with neuroblastoma form a normal group.[103]

On the other hand, von Studnitz[71] found elevated VMA excretion as the most common biochemical abnormality in association with neuroblastoma. Similarly, Käser[20] observed elevated VMA excretion in 94 percent of 73 patients with neuroblastoma, a figure in close agreement with the data of Gitlow et al.[13] Although Voorhess, Pickett, and Gardner failed to detect 20 percent of their first 25 patients with neuroblastoma[116] by assay of dopamine, norepinephrine, total metanephrines and VMA, there is almost universal agreement[13,20,43,51,71,117] that abnormalities in catecholamine excretion may be demonstrated in over 95 percent of these patients. The present authors found that almost every one of these patients may be detected by a single simultaneous bi-directional paper chromatographic determination of VMA and HVA. It is still unclear as to whether or not the few percent of patients with neuroblastoma who fail to excrete excessive quantities of dopamine, norepinephrine, VMA, HVA, MHPG, and total metanephrines might indeed be detectable on the basis of 3-methoxy-4-hydroxyphenylalanine (VA),[69] vanillactic acid,[75] vanilpyruvic acid,[74] N-acetyldopamine,[77] N-acetyl-norepinephrine,[78] or some other more exotic catabolite.[79] Measurement of epinephrine excretion, almost always normal in the presence of neuroblastoma, has been abandoned as a diagnostic procedure for these tumors.[103,113]

Although we lack statistically significant evidence, it has been our impression that those few patients with neuroblastoma whose catecholamine metabolite excretion is uniformly normal had a high incidence of intrathoracic lesions. This casual observation may indeed be related to the infrequency with which neuroblastomas of dorsal root origin synthesize excessive catecholamines.[118] Interestingly, the coincidence of neuroblastoma with abnormalities in central nervous system function (opsoclonus, etc.) reveals a marked preponderance of an intrathoracic origin of such tumors.[119] Since resection of these tumors often results in the relief of the cerebellar dysfunction, it is tempting to postulate a correlation of the intrathoracic location with the formation of an unusual catecholamine metabolite capable of producing central nervous system dysfunction.[120]

Many studies have pointed out the difficulty in differentiating the neural crest lesions by the pattern of their catecholamine metabolism alone. Thus, ganglioneuroma and even pheochromocytoma occurring during childhood may reveal catecholamine metabolite excretion similar in every respect to that noted with a neuroblastoma. On the other hand, normal catecholamine metabolite excretion is more commonly associated with ganglioneuroma than neuroblastoma, and subjects with pheochromocytoma tend to excrete a proportion of catecholamines, total metanephrines, and phenolic acids unlike those seen in neuroblastomas. Markedly elevated excretion of HVA is pathognomonic of a malignant neural crest lesion in the adult, but may be occasionally noted in association with a benign pheochromocytoma or ganglioneuroma in childhood.[121]

In view of the rapid transfer of catecholamines across the placental barrier,[122] it should not be surprising that instances have been described in which neuroblastoma was associated with maternal symptomatology.[123] Indeed, a prenatal urine specimen from a mother whose child has a congenital neuroblastoma may not only contain elevated quantities of catecholamine metabolites, but Chatten and Voorhess have even described an asymptomatic mother whose urinary abnormalities remained present during the intervals between the births of four offspring with neuroblastoma.[111] Although the maternal role in the etiology of this tumor is still unclear, familial cases have not been infrequent,[124] and diagnostic suspicion might exist in the presence of high maternal catecholamine excretion. Care must be exercised in the interpretation of such data since pregnancy may be associated with an increase in the excretion of certain of the catecholamine metabolites.[125]

The concentration of dopamine-beta-hydroxylase (DBH) is normally the result of a balance between its release from sympathetic nerves by exocytosis and its degradation by as yet unknown mechanisms. Its concentration is extremely low in the first year of life, achieving adult normal levels by 16 years of age.[33] Goldstein et al. noted that about one-half of their patients with neuroblastoma had elevated serum levels of DBH, an observation which they correlated with evidence of increased norepinephrine synthesis.[34]

RELATIONSHIP OF THERAPY TO CATECHOLAMINE METABOLISM

Voorhess and Gardner in 1962 were the first to draw attention to the value of serial catecholamine determinations for a patient with a neuroblastoma.[127] Additional cases were reported during the following few years.[83,128,129] Although radiotherapy occasionally resulted in temporary elevation in urinary catecholamine excretion,[130] effective therapy of various modalities was usually promptly followed by a reduction of catecholamine metabolite excretion in the great majority of patients. Precise correlation was occasionally lacking between the course of biochemical and clinical findings in individual subjects. In the child whose clinical abnormalities were minimal, objective biochemical observations would occasionally represent the most useful guide for the long-term management of therapeutic resources. Indeed, patients occasionally presented biochemical evidence of relapse in advance of the clinical observation of a recurrent mass, bone lesion, anemia or diverse symptoms.

Figures 11 through 15 depict individual examples of ways in which the clinical and biochemical data may correlate with therapy.

Although one might occasionally require alpha-adrenergic blockade for the clinical treatment of a patient with a neuroblastoma, such therapy is unlikely to alter the ultimate outcome of patients with this tumor. Fortunately, malignant pheochromocytoma often progresses slowly enough to allow a marked prolongation of useful life to result from the administration of alpha-blocking drugs.

RELATIONSHIP OF CATECHOLAMINE METABOLISM TO PROGNOSIS OF NEUROBLASTOMA

Whereas the usefulness of measurements of catecholamine metabolism in the detection and therapy of patients with neuroblastoma was fully appreciated a decade ago,[127] there are still questions concerning the usefulness of these biochemical assays in anticipating the ultimate course of a patient with this tumor.[131] By 1971, Barontini et al.[132] and Gitlow et al.[133] had attempted to correlate the pattern of excretion of the catecholamines and their metabolites with the prognosis of patients with neuroblastoma. Barontini et al. failed to observe any such correlation but did draw attention to the association of a good prognosis with the return of catecholamine metabolism to a normal pattern during initial treatment.[132]

A more detailed statistical evaluation of a group of 98 subjects with neuroblastoma was presented by Gitlow et al. in 1973.[10] Contingency table analysis of the excretion of VMA, MHPG, total metanephrines, and HVA at the time of initial diagnosis revealed significant positive correlations among the individual norepinephrine catabolites (VMA, MHPG, and total metanephrines) but not between these and the dopamine catabolite, HVA. Statistical evaluation (chi square) of the data revealed significant association between normal HVA excretion at the time of initial diagnosis and survival. Initial excretion of total metanephrines and MHPG failed to relate to prog-

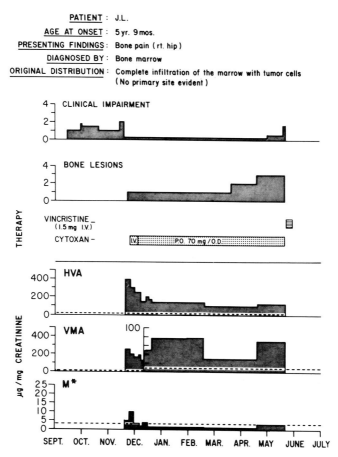

Figure 11. Therapy, although followed by a rapid clinical and biochemical improvement, failed to achieve normality in either parameter. Increasing catecholamine metabolite excretions and bone lesions were evident prior to his eventual demise.

138

nosis, whereas that for VMA approached statistical significance. Similarly, when patients were separated on the basis of initial catecholamine metabolite excretion more or less than 5 times the 3 sigma upper limit of normal, only HVA correlated with prognosis. It was of interest that the excretion of the catecholamine catabolites—VMA and total metanephrines—failed to correlate with age at diagnosis, whereas lower HVA and higher MHPG excretions were

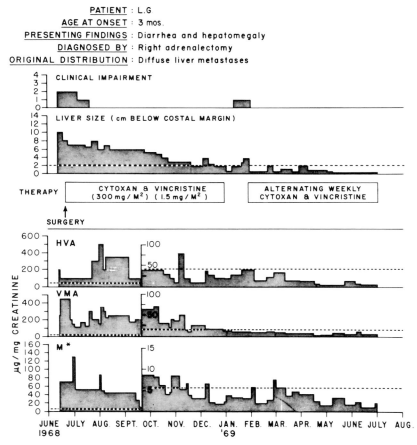

Figure 12. A gradual but progressive parallel response in clinical and biochemical abnormalities resulting in completely normal parameters at the present time (five years old).

more commonly noted in the younger patients. The implication of this observation was that those tumors failing to produce excessive quantities of dopamine but rather favoring the formation of the norepinephrine metabolite, MHPG, were associated with that group of patients (under two years of age) possessing a better prognosis.

Although the initial catecholamine metabolite excretion pattern was of limited prognostic import, the modification of catecholamine

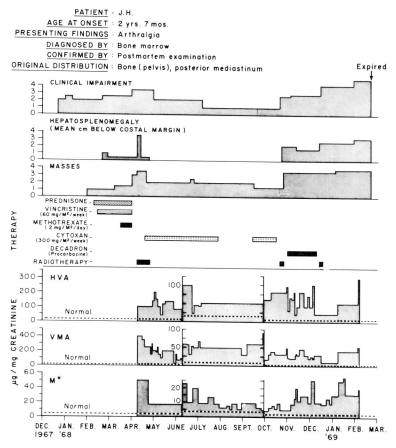

Figure 13. A minimal clinical and biochemical improvement following therapy, resulted in ultimate increases in catecholamine metabolite excretion about one month prior to exacerbation of the clinical evidence of the disease.

metabolism during initial therapy proved to be a critical determinant of ultimate course of the disease. In a group of 54 patients divided into survivor and non-survivor sub-groups on the basis of their course during a potential two-year minimum follow-up, 86 percent of those whose catecholamine metabolite excretion returned to normal during therapy were classified as survivors, whereas 100 percent of those whose catecholamine metabolism remained abnormal ultimately ex-

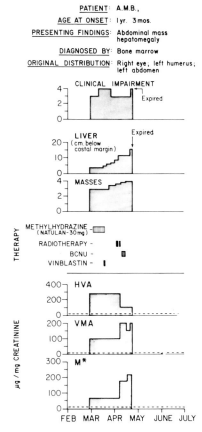

Figure 14. A rapid and progressively downhill clinical course without therapeutic response correlated with sustained elevations of the catecholamine metabolites. A fall in HVA excretion during the few weeks prior to death was not accompanied by a similar change in VMA and TM excretion.

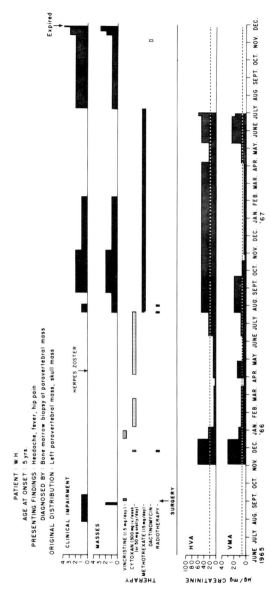

Figure 15. A complete clinical remission following surgery failed to be reflected in the biochemical parameters, but medical therapy ultimately resulted in near-normal HVA and VMA excretion. Catecholamine metabolite excretion increased concomitantly with clinical relapse and persisted throughout the second remission accurately forecasting the ultimate demise of this patient.

pired. The return to normal catecholamine metabolism occurred within five months of initiation of therapy, often within the first few weeks of such treatment, and in the majority of instances the excretion of the various metabolites fell in parallel. In the same study, histologic parameters were also found to correlate closely with the prognosis of neuroblastoma, but a statistical relationship between the initial biochemical data and these pathological criteria could not be demonstrated. Trends were noted in which neuroblast differentiation and the presence of ganglion cells were related to HVA excretion, whereas the presence of hemorrhage or mitoses were related to the excretion of the norepinephrine catabolites.

Just as age at onset, histology, site of origin, and tumor distribution are of importance in structuring a prognostic classification for neuroblastoma, the biochemical pattern of catecholamine metabolism at the time of initial diagnosis, as well as its response to initial therapy, represent major determinants in such a classification.

CATECHOLAMINE METABOLISM WITHIN NEUROBLASTOMA TISSUE

There is a striking discrepancy between clinical signs and symptoms resulting from increased catecholamine synthesis in association with pheochromocytoma, as opposed to the relative absence of such manifestations when there is increased catecholamine synthesis in association with neuroblastoma. This discrepancy demanded investigation of the detailed means by which these tumors metabolized catecholamines. Page and Jacoby[131] were the first to demonstrate the relative absence of catecholamine storage vesicles in neuroblastoma tissue as opposed to the relatively frequent dense core vesicles apparent in ultramicroscopic studies of pheochromocytoma. Since the presence of storage vesicles is a prerequisite for the protection of catecholamines from the action of degradative enzymes, it was not surprising that norepinephrine and epinephrine concentrations were found to be much higher in pheochromocytoma than in neuroblastoma.[20,104] The ratio of the unchanged catecholamines to VMA in the urine, originally observed to be 1:100 under normal circumstances and 1:10 in the presence of pheochromocytoma,[134] was observed by Itoh and Omori to approach the normal levels in the presence of neuroblastoma.[135] These circumstances could conceivably result from the action of degradative enzymes within the neuroblastoma and/or the absence of periodic massive catecholamine release by tumor vesicles.

Although the levels of catecholamine catabolites within neuroblastoma tissue are low, these data may result from rapid transport of the neutral and acidic metabolites of the catecholamines from the tumor tissue. LaBrosse and Karon observed catechol-O-methyltransferase (COMT) activity[136] and Lurvey et al., [137] as well as Dziedzic et al., [138] observed HVA in neuroblastoma tissue. Continuous as opposed to discrete discharge of catecholamines by tumor tissue may also result in increased alpha-adrenergic tolerance. One may, therefore, hypothesize any one or all of a number of mechanisms whereby the patient with neuroblastoma or the mother harboring a fetus with neuroblastoma might be less likely to exhibit the alpha-adrenergic signs and symptoms than might be observed in the presence of a pheochromocytoma synthesizing comparable quantities of catecholamines.

Although all of the major catecholamine metabolites were not measured and the volume of neuroblastoma tumor tissue could only be estimated, attempts to evaluate catecholamine metabolism in neural crest lesions have shown that catecholamine synthesis per gram of tumor tissue is somewhat less in neuroblastoma despite similar catecholamine turnover rates in pheochromocytoma.[139] The massive quantity of neuroblastoma tissue may well explain the marked elevation of catecholamine metabolite excretion often associated with neuroblastoma. Certainly, neuroblastoma possesses the necessary enzymatic mechanisms for synthesizing catecholamines. Tyrosine hydroxylase as well as dopa decarboxylase are present in neuroblastoma tissues in quantities comparable to those observed in pheochromocytoma and normal adrenal medullae.[135,140] Only dopamine-beta-hydroxylase and phenylethanolamine-N-methyltransferase may be found in levels lower than those noted in other tissues of neural crest origin.[34]

CONCLUSION

Within 15 years, the biochemical study of neural crest lesions has assumed major clinical significance. Diagnostic, prognostic, and therapeutic evaluation of each patient with a neuroblastoma has necessitated a detailed and reliable measurement of the patient's catecholamine metabolism. Clinical laboratories have fallen seriously behind in this drive to improve the care of children with this malignancy. The clinician must be the ultimate judge of the adequacy of those biochemical assays upon which patient care may rest.

APPENDIX A

Abbreviations Used

Enzymes and Cofactors

TH	tyrosine hydroxylase
DDC	dopa decarboxylase (aromatic L-amino acid decarboxylase)
PNMT	phenylethanolamine-N-methyltransferase
DBH	dopamine-β-hydroxylase
ADH	aldehyde dehydrogenase
MAO	monoamine oxidase
COMT	catechol-O-methyltransferase
PAH	phenylalanine hydroxylase
SAM	S-adenosylmethionine
FAD	flavin adenine dinucleotide

Catecholamine Metabolites and Precursors

PA	phenylalanine
TYR	tyrosine
DOPA	3,4-dihydroxyphenylalanine
DA	dopamine
NE	norepinephrine
E	epinephrine
VMA	vanillylmandelic acid
HVA	homovanillic acid
NM	normetanephrine
M	metanephrine
MT	3-methoxytyramine
DOPAC	3,4-dihydroxyphenylacetic acid
DOMA	3,4-dihydroxymandelic acid
MHPG	3-methoxy-4-hydroxyphenylethyleneglycol
MHPE	3-methoxy-4-hydroxyphenylethanol
DOPEG	3,4-dihydroxyphenylethyleneglycol
DOPET	3,4-dihydroxyphenylethanol
TM or M*	total metanephrines (NM + M)
VA	vanilalanine
VLA	vanillactic acid
VPA	vanilpyruvic acid
DOPLA	3,4-dihydroxyphenyllactic acid
DOPPA	3,4-dihydroxyphenylpyruvic acid

REFERENCES

1. Mason, G.H., Hart-Mercer, J., Miller, E.J., et al.: Adrenaline-secreting neuroblastoma in an infant. *Lancet* 2: 322–325, 1957.

2. Isaacs, H., Medalie, M., and Politzer, W.M.: Noradrenaline-secreting neuroblastoma. *Brit. Med. J.* 1: 401–404, 1959.

3. Greenberg, R.E., and Gardner, L.I.: New diagnostic test for neural tumors of infancy, increased urinary excretion of 3-methoxy-4-hydroxy-mandelic acid and norepinephrine in a ganglioneuroma with chronic diarrhea. *Pediatrics* 24: 683–684, 1959.

4. Stickler, G.B., Hallenbeck, G.A., and Flock, E.V.: Ganglioneuroblastoma associated with chronic diarrhea and increased excretion of catecholamines. *Proc. Staff Meet. Mayo Clin.* 34: 548–549, 1959.

5. Armstrong, M.D., McMillan, A., and Shaw, K.: 3-Methoxy-4-hydroxy-D-mandelic acid, a urinary metabolite of norepinephrine. *Biochem. Biophys. Acta* 25: 422–423, 1957.

6. Greenberg, R.E., and Gardner, L.I.: Catecholamine metabolism in a functional neural tumor. *J. Clin. Invest.* 39: 1729–1736, 1960.

7. von Studnitz, W.: Occurrence, isolation and identification of 3-methoxy-4-hydroxyphenylalanine. *Clin. Chim. Acta* 6: 525–530, 1961.

8. Everson, T.C., and Cole, W.H.: *Spontaneous Regression of Cancer.* Philadelphia: W.B. Saunders Company, 1966.

9. Sutow, W.W., Gehan, E.A., Heyn, R.M., et al.: Comparison of survival curves, 1956 versus 1962 in children with Wilms' tumor and neuroblastoma. *Pediatrics* 45: 800–811, 1970.

10. Gitlow, S.E., Dziedzic, L.B., Strauss, L., et al.: Biochemical and histological determinants in the prognosis of neuroblastoma. *Cancer* 32: 898–905, 1973.

11. Koop, C.E., and Hernandez, J.R.: Neuroblastoma: experience with 100 cases in children. *Surgery* 56: 726–733, 1964.

12. Marsden, H.B., and Steward, J.K.: Neuroblastoma. In *Tumours in Children.* New York: Springer-Verlag,1968, pp. 131–170.

13. Gitlow, S.E., Bertani, L.M., Rausen, A., et al.: Diagnosis of neuroblastoma by qualitative and quantitative determination of catecholamine metabolites in urine. *Cancer* 25: 1377–1383, 1970.

14. Alpert, J.N., and Mones, R.: Neurologic manifestations of neuroblastoma. *J. Mount Sinai Hosp.* 36: 35–47, 1969.

15. Grant, H., and Pulvertaft, R.J.V.: Differential diagnosis of neuroblastoma and Burkitt's tumor. *Arch. Dis. Childh.* 41: 193–197, 1966.

16. Dargeon, H.W.: Neuroblastoma. *J. Pediatr.* 61: 456–471, 1956.

17. Marsden, H.B., and Steward, J.K.: Ewing's tumours and neuroblastoma. *J. Clin. Path.* 17: 411–417, 1964.

18. Willis, R.A.: Neuroblastoma and ganglioneuroma. In *Pathology of Tumours.* (2d Ed.) London: Butterworths, 1953, pp. 843–871.

19. Bohuon, C.: Catecholamine metabolism in neuroblastoma. *J. Pediatr. Surg.* 3: 114–118, 1968.

20. Käser, H.: Catecholamine-producing neural tumors other than pheochromocytoma. *Pharmacol. Rev.* 18: 659–665, 1966.

21. Holtz, P., Heise, R., and Ludtke, K.: Fermentativer Abbau von 1-Dioxyphenylalanine (DOPA) durch Niere. *Arch. Exp. Path. Pharmak.* 191: 87–118, 1938.

22. Blaschko, H.: The specific action of l-dopa decarboxylase. *J. Physiol.* (London); 96: 50P–51P, 1939.

23. Ikeda, M., Fahien, L.A., and Undenfriend, S.: A Kinetic study of bovine adrenal tyrosine hydroxylase. *J. Biol. Chem.* 241: 4452–4456, 1966.

24. Nagatsu, T., Levitt, B.G., and Udenfriend, S.: Tyrosine hydroxylase: the initial step in norepinephrine biosynthesis. *J. Biol. Chem.* 238: 2910–2917, 1964.

25. Weiner, N., Cloutier, G., Bjur, R., and Pfeffer, R.I.: Modification of norepinephrine synthesis in intact tissue by drugs and during short-term adrenergic stimulation. *Pharmacol. Rev.* 24: 203–221, 1972.

26. Lovenberg, W., Weissbach, H., and Udenfriend, S.: Aromatic-l-amino acid decarboxylase. *J. Biol. Chem.* 237: 89–93, 1962.

27. Weiner, N.: Regulation of norepinephrine biosynthesis. *Annual Rev. Pharmacol.* 10: 273–290, 1970.

28. Goldstein, M., Lauber, E., and McKereghan, M.R.: Studies on the purification and characterization of 3,4-dihydroxyphenylethylamine-B-hydroxylase. *J. Biol. Chem.* 240: 2066–2072, 1965.

29. Levin, E.Y., Levenberg, B., and Kaufman, S.: The enzymatic conversion of 3,4-dihydroxyphenylethylamine to norepinephrine. *J. Biol. Chem.* 236: 2043–2049, 1961.

30. Viveros, O.H., Arqueras, L., Connett, R.J., and Kirschner,

N.: Mechanism of secretion from the adrenal medulla. III. Studies of dopamine-B-hydroxylase as a marker for catecholamine storage vesicle membranes in rabbit adrenal glands. *Molec. Pharmacol.* 5: 60–68, 1969.

31. Kirschner, N., Roric, M., and Kamin, D.L.: Inhibition of dopamine uptake *in vitro* by reserpine administered *in vivo. J. Pharmacol. Exp. Ther.* 141: 285–289, 1963.

32. Weinshilbaum, R.M., Thoa, N.B., Johnson, D.G., et al.: Proportional release of norepinephrine and dopamine-B-hydroxylase from sympathetic nerves. *Science* 174: 1349–1351, 1971.

33. Freedman, L.S., Ohuchi, T., Goldstein, M., et al.: Changes in human serum dopamine-B-hydroxylase activity with age. *Nature* (London) 236: 310–311, 1972.

34. Goldstein, M., Fuxe, K., and Hökfelt, T.: Characterization and tissue localization of catecholamine synthesizing enzymes. *Pharmacol. Rev.* 24: 293–309, 1972.

35. Hartman, B.K., and Udenfriend, S.: The application of immunological techniques to the study of enzymes regulating catecholamine synthesis and degradation. *Pharmacol. Rev.* 24: 311–330, 1972.

36. Axelrod, J.: Metabolism of epinephrine and other sympathomimetic amines. *Physiol. Rev.* 39: 751–776, 1959.

37. Axelrod, J.: Methylation reactions in the formation and metabolism of catecholamines and other biogenic amines. *Pharmacol. Rev.* 18: 95–113, 1966.

38. Molinoff, P.B., and Axelrod, J.: Biochemistry of catecholamines. *Ann. Rev. Biochem.* 40: 465–500, 1971.

39. Zeller, E.A.: Oxidation of amines. In (Sumner, J.B., and Myrboin, K., Eds.): *The Enzymes, Chemistry and Mechanism of Action.* (Vol. 2). New York: Academic Press, 1951, pp. 536–538.

40. Schnaitman, G., Erwin, V.G., and Greenwalt, J.W.: Submitochondrial localization of monoamine oxidase. *J. Cell. Biol.* 34: 718–735, 1967.

41. Gitlow, S.E., Ornstein, L., Mendlowitz, M., et al.: A. simple colorimetric urinary analysis for the diagnosis of pheochromocytoma. *Amer. J. Med.* 28: 921–926, 1960.

42. Bell, M., and Steward, J.K.: Neuroblastoma and catecholamine excretion. *Lancet* 1: 1061, 1961.

43. Bell, M.: Observations on the biochemical diagnosis of neuroblastoma. (Bohuon, C. Ed.): In *Neuroblastoma Biochemical Studies.* New York: Springer-Verlag, 1966, pp. 42–51.

44. Young, R.B., Steiker, D.D., Steiker, D.D., et al.: Urinary

vanilmandelic acid (VMA) excretion in children. Use of a semiquantitative test. *J. Pediatr.* 62: 844–854, 1963.

45. LaBrosse, E.H.: Biochemical diagnosis of neuroblastoma: use of a urine spot test. *Proc. Amer. Assoc. Cancer Res.* 9: 39, 1968.

46. Evans, A.E., Blore, J., Hadley, R., and Tanindi, S.: The LaBrosse spot test, a practical aid in the diagnosis and management of children with neuroblastoma. *Pediatrics* 47: 913–915, 1971.

47. Leonard, A.S., Roback, S.A., Nesbit, M., and Freier, E.: The VMA test strip, a new tool for mass screening, diagnosis and management of catecholamine-secreting tumors. *J. Pediatr. Surg.* 7: 528–531, 1972.

48. von Studnitz, W.: Methodische und klinische Untersuchungen über die Ausscheidung der 3-methoxy-4-hydroxymandelsäure im Urin. *Scandinav. J. Clin. Lab. Invest.* (Suppl. 48) 12: 3–73, 1960.

49. Pisano, J.J., Crout, J.R., and Abraham, D.: Determination of 3-methoxy-4-hydroxymandelic acid in urine. *Clin. Chim. Acta* 7: 285–291, 1962.

50. McKendrick, T., and Edwards, R.W.H.: The excretion of 4-hydroxy-3-methoxymandelic acid by children. *Arch. Dis. Childh.* 40: 418–425, 1965.

51. Williams, C.M., and Greer, M.: Homovanillic acid and vanilmandelic acid in diagnosis of neuroblastoma. *J.A.M.A.* 183: 836–840, 1963.

52. Wilk, S., Gitlow, S.E., Franklin, M.J. et al.: A quantitative assay for vanillylmandelic acid (VMA) by gas-liquid chromatography. *Analyt. Biochem.* 13: 544–551, 1965.

53. Dziedzic, S.W., Bertani, L.M., Clarke, D.D., and Gitlow, S.E.: A new derivative for the gas-liquid chromatographic determination of homovanillic acid. *Analyt. Biochem.* 47: 592–600, 1972.

54. Laasberg, L.H., and Shimosato, S.: Paper chromatographic identification of catecholamines. *J. Appl. Physiol.* 21: 1929–1934, 1966.

55. Gutteridge, J.M.C.: Thin-layer chromatographic techniques for the investigation of abnormal urinary catecholamine metabolite patterns. *Clin. Chim. Acta* 21: 211–216, 1968.

56. Garrettson, L.K., Turpin, D.L., Hvidberg, E.F., and Mellinger, T.J.: Para-hydroxyphenylacetic and homovanillic acid excretion: variation during growth and in cystic fibrosis and other pulmonary diseases. *J. Clin. Path.* 55: 318–324, 1971.

57. Sato, T.L.: The quantitative determination of 3-methoxy-4-hydroxy phenylacetic acid (homovanillic acid) in urine. *J. Lab. Clin. Med.* 66: 516–525, 1965.

58. Geissbühler, P.: Dosage fluorimetrique de l'acide homovanillique dans le liquide cephalorachidien l'urine et le sang. *Clin. Chim. Acta* 26: 231–234, 1969.

59. Ruthven, C.R.J., and Sandler, M.: Estimation of homovanillic acid in urine. *Analyt. Biochem.* 8: 282–292, 1964.

60. Axelrod, J., Kopin, I.J., and Mann, J.D.: 3-Methoxy-4-hydroxy-phenylglycol sulfate, a new metabolite of epinephrine and norepinephrine. *Biochim. Biophys. Acta* 36: 576–577, 1959.

61. Gitlow, S.E., Mendlowitz, M., Kruk, E., et al.: Excretion of catecholamines and their metabolites in hypertension. *Fed. Proc.* 22: 389, 1963.

62. Wilk, S., Gitlow, S.E., Clarke, D.D. and Paley, D.H.: Determination of urinary 3-methoxy-4-hydroxyphenylethyleneglycol by gas-liquid chromatography and electron capture detection. *Clin. Chim. Acta* 16: 403–408, 1967.

63. Pisano, J.J.: A simple analysis for normetanephrine and metanephrine in urine. *Clin. Chim. Acta* 5: 406–414, 1960.

64. Crout, J.R., Pisano, J.J., and Sjoerdsma, A.: Urinary excretion of catecholamines and their metabolites in pheochromocytoma. *Amer. Heart J.* 61: 375–381, 1961.

65. Gitlow, S.E., Mendlowitz, M., and Bertani, L.M.: The biochemical techniques for detecting and establishing the presence of a pheochromocytoma. *Amer. J. Cardiol.* 26: 270–279, 1970.

66. Bertani, L.M., Dziedzic, S.W., Clarke, D.D., and Gitlow, S.E.: A gas-liquid chromatographic method for the separation and quantitation of normetanephrine and metanephrine in human urine. *Clin. Chim. Acta* 30: 227–233, 1970.

67. Stott, A.W., and Robinson, R.: Urinary normetadrenaline excretion in essential hypertension. *Clin. Chim. Acta* 16: 249–252, 1967.

68. Taniguchi, K., Kakimoto, Y., and Armstrong, M.D.: Quantitative determination of metanephrine and normetanephrine in urine. *J. Lab. Clin. Med.* 64: 469–484, 1964.

69. Sourkes, T.L., Denton, R.L., Murphy, G.F., et al.: The excretion of dihydroxyphenylanine, dopamine and dihydroxyphenylacetic acid in neuroblastoma. *Pediatrics* 31: 660–668, 1963.

70. Williams, C.M., and Leonard, R.H.: Microanalytical determination of dihydroxy aromatic acids by gas chromatography. *Analyt. Biochem.* 5: 362–366, 1963.

71. von Studnitz, W., Käser, H., and Sjoerdsma, A.: Spectrum of catecholamine biochemistry in patients with neuroblastoma. *N. Engl. J. Med.* 269: 232–235, 1963.

72. Gjessing, L.R.: Studies of functional neural tumors. I. urinary 3-methoxy-4-hydroxyphenyl metabolites. Scandinav. *J. Clin. Lab. Invest.* 15: 463–473, 1963.

73. LaBrosse, E.H., and Karon, M.: Metabolism of catecholamines in patients with neuroblastoma. *Excerpta Medica, Intern. Cong. Series* #48, 1962.

74. Gjessing, L.R., and Borud, O.: Urinary vanilpyruvic acid in neuroblastoma. *Lancet* 2: 818, 1964.

75. Smith, P.: Pathological excretion of 4-hydroxy-3-methoxyphenyllactic acid. *Nature* 205: 1236, 1965.

76. von Studnitz, W., and Hanson, A.: Demonstration of urinary N-acetyltyramine in patients with neuroblastoma. *Clin. Chim. Acta* 16: 180–183, 1967.

77. Hanson, A., and von Studnitz, W.: Demonstration of urinary N-acetyl-dopamine in patients with neuroblastoma. *Clin. Chim. Acta* 11: 384–385, 1965.

78. Herrlich, P., and Sekeris, C.E.: Identifizierung von N-acetylnoradrenalin im Urin eines Patienten mit Neuroblastom. *Hoppe-Segl. Z.* 19: 249–250, 1964.

79. Gjessing, L.R.: Biochemistry of functional neural crest tumors. *Advances Clin. Chem.* 11: 82–131, 1968.

80. von Euler, U.S., and Floding, I.: Diagnosis of pheochromocytoma by fluorimetric estimation of adrenaline and noradrenaline in urine. *Scandinav. J. Lab. Clin. Invest.* 8: 288–295, 1956.

81. von Euler, U.S. and Lishjko, F.: The estimation of catecholamines in urine. *Acta Physiol. Scand.* 45: 122–132, 1959.

82. Anton, A.H., and Sayre, D.F.: A study of the factors affecting the aluminum oxide trihydroxyindole procedure for the analysis of the catecholamines. *J. Pharmacol. Exp. Therap.* 138: 360–375, 1962.

83. Clarkson, P.M.: Neuroblastoma and catecholamine metabolism. *Clin. Pediatr.* 4: 397–403, 1965.

84. Carlsson, A., and Waldeck, B.: A fluorimetric method for the determination of dopamine (3-hydroxytyramine). *Acta Physiol. Scand.* 44: 293–298, 1958.

85. Clarke, D.D., Wilk, S., Gitlow, S.E., and Franklin, M.J.: Gas chromatographic determination of dopamine at the nanogram level. *J. Gas Chrom.* 5: 307–310, 1967.

86. Kawai, S., and Tamura, Z.: Gas chromatography of catecholamines as their trifluoroacetates. *Ch. Pharm. Bull.* 16: 699–701, 1968.

87. Kawai, S. and Tamura, Z.: Gas chromatography of

catecholamines as their trifluoroacetates in urine and tumor. *Chem. Pharm. Bull.* 16: 1091–1194, 1968.

88. Häggendal, J.: Newer developments in catecholamine assay. *Pharmacol. Rev.* 18: 325–330, 1966.

89. Lurvey, A., Yusin, A., and DeQuattro, V.: Pseudopheochromocytoma after self-administered isoproterenol. *J. Clin. Endocrinol. Metab.* 36: 766–769, 1973.

90. Skopin, N., Tatarinova, T.E., Friedman, S.L. and Binder, K.I.: Stimulation of arterial hypertension with large doses of ephedrine and theophedrine. *Ter. Arkh.* 32: 64–65, 1960.

91. Aquilar-Parada, E., Rivadeoneyra, J., Torres-Leon, A.F. and Serrano, P.A.: Pseudopheochromocytoma. *J.A.M.A.* 218: 884–885, 1971.

92. Gifford, R.W., and Tweed, D.C.: Spurious elevation of urinary catecholamines during therapy with alpha-methyldopa: a diagnostic pitfall. *J.A.M.A.* 182: 493–495, 1962.

93. Gitlow, S., Bertani, L., Wong, B.L., and Dziedzic, S.: Effects of debrisoquin (D), pargyline (P), amitriptyine (A) and Phenoxybenzamine (PB) upon human norepinephrine (NE) metabolism. *Fed. Proc.* 30: 678, 1971.

94. Smith, A., Gitlow, S.E., Gall, E., et al.: Effect of disulfiram and ethanol on the metabolism of d, 1-B-H³- norepinephrine. *Clin. Res.* 8: 367, 1960.

95. Gitlow, S., Mendlowitz, M., Wilk, E.K., et al.: Excretion of catecholamine metabolites by normal children and those with familial dysautonomia. *J. Clin. Invest.* 44: 1049, 1965.

96. Voorhess, M.L.: Urinary catecholamine excretion by healthy children. *Pediatrics* 39: 252–257, 1967.

97. Gitlow, S.E., Mendlowitz, M., Wilk, E.K., et al.: Excretion of catecholamine catabolites by normal children. *J. Lab. Clin. Med.* 72: 612–620, 1968.

98. Stickler, G.B., and Flock, E.V.: Neuroblastoma and ganglioneuroblastoma; associated increased urinary excretion of catecholamines. *Cancer Chemotherap. Rep.* 16: 439–442, 1962.

99. von Studnitz, W.: Uber die ausscheidung der 3-methoxy-4-hydroxy-phenylessigsaure (Homovanillinsäure) beim neuroblastom und anderen neuralen tumoren. *Klin. Wschr.* 40: 163–167, 1962.

100. Voorhess, M.L., and Gardner, L.I.: The value of serial catecholamine determinations in children with neuroblastoma. *Pediatrics* 30: 241–246, 1962.

101. Perry, T.L., Shaw, K.N.F., Walker, D., and Redlich, D.:

Urinary excretion of amines in normal children. *Pediatrics* 30: 576–584, 1962.

102. Gjessing, L.R.: Studies on urinary phenolic compounds in man. V. Homovanillic acid vanillylmandelic acids in children without functional neural tumors. *Scandinav. J. Clin. Lab. Invest.* 18: 540–542, 1966.

103. Barontini de Gutierrez-Moyano, M., Bergada, C., and Becu, L.: Catecholamine excretion in 40 children with sympathoblastoma. *J. Pediatr.* 77: 239–244, 1970.

104. Voorhess, M.L., and Kirkland, I.: In discussion in: The catecholamines in tumor and urine from patients with neuroblastoma and ganglioneuroblastoma. *J. Pediatr. Surg.* 3: 151–152, 1968.

105. Kontras, S.B.: Urinary excretion of 3-methoxy-4-hydroxy-mandelic acid in children with neuroblastoma. *Cancer* 15: 978–986, 1962.

106. Voorhess, M.L.: Urinary excretion of dopa and metabolites by patients with melanoma. *Cancer* 26: 146–149, 1970.

107. Beckwith, J.B., and Perrin, E.V.: In situ neuroblastomas, A contribution to the natural history of neural crest tumors. *Amer. J. Pathol.* 43: 1089–1104, 1963.

108. Shanklin, D.R., and Sotelo-Avila, C.: In situ tumors in fetuses, newborns and young infants. *Biol. Neonat.* 14: 286–316, 1969.

109. Guin, G.H., Gilbert, E.F., and Jines, B.: Incidental neuroblastoma in infants. *Amer. J. Clin. Path.* 51: 126–136, 1969.

110. Gitlow, S., Dziedzic, S., Dziedzic, L.B., and Gitlow, H.: Elevated catecholamine metabolite excretion by a sub-group of normal children. *Clin. Res.* 21: 464, 1973.

111. Chatten, J., and Voorhess, M.L.: Familial Neuroblastoma. *N. Engl. J. Med.* 277: 1230–1236, 1967.

112. Gitlow, S.E.: Unpublished Observations.

113. Voorhess, M.L.: The catecholamines in tumor and urine tissue from patients with neuroblastoma, ganglioneurobalstoma and pheochromocytoma. *J. Pediatr. Surg.* 3: 146–148, 1968.

114. Voorhess, M.L.: Discussion of Treatment of Neuroblastoma. *J. Pediatr. Surg.* 3: 151–152, 1968.

115. Voorhess, M.L., and Gardner, L.I.: Studies of catecholamine excretion by children with neural tumors. *J. Clin. Endocrinol. Metab.* 22: 126–133, 1962.

116. Voorhess, M.L., Pickett, L.K., and Gardner, L.I.: Functioning tumors of neural crest origin in childhood. *Amer. J. Surg.* 106: 33–35, 1963.

117. Marsden, H.B., and Steward, J.K.: Neuroblastoma. In *Tumors in Children*. New York: Springer-Verlag, 1968.

118. Voorhess, M.L.: Neuroblastoma with normal urinary catecholamine excretion. *J. Pediatr.* 78: 680–683, 1971.

119. Bray, P.F., Ziter, F., Lahey, M.E., and Myers, G.G.: The coincidence of neuroblastoma and acute cerebellar encephalopathy. *J. Pediatr.* 75: 983–990, 1969.

120. Barass, B.C., Coult, D.B., and Pinder, R.M.: 3-Hydroxy-4-methoxy phenylethylamine: the endogenous toxin of parkinsonism. *J. Pharm. Pharmacol.* 2: 499–501, 1972.

121. Gitlow, S.E., Bertani, L.M., Greenwood, S., et al.: Benign pheochromocytoma in association with elevated homovanillic acid excretion. *J. Pediatr.* 81: 1112–1116, 1972.

122. Morgan, C.D., Sandler, M., and Panigel, M.: Placental transfer of catecholamines in vitro and in vivo. *Amer. J. Obstet. Gynec.* 112: 1068–1075, 1972.

123. Vouté, P.A., Jr., Wadman, S.K., and Van Putten, W.J.: Congenital neuroblastoma. *Clin. Pediatr.* 9: 206–207, 1970.

124. Hardy, P.C., and Nesbit, M.E., Jr.: Familial neuroblastoma; report of a kindred with a high incidence of infantile tumors. *J. Pediatr.* 80: 74–77, 1972.

125. Gitlow, S.E.: Unpublished Observations.

126. Goldstein, M., Freedman, L.S., Bohuon, A.C., and Guerinot, F.: Serum dopamine-B-hydroxylase activity in neuroblastoma. *N. Engl. J. Med.* 286: 1123–1125, 1972.

127. Voorhess, M.L., and Gardner, L.I.: The value of serial catecholamine determinations in children with neuroblastoma. *Pediatrics* 30: 241–246, 1962.

128. Voorhess, M.L., and Whalen, J.P.: The role of catecholamine excretion in diagnosis and treatment of neuroblastoma; report of two cases. *Radiology* 83: 92–97, 1964.

129. Brett, E.M., Oppé, T.E., Ruthven, C.R.J., and Sandler, M.: Congenital dopamine-secreting neuroblastoma with clinical and biochemical remission. *Arch. Dis. Childh.* 39: 403–405, 1966.

130. Voorhess, M.L.: Functioning neural tumors. *Pediatr. Clin. N. Amer.* 13: 3–18, 1966.

131. Page, L.B., and Jacoby, G.A.: Catecholamine metabolism and storage granules in pheochromocytoma and neuroblastoma. *Medicine* 43: 379–383, 1964.

132. Barontini de Gutierrez-Moyano, M., Bergada, C., and Becu, L.: Significance of catecholamine excretion in the follow-up of sympathoblastomas. *Cancer* 27: 228–232, 1971.

133. Gitlow, S.E., Bertani, L.M., Dziedzic, S.W., et al.: Relationship of catecholamine catabolite excretion to prognosis in neuroblastoma. *Meeting of American Pediatr. Society.* 1971. (Abstracts), p. 216.

134. Gitlow, S.E., Mendlowitz, M., Khassis, S., et al.: The diagnosis of pheochromocytoma by determination of urinary 3-methoxy-4-hydroxymandelic acid. *Clin. Invest.* 39: 221–226, 1960.

135. Itoh, T., and Ohmori, K.: Biosynthesis and storage of catecholamines in pheochromocytoma and neuroblastoma cells. *J. Lab. Clin. Med.* 81: 887–896, 1973.

136. LaBrosse, E.H., and Karon, M.: Catechol-O-methyl-transferase activity in neuroblastoma tumour. *Nature* 196: 1222–1223, 1962.

137. Lurvey, A.N., Kathan, R.H., and Rosenthal, I.M.: Homovanillic acid content in neuroblastomas. *Proc. Soc. Exp. Med.* 130: 972–975, 1969.

138. Dziedzic, S.W., and Gitlow, S.E.: Unpublished Observations.

139. Greenberg, R., Rosenthal, I., and Falk, G.S.: Electron microscopy of human tumors secreting catecholamines: correlation with biochemical data. *J. Path. Exp. Neurol.* 28: 475–500, 1969.

140. Imashuku, S., Takada, H., Sawada, T., and Nakamura, T.: Tyrosine hydroxylase activity in neuroblastoma and human adrenal glands. *J. Lab. Clin. Med.* 80: 190–199, 1972.

6 Histogenesis and Pathology of Neuroblastoma

Carl Pochedly, M.D.
Lotte Strauss, M.D.

1. History
2. Anatomy of the sympathetic nervous system
3. Embryological development of the autonomic nervous system
4. Histogenesis of neuroblastomas
5. Pathological findings
   a. Neuroblastoma
   b. Ganglioneuroblastoma
   c. Ganglioneuroma
6. Tumors that resemble neuroblastomas histologically

The first description of a neuroblastoma is ascribed to Rudolf Virchow in 1864.[1] He classified it as a glioma. Neurofibrils were observed in an adrenal neoplasm by Morgan[2] as early as 1879, and in 1884 Dalton described a case of adrenal neuroblastoma with metastases to the liver.[3] He also described rosette formation, which is still recognized as an important diagnostic feature of this neoplasm. In 1891 Marchand[4] noted the resemblance of this tumor to the embryonic central nervous system. He also called attention to the histological similarity between adrenal medulla and sympathetic nervous tissue. Thus, common features were noted between neuroblastoma and the developing sympathetic ganglia.

In 1910 Wright[5] reaffirmed the origin of neuroblastomas from the developing sympathetic nervous system, when he showed that the microscopic pattern of this tumor was similar to that seen in the embryonic adrenal medulla. He proposed the term neuroblastoma for

155

these neoplasms. Prior to that time they had generally been classified as gliomas or sarcomas.[6] Herxheimer[7] in 1914 demonstrated, by Bielschowsky's silver impregnation technique, that the fibrils in neuroblastomas were primitive nerve fibers and that these were similar to those seen in normal neuroblasts. These findings were later confirmed by Murray and Stout[8] in studies of neuroblastoma cells cultured in vitro.

These early studies showed that neuroblastomas are composed of cells identical with the neuroblasts of the developing embryo. Not only do the cells resemble the normal embryonic precursors of the central nervous system, but in many of the tumors the microscopic architecture, through the formation of rosettes, is very similar to the arrangement of the neuroblasts in the developing sympathetic ganglia. It was not until 1891 that the origin of these tumors was recognized and not until 1914 that confirmation of their histogenesis by the demonstration of neurofibrils within the tumor was accomplished.[9]

ANATOMY AND PHYSIOLOGY OF THE SYMPATHETIC NERVOUS SYSTEM

The autonomic nervous system consists of the sympathetic and parasympathetic divisions. Neuroblastomas arise from the sympathetic division. Although the autonomic nervous system is usually defined as a distinct portion of the peripheral nervous system, anatomically it is distinct only in part, since it lies partially within the central nervous system. This is a functionally rather than an anatomically distinct system.[10] The autonomic nervous system supplies smooth muscle, cardiac muscle, and certain glands, structures over which there is ordinarily no voluntary control.

The sympathetic system is designed for emergencies, preparing the individual for flight or fight when faced with danger. The sympathetic system, for example, dilates the pupil of the eye, thus providing a wider field of vision and a better opportunity to see a dangerous object approaching from the side. It speeds up the rate and increases the strength of the heart beat. It constructs blood vessels especially in the skin and digestive tract, allowing blood to be diverted from these structures for circulation to the voluntary muscles. It tends also to slow down the peristaltic action of the digestive tract, a function appropriate to the decreased circulation to that part. Through its action on the adrenal medulla, the sympathetic system activates the release of adrenalin into the blood stream. Adrenalin has the same effect on smooth muscle and cardiac muscle as stimulation by sympathetic fibers.[10] The sympathetic chains are paired, each consisting of a series of ganglia connected by intervening fibers, so that the ganglia appear somewhat like beads strung some distance apart on a string. Each trunk extends from the level of the first cervical vertebra to the tip of the sacrum. They are not strictly segmental, one for each spinal nerve. Thus, there are usually only 3 cervical ganglia rather than 8, 11 thoracic ganglia rather than 12, 4 lumbar ganglia, and less than 5 ganglia in the sacrococcygeal region.[10]

Preganglionic fibers of the sympathetic system leave the spinal cord through the ventral roots of all 11 thoracic and of the upper 2 lumbar nerves. They leave these nerves as white rami communicantes to join the sympathetic trunk. Some preganglionic fibers end within the trunk, many running up or down within it for some distance; others simply traverse the trunk and form visceral or splanchnic nerves.[10]

EMBRYOLOGICAL DEVELOPMENT OF THE AUTONOMIC NERVOUS SYSTEM

During embryonic development the neural tube gives rise to all nervous elements whose cell bodies lie within the brain and spinal cord. It also furnishes the neuroglial cells. The lateral margins of the neural plate are not incorporated into the neural tube. Instead, each becomes a band of cells called the *neural crest* (Figure 1). From this differentiate all ganglion cells (cranial, spinal, autonomic) as well as various other derivatives.[11]

When the neural folds become a tube and the ectoderm detaches from it, the crest-substance separates into right and left linear halves, distinct from the neural tube. These portions settle to a position between the tube and the myotomes. Each half of the original crest-substance is a cellular band extending the full length of spinal cord and far rostrad along the brain wall. While the neural tube grows caudad, new crest-tissue is added progressively to these bands.[11] Certain neuroblasts of crest origin migrate ventrad and differentiate into cells of the autonomic ganglia.

In the fifth week, some of the crest cells migrate along the dorsal roots of the spinal nerves. Leaving the nerve trunk, they take position in paired masses dorsolateral to the aorta. Growth quickly merges them into continuous longitudinal strands, with segmental enlargements representing primordial autonomic ganglia, each containing an aggregation of neuroblasts. These soon differentiate into multipolar ganglion cells, encapsulated by satellite cells also of neural crest origin.[11] In the fetal lumbar region, certain sympathetic ganglion precursors detach themselves and become glandular cells of the adrenal medulla. The adrenal medulla and the sympathetic nervous system thus share a common cell of origin, the sympathogon. This explains how retroperitoneal neuroblastomas may arise from the adrenal medulla as well as from the sympathetic ganglia in close proximity to the adrenal glands.[12]

Nearly all of the retroperitoneal neurogenic neoplasms in infants and children arise in the sympathetic nervous system or the adrenal medulla. The development of the sympathetic cell line comprises four stages: the *sympathogon,* which is the precursor cell and forms the ganglionic anlage; the *sympatheticoblast,* a result of somewhat further differentiation. These are undifferentiated pluripotential cells derived from the neural crest. They migrate into the visceral areas to form the anlage of the sympathetic nervous system and finally differentiate into *unipolar* and *multipolar* neuroblasts; further differentiation occurs into mature *ganglion* cells.[13]

Not all of the cells of the primitive autonomic ganglia differentiate into neurons. Some become satellite and neurolemmal cells, associated with the neurons. Still others become distinctive

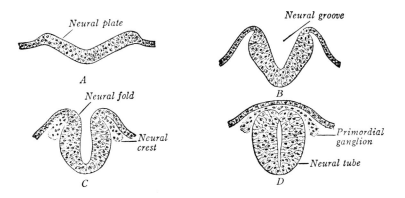

Figure 1. Origin of neural tube and neural crest, illustrated by transverse sections from early human embryos. (Courtesy of Dr. L.B. Arey and the W.B. Saunders Company[11])

endocrine elements that stain brown with chrome salts and hence are designated chromaffin cells. This reaction is due to the presence of adrenalin within the cells. Cells of this type constitute the chromaffin system, the most conspicuous member of which is the medulla of the adrenal gland.[11]

Some chromaffin cells collect in rounded masses in close relation to autonomic ganglia and plexuses. Because of this association they have received the appropriate name paraganglia. They begin to organize at two months and before birth attain a diameter of 1.0 mm or more. Other chromaffin masses, similar in nature, occur along the course of the aorta (Figure 2). The largest, found in the abdominal sympathetic plexus, is the pair of aortic chromaffin bodies of Zuckerkandl. These are first recognizable toward the end of the second month about the root of the inferior mesenteric artery. At birth they are about 1.0 cm long. All representatives of this group are composed of cords of chromaffin cells intermingled with strands of connective tissue; the whole mass is surrounded by a connective-tissue capsule. After birth the chromaffin bodies decline but do not disappear entirely until puberty.[11] These chromaffin bodies may be sites of origin of neuroblastomas, in addition to the adrenal medulla.

Other paraganglia are associated with the vessels derived from

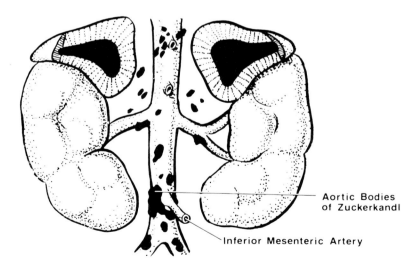

Aortic Bodies
of Zuckerkandl

Inferior Mesenteric Artery

Figure 2. Distribution of chromaffin bodies in the adrenal medulla and along the abdominal aorta in the six-month human embryo. These bodies contain both chromaffin and non-chromaffin cells. (Adapted from Arey[11])

the aortic arches. Among these are the carotid bodies which organize in the seventh week from a mesodermal condensation on the wall of each internal carotid artery. They are invaded by non-chromaffin cells from a nearby cervical autonomic ganglion and receive afferent fibers chiefly from the glossopharyngeal nerves. The invading neuroblasts presumably become the chemoreceptive cells of the mature organ which serves as a reflex system in the regulation of blood pressure.[11]

HISTOGENESIS OF NEUROBLASTOMAS

Neuroblastoma is a dysontogenetic malignant tumor. Dysontogenesis is manifested by a disturbance in the normal maturation or differentiation of the sympathogonia. The origin of neuroblastomas from the sympathetic nervous system or its precursors is well established. Since these tumors histologically resemble embryonic adrenal medullary tissue, Wright concluded as early as 1910 that they originate from the sympathetic nervous system.[5] Demonstration of neurofibrils established their nervous origin. The discovery that a vast majority of these tumors secrete catecholamines further established neuroblastomas as being of sympathetic nervous system origin.

Neuroblastomas arise from primitive sympathetic neuroblasts (sympathogonia), one of several derivatives of the neural crest (Figure 3). It has recently been proposed that this group of neoplasms should be considered as one variant of "neurocristopathy."[14] Early in embryonic life neural crest cells migrate ventrally to form a syncytium form which develop the sympathetic chain and ganglia and the celiac plexus. Cells from the celiac plexus then migrate further to enter the mesodermal anlage of the developing adrenal gland to form the primitive adrenal medulla. These migrating cells, sympathogonia, ultimately give rise to two distinct cell lines—the non-chromaffin and the chromaffin cells.[15] The chromaffin cells are responsible for the elaboration of the adrenal medullary hormones. Tumors derived from the pheochromocytic cell line are of two types: the pheochromocytoma, which is hormonally active, and the paraganglioma, which is hormonally inactive. According to this concept, cells of the sympathoblastic line give rise to neuroblastomas (Figure 4).

Thus, neuroblastomas, pheochromocytomas, and paragangliomas are derived from common precursor cells of the sympathetic nervous system. This may account for the occasional occurrence of tumors containing both chromaffin and non-chromaffin components.[16] Generally, however, it appears that pheochromo-cytomas and neuroblastomas occur as distinct neoplasms, each resulting from the proliferation of cells having differentiated along a specific line, but going back to common precursors.

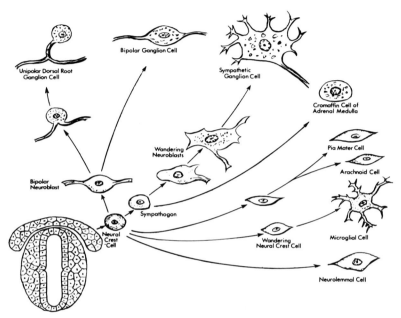

Figure 3. Primitive cells of the neural crest differentiate into somatic sensory cells, visceral sensory cells, postganglionic autonomic motor neurons, and the chromaffin cells of the adrenal medulla. Neuroblastomas originate from sympathogonia.

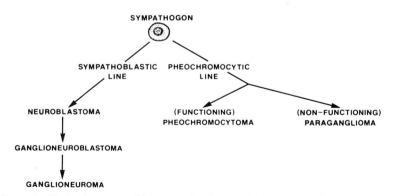

Figure 4. Probable routes of histogenesis of sympathetic nerve cell tumors.

Neuroblastoma is the currently accepted name for tumors of immature neuroblasts. Other names which have been used are *neurocytoma, sympathoma embryonale, sympathoblastoma,* and *sympathogonioma.* It is possible that sympathoblastoma may yet prove to be a more valid name than neuroblastoma.[16] In rare neuroblastomas, chromaffin as well as non-chromaffin cells may be encountered. In some undifferentiated neuroblastomas, sympathoblasts with more prominent cytoplasm are found. In a few examples, some of these larger cells have been shown to give an indefinite chromaffin reaction. The question has been raised that these cells may not be neuroblasts but incompletely differentiated chromaffin cells. It is well known that fetal chromaffin tissue is secreting pressor amines as early as the third or fourth month of fetal life, at a stage when the cells are morphologically indistinguishable from neuroblasts and before they give an unequivocal chromaffin reaction.[16]

It may well be that chromaffin cells occur in a much higher proportion of neuroblastomas than we have supposed. It is possible that meticulous fine structural and histochemical study (especially for mild degrees of chromaffinity) will establish the dual or mixed (chromaffin and non-chromaffin) character of many neuroblastomas. Such a finding would be consistent with the embryogenesis of this tumor. If this is so, it will enhance the validity of the name sympathoblastoma, in preference to neuroblastoma. The name sympathoblastoma would acknowledge that the tumor originates from sympathoblasts rather than from neuroblasts. However, maturation of these tumors usually produces ganglioneuromatous tissue only, and rarely well-differentiated chromaffin tissue.[16]

PATHOLOGICAL FINDINGS

Three major variants of tumors of the sympathetic nervous system are recognized: (1) neuroblastoma, comprised entirely of sympathogonia or sympathoblasts; (2) ganglioneuroblastoma (or differentiated neuroblastoma), combining both primitive cells and differentiated cells; and (3) ganglioneuroma, composed of fully differentiated elements. Although these tumors comprise a biological spectrum,[17,18] as reflected in morphological features, comparisons and contrasts can be more effectively drawn by considering the three variants individually.

Neuroblastoma

This is the least differentiated of the three variants. It is a neoplasm of infancy, one-half of all cases appearing in the first year of life. It is rarely encountered after the age of eight years, and only exceptionally in adults. Neuroblastomas vary in size and appearance and may be bulky when first discovered. There is no correlation between size and degree of differentiation or presence of metastases. The primary tumor may remain well demarcated though usually devoid of a true capsule (Figure 5). The consistency of the intact tumor is fairly firm, and the color is light gray or yellowish. Often there is a violaceous tinge to the surface, indicative of marked vascularity or, more often, of hemorrhage. Larger tumors are often multinodular. The cut surface, which is rarely uniform in larger tumors, reveals a multilobular, cellular, yellowish gray tissue with areas of hemorrhage (Figure 6), and with foci of necrosis which may become cystic.

Calcification which is frequently demonstrated radiographically can at times be appreciated with the naked eye (Figure 7). Ossification may occur, especially in clinically silent tumors which regress.

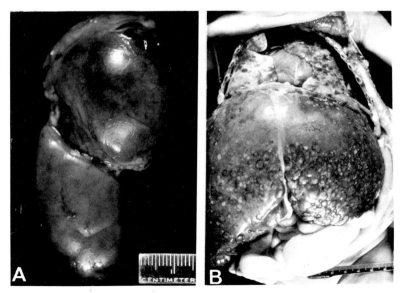

Figure 5. A: Neuroblastoma of right adrenal gland compressing upper pole of kidney, in an infant six weeks of age. **B:** The spherical tumor is completely confined within the adrenal capsule, though it had metastasized widely throughout the liver.

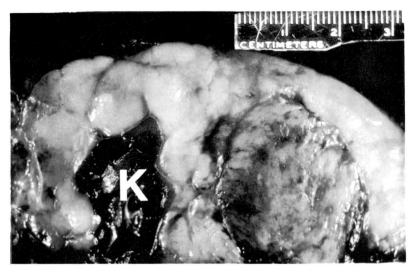

Figure 6. Cut surface of large adrenal neuroblastoma in a newborn infant; the tumor completely surrounds the kidney (K) without invading it. Note the lobular structure and dark foci of hemorrhage in the solid, otherwise intact, neoplasm. The tumor had metastasized to skin and bone marrow prior to birth.

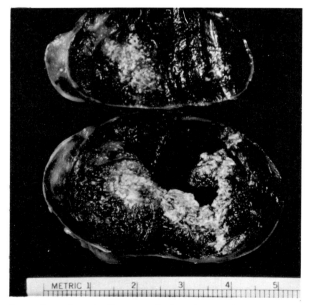

Figure 7. Cut surface of surgically resected adrenal neuroblastoma showing extensive hemorrhage, necrosis, and conspicuous calcific deposits (white areas).

Neuroblastomas of the adrenal medulla expand and attenuate the cortex at first and eventually tend to infiltrate and interrupt its continuity. Remnants of adrenal cortical tissue are usually found on the surface of even large tumors. Occasionally a tumor may spread to envelop the kidney, mimicking a renal neoplasm (Figure 6), or it may encroach on major blood vessels such as the renal vessels, the inferior vena cava, or the abdominal aorta. Often the tumor has invaded neighboring structures when first seen.[18] By contrast, small adrenal tumors or in situ neuroblastomas are well confined within the adrenal medulla causing little or no distortion of the gland (Figure 8). Tumors arising in extraadrenal sites similarly tend to encroach on adjacent structures. A tumor may be discovered on routine radiological examination because of pressure effects on adjacent bone, or it may give rise to neurological symptoms because of its growth through an intervertebral foramen. The larger the tumor, the greater the chance that it becomes softened, hemorrhagic, and necrotic. Degenerative changes may be encountered in encapsulated as well as in invasive tumors.

Histopathologically, undifferentiated neuroblastoma consists of nests or sheets of primitive cells with scant cytoplasm and dark-staining nuclei, usually spherical, somewhat resembling lymphocytes (Figure 9).[19] The tumor tends to be subdivided into lobules by delicate connective tissue septa carrying small blood vessels (Figure 10). The tumors rarely are completely uniform, as there may be a variable proportion of more or less differentiated cells. Maturation is manifested by increasing size of the nucleus which may become more vesicular, by more abundant cytoplasm, and by the presence of eosinophilic neurofibrillar processes (Figure 11). The tumor cells and their fibrillar processes may form so-called rosettes (Figure 12) which are considered diagnostic of neuroblastoma but do not occur in all tumors. More often the fibrils form a feltwork between nests of cells, or lakes in which scattered cells may be seen.[20] Silver impregnation and electron microscopy have demonstrated that the fibrils are neurites.[9,21]

The number of mitoses is variable, but rarely are they very numerous.[17] Secondary changes such as hemorrhage, necrosis, and calcium deposits are common. Lymphocytic aggregates may be present, especially in the more differentiated tumors (Figure 13). Evidence of maturation towards ganglion cells is detected in about half the specimens. This may involve a large proportion of the cells of a given tumor or only scattered cells in an otherwise rather undifferentiated neoplasm. Even tumors which are predominantly undifferentiated contain occasional cells with large nuclei, prominent nucleoli, and an increase in the amount of cytoplasm.[20] The lack of uniformity of the cells in some tumors makes it advisable to sample many areas of a surgically resected tumor. Metastatic lesions may differ from the primary tumor in the degree of differentiation of the cells, but this is uncommon. It is well known that occasionally

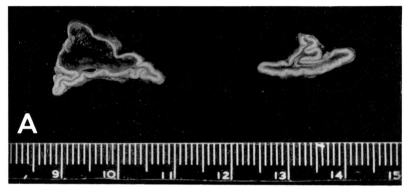

Figure 8. **A:** Cut surface of slightly enlarged right and normal left adrenal gland of one-month-old infant, showing in situ neuroblastoma of right adrenal, discovered at autopsy. The small medullary tumor is completely surrounded by intact, slightly expanded cortex.

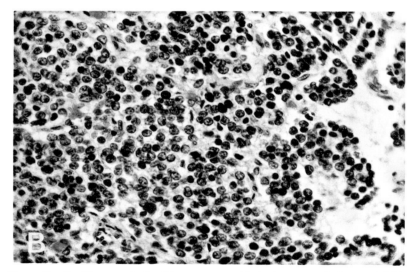

Figure 8. **B:** Microscopically this tumor consisted of nests and sheets of fairly uniform sympathogonia with round nuclei, scant cytoplasm and little neurofibrillar material. (H and E stain, ×430)

primary neuroblastomas, as well as metastatic deposits, may undergo spontaneous maturation to benign ganglioneuroma.[23]

Histologic grading Attempts have been made to correlate histologic grading of neuroblastomas with biological behavior. It has been noted that vesicular nuclei, abundant cytoplasm, formation of cytoplasmic processes, rosette formation, and presence of ganglion cells suggest a more favorable prognosis (Table 1).[24] Beckwith and Martin[25] noted that the prognosis appears to be more favorable if at

Table 1
Histological Features of Neuroblastoma Which May
Be Considered Signs of Maturation.[24,26]

1. Enlargement of the nuclei and presence of single, large vesicular nuclei.
2. Appearance of nucleoli or increased prominence of nucleoli.
3. Development of cytoplasm.
4. Formation of cytoplasmic fibrillar processes.
5. Clumping of the cells.
6. Arrangement of cells into rosette-like formation.
7. Bands of stroma separating the tumor cells into units of different diameter.
8. Presence of ganglion cells.

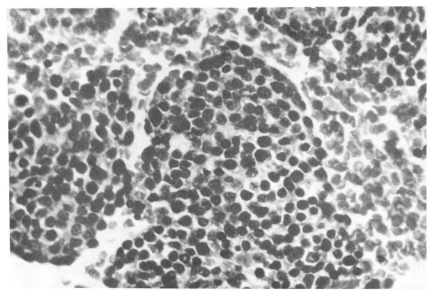

Figure 9. Undifferentiated neuroblastoma with hemorrhage. Tumor cells are tightly packed and uniform, with scant cytoplasm, hyperchromatic nuclei and no visible fibrillar processes. (H and E stain, ×430)

168

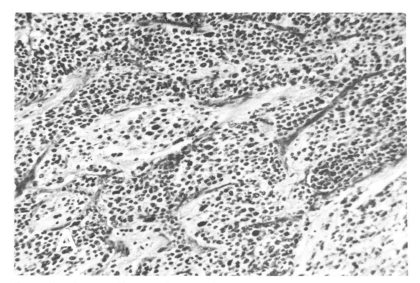

Figure 10. **A:** Neuroblastoma showing characteristic arrangement of cells in nests separated by delicate connective tissue septa. Tumor cells are tightly packed in places, or loosely scattered within a pale, finely fibrillar background in others. (H and E stain, ×160)

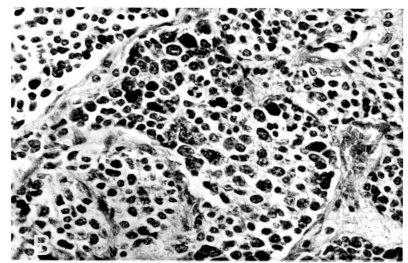

Figure 10. **B:** Higher magnification of a different area from the same specimen showing the delicate vascularized connective tissue framework of the tumor, dividing it into nests or lobules. The tumor cells show considerable variation in size and chromatin pattern of the nuclei. The cytoplasm is inconspicuous, and relatively few neurofibrils are seen. (H and E stain, ×430)

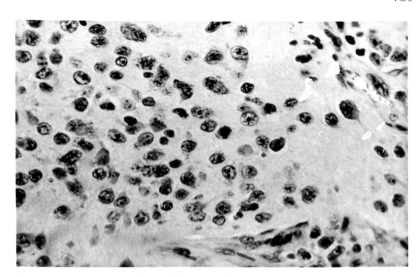

Figure 11. Retroperitoneal neuroblastoma, showing relatively high degree of differentiation of the tumor cells (compare with Figure 12) which do not form rosettes but are loosely scattered in a fibrillar background. The nuclei are larger, have a distinct chromatin pattern and nucleoli. Some of the cells have distinct cytoplasm and a unipolar process. (H and E stain, ×430)

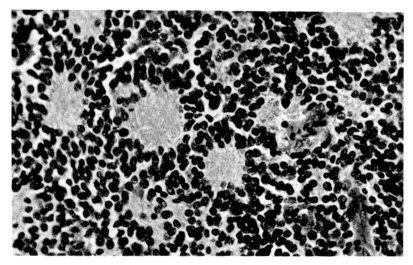

Figure 12. Neuroblastoma with rosettes. These are produced by arrangement of tumor cells around fibrillar cytoplasmic processes. (H and E stain, ×430)

least 5 percent of the cellular elements showed evidence of maturation (see Chapter 13). It should be noted that the histologic grade of the tumor has no consistent relation to the better prognosis in children under one year of age, while it may correlate with the outcome in older children with primary adrenal neuroblastomas.

Attempts have been made to establish subtypes of neuroblastoma depending upon their degree of differentiation. But this tumor does not lend itself to further categorization, since a given tumor may contain poorly differentiated as well as moderately well differentiated cells in different areas. By the same token, metastatic deposits may be less differentiated than the primary tumor. Further histologic subclassification thus is not only impractical and subject to error, but it has no clinical usefulness. In general, presence of histologic signs of maturation in a neuroblastoma is correlated with a slightly better prognosis. This conclusion does not apply to neuroblastoma in very young children in whom the prognosis is vastly better than after the age of one year, regardless of the histological grade.[26]

Ganglioneuroblastoma (Differentiated Neuroblastoma)

In this variant partial differentiation is reflected in the presence of ovoid or fusiform bipolar ganglion cells. Ganglioneuroblastomas are

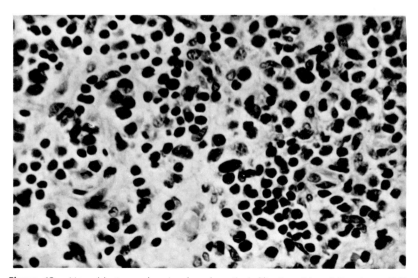

Figure 13. Neuroblastoma showing lymphocytic infiltration (H and E stain, ×430)

encountered predominantly in older children and adolescents rather than in infants, and less than one-half of cases originate in the adrenal medulla. The posterior mediastinum is the commonest extra-adrenal site.[18] Ganglioneuroblastomas are spherical bosselated, partially or totally encapsulated tumors that may reach large size before producing symptoms. Granular calcification is often demonstrable radiographically. Grossly, these lesions are firmer and more homogeneous than neuroblastomas. In examining such tumors, areas of capsular infiltration, foci of necrosis, or soft cellular lobules of tissue should be sought and subjected to microscopic examination for neuroblastoma tissue and invasion.[18] Hemorrhage and calcification are not uncommon. This tumor may infiltrate locally, as well as metastasize by way of hematogenous and lymphatic channels, as does the neuroblastoma.

Ganglioneuroblastomas may be composed of undifferentiated neuroblasts interspersed with mature ganglion cells (Figure 14). Areas that have undergone a considerable degree of maturation look strikingly different from the neuroblastoma. Mature ganglion cells, many times larger than neuroblasts, possess eccentric nuclei with distinct nucleoli and abundant cytoplasm. The ganglion cells, some of which may be multinucleated, are set in a background of abundant fibrillar tissue surrounded by tangled or parallel bundles of neurites, and more or less abundant Schwann cells. Because the histologic pattern may vary from one portion of the tumor to the other, one must examine multiple areas to avoid erroneously labeling a tumor with malignant elements as a benign ganglioneuroma.[17]

These tumors vary in their histologic characteristics to a very high degree. At one extreme they resemble the neuroblastoma and at the other the ganglioneuroma. Histologically they may present a fairly uniform appearance, but there may also be great variation from one part to another. Large areas may appear to be identical with neuroblastomas and the identity of the tumor may only be revealed by the presence of occasional large cells with abundant cytoplasm and a distinct resemblance to ganglion cells. In other tumors most of the cells may appear quite mature and only varying nuclear characteristics may serve to differentiate it from the benign ganglioneuroma. These different cell types may not be distributed throughout the tumor, and sections from one area alone may be misleading.

The ultrastructure of neuroblastoma and ganglioneuroblastoma is thought to reflect synthesis and storage of catecholamines. Misugi and co-workers have demonstrated a correlation between increased excretion of vanillylmandelic acid (VMA) and the cytoplasmic con-

172

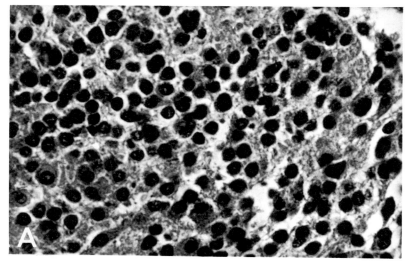

Figure 14. Ganglioneuroblastoma. **A:** Area showing relatively undifferentiated cells, indistinguishable from undifferentiated neuroblastoma.

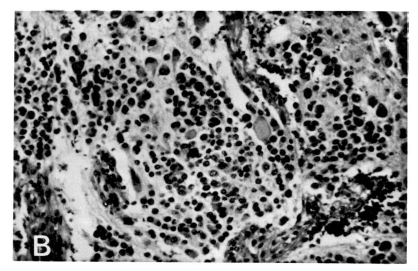

Figure 14. **B:** Another area in the same tumor showing mixture of more and less differentiated tumor cells.

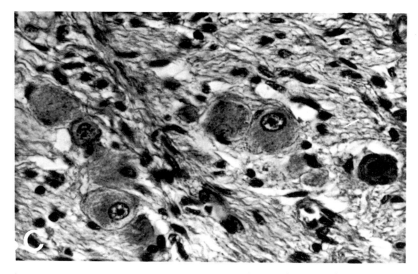

Figure 14. **C:** Same tumor with mature ganglion cells and Schwann cells. (H and E stain, ×430)

centration of membrane-bound granules approximately 100 mμ in size.[27] These were labeled "catechol" granules because of their similarity to the catecholamine granules in the normal adrenal medulla. Similar but larger electron-dense granules 500 mμ in size were thought to be derived from these smaller granules. Such granules were observed in bone marrow and lymph node metastases from a ganglioneuroblastoma, and histochemical studies were consistent with the presence of catecholamines in those tumor cells. It is suggested that these granules may be storage sites for catecholamines, although conclusive proof is lacking.[27]

Ganglioneuroma

Ganglioneuroma is the benign member of this group of neural crest neoplasms. The ratio of neuroblastomas to ganglioneuromas in one series was 8:1.[22] Ganglioneuroma occurs primarily in older children, adolescents, and young adults; it is rare in young children and only occasionally found in infants.[9] Thus, it occurs in patients of greater age than those with neuroblastoma. In one series of over 200 ganglioneuromas, 90 percent occurred in patients over the age of 10 years. Ganglioneuroma is found uncommonly in the adrenal gland; it occurs most frequently in the posterior mediastinum or in paravertebral areas.[18] The tumor may be solitary or multiple. By definition it does not metastasize; however, it may develop extensions and intimately circumscribe and compress vital structures. Occasionally it extends through an intervertebral foramen to produce neurologic symptoms.

The tumors are well circumscribed, firm, rubbery, and usually spherical, ovoid or lobulated; although the shape to a certain extent is determined by the pressure applied by the surrounding tissues. The cut surface has a fibrous texture and may vary in appearance from opaque, dense white to translucent yellow, resembling neurofibromas (Figure 15). Flecks of calcium are seen in about 20 percent. Hemorrhage is uncommon.[18]

Microscopically, ganglioneuromas contain mature ganglion cells with one or two nuclei, distinct nucleoli, abundant cytoplasm which may show Nissl granules and prominent cytoplasmic processes (axons) (Figure 16). The cells may be indistinguishable from normal ganglion cells. Satellite cells may be present. The ganglion cells are

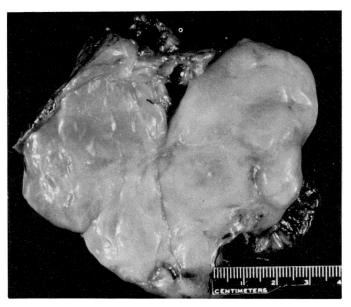

Figure 15. Ganglioneuroma. Cut surface of the tumor which is slightly lobulated, and has a fibrous texture, grossly resembling a neurofibroma. It has no true capsule and is adherent to tissue from the posterior mediastinum.

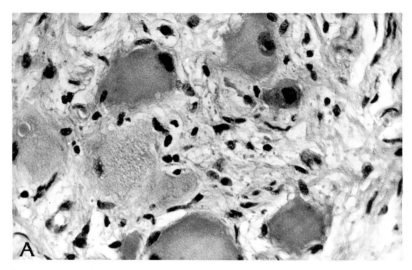

Figure 16. Ganglioneuroma. **A:** Group of ganglion cells with large cytoplasmic body, eccentric nucleus and prominent nucleolus. Several ganglion cells are undergoing degeneration manifested by pyknotic nucleus and poor definition of cytoplasmic outlines and texture. (H and E stain, ×430)

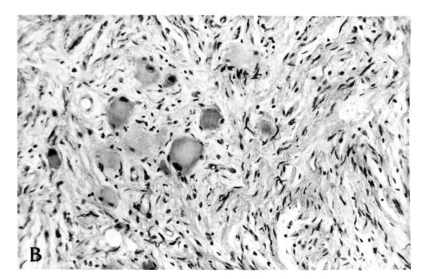

Figure 16. **B:** Lower magnification of the same tumor showing the relation of the ganglion cells to the Schwann cells and fibrous component of the tumor. (H and E stain, ×160)

scattered through a fibrous background which contains interlacing bundles of neurites, neurolemmal sheaths, and fibrous connective tissue.[18]

Ganglion cells vary considerably in number, with scanty cells rather diffusely scattered in some tumors and numerous clustered cells having the lobular arrangement of the neuroblastoma in others. The ganglion cells show variation in size with relatively normal cells and large multipolar and multinucleate forms. Swollen, degenerate, eosinophilic granular neurones are also seen. Lymphocytic infiltration is noted in some of the tumors and the resemblance of such infiltrates to immature neuroblasts can cause confusion (Figure 17). A fibrous capsule is present in some parts but this is not a constant feature, although the tumors are circumscribed and do not show invasive tendencies.[22]

The histologic hallmark of ganglioneuromas is the ganglion cell. This appears normal in most respects except that Nissl substance is not always present. Variations are common and bi-nucleated cells may be encountered. Mitoses are not seen, and if found must arouse suspicion that the tumor is a ganglioneuroblastoma. In some tumors, ganglion cells may be scarce, the bulk of the tumor being composed of Schwann cells, endoneurium, reticulum and fibrovascular stroma.

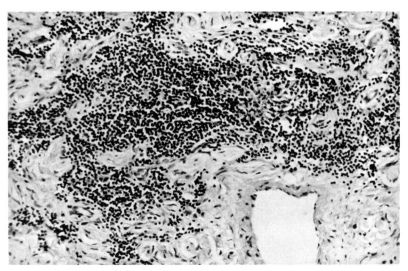

Figure 17. Focus of lymphocytic infiltration in a ganglioneuroma. These must not be mistaken for neuroblasts. (H and E stain, ×160)

Such tumors are difficult to distinguish from neurofibroma or neurolemoma. Small cystic areas of degeneration, hemorrhage and calcification may occur, but are much less extensive than in neuroblastoma.[9]

TUMORS THAT MAY RESEMBLE NEUROBLASTOMAS HISTOLOGICALLY

Several childhood tumors, by virtue of their embryonal nature, may resemble neuroblastoma and must be distinguished by careful histological study correlated with clinical behavior and tests for biological activity.

Lymphosarcoma   May occur in many of the same locations as neuroblastomas—in the neck, mediastinum, and retroperitoneal space. Lymphosarcoma cells may resemble the primitive neuroblasts of a highly undifferentiated neuroblastoma. Diagnostic difficulties may arise, especially when one must differentiate neuroblastoma without excretion of catecholamines from lymphosarcoma.

Burkitt's tumor   May occur in some of the same locations as neuroblastoma—for example, in the submandibular area or in the abdomen. As in lymphosarcoma, histological differentiation from neuroblastoma may occasionally be difficult. The urinary catecholamine determination in such cases is crucial in differential diagnosis.

Acute leukemia   May present with an abdominal mass (splenomegaly), fever, and bone pain, which may mimic the clinical picture of neuroblastoma. Leukemic cells in the bone marrow smears, if they are present in clusters, may resemble the bone marrow appearance of disseminated neuroblastoma. The same applies to tumor deposits in the skin.

Embryonal rhabdomyosarcoma   May occur in many of the same locations as neuroblastomas—in the neck, mediastinum, and retroperitoneum. Embryonal rhabdomyosarcoma, when made up of small round cells, may mimic the histological picture of neuroblastoma. Determination of urinary catecholamines is an important aid in differential diagnosis.

Ewing's tumor   Neuroblastoma with metastasis to bone may present x-ray findings closely resembling those of a primary bone tumor. When one finds isolated bony lesions by x-ray examination in small children, careful search for an abdominal tumor, especially

178

one retroperitoneal in origin, should be performed. Urinary catecholamines should be determined. Histological and radiographic appearance of Ewing's tumor and neuroblastoma with metastasis to bone may be quite similar. The distinction between the two tumors often must be made by clinical and biochemical studies of the patient.

Sometimes in clinical practice the differential diagnosis cannot be established with certainty between a catecholamine-negative neuroblastoma and a lymphosarcoma, Burkitt's tumor, embryonal rhabdomyosarcoma, or Ewing's tumor. Problems in histological diagnosis may arise especially in biopsy material such as a lymph node, liver, bone marrow, or a skin nodule, and tissue from the primary tumor itself is not available for direct examination. In such situations histological examination and the usual biochemical and clinical studies may not be able to produce an unequivocal diagnosis. Occasionally, study of the tumor by growth in tissue culture may provide the diagnosis.

SUMMARY

Virchow first described the histological appearance of a neuroblastoma in 1864, but the complex embryological and histogenetic origin of these tumors was not understood until about 50 years later. Neuroblastomas originate from primitive anlage in the sympathetic nervous system. The embryological origin of sympathetic ganglia and, thus, of neuroblastomas, is from the neural crest. The primary cells of origin are the sympathogonia and sympathoblasts.

Neuroblastoma, ganglioneuroblastoma, and ganglioneuroma constitute a histological spectrum. Neuroblastomas are composed of small, round or polyhedral cells, with scant cytoplasm and a central, densely chromatic nucleus. However, the histological appearance may be quite variable due to cellular maturation. Rosette formation is a sign of differentiation. Ganglioneuroblastomas contain greater evidence of maturation, with areas resembling ganglioneuroma. The degree of relative histological maturity is slightly correlated with the prognosis. Ganglioneuromas are completely differentiated benign neoplasms.

Other malignant tumors may resemble neuroblastoma and may be difficult to distinguish from neuroblastoma by histological study alone.

REFERENCES

1. Virchow, R.: Hyperplasie der Zirbel und der Nebennieren. In *Die krankhaften Geschwülste* (Vol. 2). Berlin: A Hirschwald, 1864–1865.

2. Morgan, J.J.: *Trans. Path. Soc. Lond.* 30: 399, 1879. Cited by Willis, R.A.: *Pathology of Tumors* (Ed. 4). New York: Appleton-Century-Crofts, 1967, pp. 857–885.

3. Dalton, N.: Infiltrating growth in liver and suprarenal capsule. *Trans. Path. Soc.* 36: 247, 1884.

4. Marchand, F.: Beiträge zur Kenntnis der normalen und pathologischen Anatomie der Glandula carotica und der Nebennieren. *Virchows Arch.* 5: 578, 1891.

5. Wright, J.H.: Neurocytoma or neuroblastoma, a kind of tumor not generally recognized. *J. Exper. Med.* 12: 556–561, 1910.

6. Griff, L., and Griff, R.: Neuroblastoma; emphasis on the mediastinal neuroblastoma. *Amer. J. Roentgenol.* 103: 19–24, 1968.

7. Herxheimer, G.: Über Tumoren des Nebennierenmarkes, Insbesondere das Neuroblastoma sympathicum. *Beitr. Pathol. Anat.* 57: 112, 1914.

8. Murray, M.R., and Stout, A.P.: Distinctive characteristics of the sympathicoblastoma cultivated *in vitro;* a method for prompt diagnosis. *Amer. J. Pathol.* 23: 429–441, 1947.

9. Stowens, D.: *Pediatric Pathology.* Baltimore: Williams and Wilkins Company, 1966, pp. 412–419.

10. Hollinshead, W.H.: *Textbook of Anatomy.* New York: Hoeber Medical Books, 1967, pp. 57–65.

11. Arey, L.B.: *Developmental Anatomy.* Philadelphia: W.B. Saunders Company, 1965, pp. 454–460, 513–519.

12. Hoffman, S., and Green, G.: Neuroblastoma with metastases to the mandible; report of a case. *J. Oral Surg.* 24: 75–81, 1966.

13. Benson, C., Mustard, W., Ravitch, M., et al. (Eds.): *Pediatric Surgery.* (Vol. II). Chicago: Year Book Medical Publishers, 1962, pp. 874–885.

14. Bolande, R.P.: The neurocristopathies; a unifying concept of disease arising in neural crest maldevelopment. *Hum. Path.* 5: 409–429, 1974.

15. Adams, L.: Neuroblastoma; review of literature and report of 18 cases. *North Carolina Med. J.* 27: 113–125, 1966.

16. Willis, R.: *Pathology of Tumours of Children.* Springfield, Ill.: Charles C Thomas, 1962, pp. 7–16.

17. Williams, T., and Donaldson, M.: Neuroblastoma. (Sutow, W., Vietti, T., and Fernbach, D., Eds.): In *Clinical Pediatric Oncology*. St. Louis: C.V. Mosby Company, 1973, pp. 384–387.

18. Kissane, J., and Smith, M.: *Pathology of Infancy and Childhood*. St. Louis: C.V. Mosby Company, 1967, pp. 706–713.

19. Abell, M.R., Hart, W.R., and Olson, J.R.: Tumors of the peripheral nervous system. *Human Pathol.* 1: 503–551, 1970.

20. Harkin, J.C., and Reed, R.J.: Tumors of the peripheral nervous system. *Atlas of Tumor Pathology*. Second series. fasc. 3. Washington, D.C.: Armed Forces Institute of Pathology, 1969, pp. 137–149.

21. Ackerman, L.V., and Rosai, J.: *Surgical Pathology* (5th Ed.). St. Louis: C.V. Mosby Company, 1974, pp. 597–599, 1959.

22. Marsden, H., and Steward, J.: *Tumours in Children*. New York: Springer-Verlag, 1968, pp. 131–137.

23. Willis, R.A.: *Pathology of Tumours* (Ed. 4). New York: Appleton-Century-Crofts, 1967, pp. 857–885.

24. Mäkinen, J.: Microscopic patterns as a guide to prognosis of neuroblastoma in childhood. *Cancer* 29: 1637–1646, 1972.

25. Beckwith, J.B., and Martin, R.F.: Observations on the histopathology of neuroblastomas. *J. Pediatr. Surg.* 3: 106–110, 1968.

26. Gitlow, S.E., Dziedzic, L.B., Strauss, L., et al.: Biochemical and histological determinants in the prognosis of neuroblastoma. *Cancer* 32: 898–905, 1973.

27. Misugi, K., Misugi, N., and Newton, W.A.: Fine structural study of neuroblastoma, ganglioneuroblastoma, and pheochromocytoma. *Arch. Pathol.* 86: 160–170, 1968.

7 Biology of the Neuroblastoma Cell

Carl Pochedly, M.D.

1. Nerve growth factor
   a. Generalities
   b. Role of NGF in pathogenesis
   c. Role of anti-NGF in pathogenesis
   d. Clinical studies of NGF levels
   e. Use of NGF in treatment
2. In vitro behavior of neuroblastoma cells
   a. Cultivation of human neuroblastoma cells
   b. Cultivation of mouse neuroblastoma cells
      (1) Inducing maturation
3. In vivo studies on implanted mouse neuroblastoma cells
4. Chromosomal abnormalities
   a. Clinical studies
   b. Double-minute chromosomes

The biology of neuroblastoma cells is as fascinating and paradoxical as the manifestations of clinically overt tumors. Intensive studies on neuroblastoma cells in vitro have been mainly motivated by efforts to explain the high rate of spontaneous regression of these tumors, especially among those cases occurring in the first year of life. Knowledge of in vitro behavior of neuroblastoma is fragmentary and its clinical relevance is often uncertain. For convenience, the biology of neuroblastoma cells will be discussed under four headings: nerve growth factor, in vitro behavior, in vivo studies, and chromosomal abnormalities.

NERVE GROWTH FACTOR

Burdman and Goldstein in 1964 investigated the relationship of the nerve growth factor to the behavior of neuroblastomas in vivo and in vitro.[1] It had previously been reported that the transplantable mouse sarcoma 180, if implanted into chick embryos, caused an enormous increase in the growth of nerve fibers in the chick embryo.[2] By tissue culture experiments it was shown that this growth of nerve fibers was caused by a diffusible substance secreted by the sarcoma 180. This substance, the nerve growth factor (NGF), appeared to be a protein and affected only nerve cells which had migrated away from the central nervous system—namely, those in sensory or sympathetic ganglia.

In trying to purify NGF, Cohen used snake venom and found, to his surprise, that this had the same effect as NGF. Reasoning that snake venom is merely modified saliva, he tested an extract of mouse submandibular glands and found that this was, by far, the richest source of NGF.[3] NGF has an effect on the sympathetic cells of many animals including man, but, by immunological methods, it has been shown that there are some species differences.

NGF is difficult to isolate from the sera of most normal animals because it is present in very low concentration. Although some children with neuroblastomas have increased amounts of NGF in their serum, significant amounts of this material cannot be detected in the tumor tissue.[1] NGF was also found in the serum of a child with fibrosarcoma and in a child with retinoblastoma but was absent from the sera of other children with tumors. In spite of the fact that neuroblastomas and sarcomas are derived from different embryonic tissues, increased amounts of nerve growth factor may be found in the sera of children with both types of tumors.

NGF is detected by its effect on cultures of 7- to 11-day chick embryo sensory ganglia which, after 24 hours incubation in the presence of NGF, became surrounded by a dense halo of nerve fibers (Figure 1).[4] An antiserum to NGF has been prepared by injecting purified preparations of NGF with Freund's adjuvant into rabbits, horses, goats, or calves. This antiserum when injected into newborn mice or rats destroys virtually all of the sympathetic nervous system, but the animals so treated thrive normally.[5]

The antibody obtained by inoculating goats with mouse NGF has no effect on cultures of human neuroblastomas; this might be due to species differences.[1] It is not known why the serum of some children with neuroblastoma have more NGF activity than that of normal children. It is unlikely that the tumor itself produces NGF since there is no growth stimulation of chick sensory ganglia even if they are cultured directly with neuroblastoma tissue. Possible explanations are

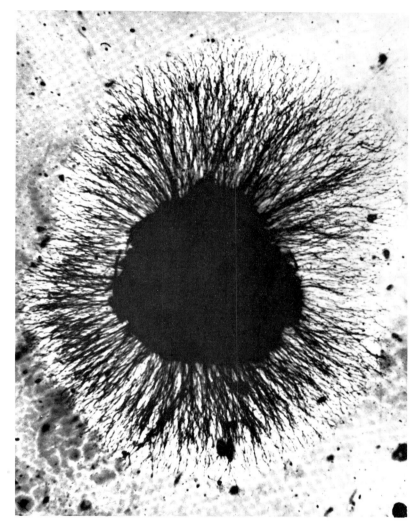

Figure 1. Stimulation of 8-day chick-embryo sensory ganglion with nerve growth factor showing a dense halo of axons. Fixed and stained with the Bodian technique. (Courtesy of Dr. J.A. Burdman and the *Journal of the National Cancer Institute*[1])

that children with neuroblastomas have an inborn error of metabolism manifesting itself by a high NGF level, or there may be a feed-back mechanism from the tumor, stimulating NGF production.[6]

Role of NGF in Pathogenesis of Neuroblastoma

It has been repeatedly suggested that neuroblastoma cells are able to mature in vivo and that the clinical course of the tumor correlates with its degree of maturation. Goldstein[7] demonstrated that neuroblastoma cells will undergo complete maturation if transferred from their host to an in vitro environment. This strongly suggested that it is the internal environment of the host, rather than intrinsic properties of neuroblastoma cells, which supports the persistence or the growth of the tumor. Thus, it is fluctuations in the host environment which are at the base of corresponding fluctuations in the morphology and the clinical manifestations of the tumor.

The simplest of possible factors in the internal environment of the host that could support growth of neuroblastomas would be a chemical agent, produced by the host and affecting the growth and/or the differentiation of the tumor cells. NGF might conceivably have such an effect on neuroblastoma cells. It affects growth and differentiation of cells which, like the neuroblastoma cells, are neural crest derivatives; it can be produced outside the responsive tissue and, furthermore, can undergo structural changes which affect quantitatively and possibly qualitatively its biological activity. However, before NGF can be accepted for such a role in the pathogenesis of neuroblastoma, evidence must be obtained to show that (a) children with neuroblastoma have NGF abnormalities, whether qualitative or quantitative or both; (b) variations of these abnormalities are paralleled by changes in the tumor; and (c) the survival, growth, or maturation of neuroblastoma cells are affected by normal or abnormal NGF.[8]

The first two conditions are necessary but not sufficient. Evidence that they are met was suggested by Burdman and Goldstein,[1] but their findings could not be confirmed. NGF activity is higher in sera of some neuroblastoma patients than in normal sera and may increase with the size of the tumor. These findings suggest an involvement, but not necessarily a role, of NGF in the pathogenesis of the tumor. For example, the neoplasm and the abnormal levels of NGF may both be caused and controlled by the same primary defect in the host without either one affecting the other. Alternatively, the NGF abnormality may be a consequence, rather than a controlling factor of the tumor, as suggested by the reported involvement of other tumors in the production of NGF. Whether the tumor itself produces NGF or induces its synthesis in other cells of the host or interferes with its normal disposal remains an important question for the understanding of NGF but not necessarily for understanding of the growth of neuroblastomas. However, such an etiological relationship between mouse NGF and growth of neuroblastomas would not exist if the NGF found in children with neuroblastomas differed not only from the mouse NGF but from normal human NGF as well.[8]

Thus, the crucial point is whether any effects can be demonstrated on neuroblastoma cells by NGF, or a substance related to it, or the lack of it. The finding that antiserum to mouse NGF did not inhibit growth or produce degeneration in neuroblastoma cultures does not exclude the requirement by the tumor cells for forms of NGF different from the one used as antigen. Also both NGF and antisera should be tested for possible effects on the maturation rather than the growth or survival of the cells. Finally, sera from neuroblastoma patients should be checked for their ability to favor or hinder maturation in vitro and tested for chemical constituents related to NGF.[8]

Nerve growth factor is essential for the development and survival of sympathetic nerve cells. In culture, normal embryonic chick and fetal human neurons also require NGF for survival. These cells die in the presence of anti-NGF serum. In contrast, neuroblastoma cells are not stimulated by NGF and are not adversely affected by its antiserum.[9]

Role of Anti-NGF Serum in Pathogenesis of Neuroblastomas

Antiserum to mouse NGF can selectively destroy immature sympathetic nerve cells in newborn mice and in newborn of other species. When antiserum is prepared in adult rabbits, it also destroys sympathetic nerve cells in these animals but not as completely as in newborn animals.[1] Antiserum prepared against mouse NGF neutralizes NGF in the sera of children with neuroblastomas.

Neuroblastoma cells explanted in vitro are morphologically similar to immature neuroblastomas and behave in tissue culture as normal nerve cells. Many of these cells mature during long-term culture in vitro and can apparently mature in vivo. On this basis, one would have predicted that immature neuroblastoma cells would be destroyed by an antiserum prepared against mouse NGF.[1] But when antiserum prepared against mouse NGF was added to cultures of human neuroblastoma, no inhibition of growth or destruction of neuroblastoma cells resulted. On the other hand, the same antiserum prevented the outgrowth of fibers and resulted in the destruction of chicken sensory ganglia and normal human sensory and sympathetic ganglia transplanted in vitro. That malignant cells were not killed is indicative of one important difference between normal sympathetic ganglion cells of the human fetus and neuroblastoma cells.[1]

Clinical Studies of Nerve Growth Factor Levels

Studies of serum levels of NGF have been carried out in children in various stages of neuroblastoma. These include cured patients and patients under treatment for active disease. Control studies have been done on the sera of normal children and on children with other malignancies.[10]

A study for nerve growth factor in the serum of children with neuroblastoma who showed prolonged survival was done. Twenty-two determinations were done on 12 children, and the values for NGF levels were compared against the sera of normal children. About 33 percent of the levels in the cured patients were in an unusually high range, as compared to only 6 percent of the normals.[10] Studies before operation of 11 infants and children with other tumors showed that the levels of NGF in the serum in 8 of these were either normal or undetectable.[10]

At present it appears unlikely that NGF is causally related to growth or regression of neuroblastomas:

1. Few children with neuroblastomas have NGF abnormalities
2. Survival, growth, and maturation of neuroblastoma cells appear to be unaffected by either NGF or anti-NGF
3. It is conceptually difficult to reconcile the fact that neuroblastomas arise as a single tumor while NGF is a systemically circulating growth stimulant
4. There is absence of hyperplasia of autonomic ganglia in cases of neuroblastoma
5. There is absence of hyperplasia of the adrenal medulla adjacent to in situ neuroblastomas.

If NGF caused growth of a neuroblastoma, it would seem more likely that something more akin to malignant neurofibromatosis would occur than activation of a single focus in the body.

Even if NGF is not important in the original genesis of the tumor, it could still play a very important role in determining the growth or maturation of the already established tumor. There are cases, particularly in young infants, of multicentric neuroblastoma that might have NGF as a pathogenetic or an etiologic factor. In the peculiar syndrome of multiple subcutaneous neuroblastomas in young infants (Figure 2), there are coexistent multicentric visceral tumors in sites where primaries are expected, such as in the mediastinum, adrenals, or pelvis. It is possible that these tumors may represent multifocal primary neuroblastomas. It would at least seem likely that a systemic stimulant might be the cause of tumors in this specific situation.[10]

However, in another series, Waghe found that none of 621 control sera or the sera from 7 children with neuroblastoma elicited a maximal response, although low levels of NGF were detected in most cases.[5] Despite the small number of patients investigated, the close correlation between their serum NGF activity and that of a much larger series of controls suggests that there is no significant abnormality in the NGF activity of children with neuroblastoma. These findings are at variance with those of Burdman and Goldstein.[1] But the series

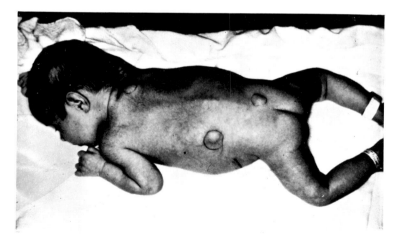

Figure 2 An eight-week-old infant with subcutaneous metastases due to neuroblastoma of the right adrenal gland. Following partial excision of the primary tumor, the child was given radiotherapy and chemotherapy with vincristine and cyclophosphamide. On follow-up six months later, the child was thriving and showed no evidence of tumor. (Courtesy of Dr. B.S. Reddy and *Consultant*)

of Waghe and associates, being much larger, may be more representative.

The main object of Waghe's study was to explore the possibility of a relationship between the NGF/anti-NGF system and the factors which initiate and determine the progress of neuroblastoma. Many children's tumors should probably be regarded not merely as groups of disorganized cells, but as manifestations of inborn abnormalities involving the whole patient and sometimes also his family. If a neuroblastoma were initiated by an inborn metabolic error involving NGF, it might be reflected in abnormal NGF activity in the serum. The observation that the NGF activity of the sera of 7 children with neuroblastoma was normal is evidence against a disturbance of NGF metabolism being the cause or the result of these tumors.[5] Thus, examination of sera from 621 normal individuals and 7 children with neuroblastoma failed to provide evidence that children with neuroblastoma had abnormally high levels of NGF activity.[5]

Use of NGF in the Treatment of Neuroblastoma

Nerve growth factor and its antibody have profound effects on sympathetic tissue. It seemed, therefore, that there might be a number of ways in which these substances could affect neuroblastomas. The possibilities were: (1) NGF might cause a neuroblastoma to mature; (2) anti-NGF might destroy a neuroblastoma just as it destroys non-neoplastic sympathetic tissue in newborn animals; and (3) if NGF and anti-NGF attached themselves to a neuroblastoma, they might be used as vehicles for cytotoxic or radioactive drugs.[11]

Both in vivo (chick embryo) and in vitro NGF cause changes in cultured sympathetic cells, including increases in neurite formation and increases in cell size, which could be interpreted as maturation. It is quite common to see groups of ganglion cells in a neuroblastoma, and sometimes a child dying from metastatic neuroblastoma is found to have a primary tumor which has completely matured into a ganglioneuroma. It appears that in such cases, maturation followed the growth of the tumor; but, unfortunately, it only rarely proceeds fast enough to catch up with the spread of the disease.[11]

It seemed possible that the administration of NGF to children with widespread neuroblastoma might accelerate maturation and thus retard or even stop the growth of the tumor. Therefore, it was decided to treat three children with disseminated neuroblastoma with intramuscular injections of NGF.[11] The injections of NGF caused a marked rise in the serum levels of NGF, but the malignant course of the neuroblastomas was unaffected. Failure to influence the clinical course or the histological appearance of the tumor by injecting sufficient amounts of NGF to cause an obvious rise in serum levels suggests that when cells of the sympathetic nervous system become neuroblastomas they cease to be affected by NGF.

No cytotoxic effect on anti-NGF on the neuroblastoma could be detected in tissue culture and no fluorescent anti-NGF could be attached to the cells. Thus, it appeared that this tumor was resistant to the antibody. Accordingly, it seems unlikely that the effect of the patients' age on the prognosis of this tumor could be due to any variations in the NGF/anti-NGF system.

It could not be demonstrated, with fluorescent anti-NGF serum, that the antibody attaches itself to neuroblastoma tissue and no effect of either NGF or anti-NGF on neuroblastoma cells could be shown in tissue culture.[11]

So far it has not been possible to demonstrate that the NGF/anti-NGF system has any relevance to the neuroblastoma. But this failure may be due to the fact that so little is known about the chemistry and biology of these substances.[11] It is possible that the particular NGF which stimulates growth of neuroblastomas is chemically and antigenically different from both normal human NGF and mouse salivary NGF. If this were true, then the clinical studies done so far would be invalid. We are left with the conclusion that the present data are tantalizing but not conclusive.

BEHAVIOR OF NEUROBLASTOMA CELLS IN VITRO

The discovery that the neuroblastoma has a very characteristic growth pattern in vitro opened up a new field of research which may well lead to a considerable increase in the knowledge of the factors governing the clinical behavior of this tumor.

Cultivation of Human Neuroblastoma Cells

The study in vitro of the growth characteristics of neuroblastoma cells reported in 1947 by Murray and Stout demonstrated that tissue culture could be used for diagnosis of this tumor.[12] Axons begin to grow out from cultures of neuroblastoma within 24 hours after these cells are explanted in vitro. The axons resemble those seen after the

190

stimulation of axon outgrowth in embryonic spinal and sympathetic ganglion cells by nerve growth factor. Use of tissue culture for diagnosis of neuroblastoma declined when urinary catecholamine assays became commonly used. But interest in in vitro cultivation of neuroblastoma was revived following reports of maturation of neuroblastoma cells during prolonged cultivation in tissue culture.

Murray and Stout,[12] using a plasma clot technique, observed long branching processes growing out from the tumor cells (Figure 3). These processes are quite unlike the shorter processes which may arise from fibroblasts and there seems little doubt that they correspond to nerve fibers. Grant and Pulvertaft described the cultural characteristics when the tumor was grown directly on glass.[13] Goldstein and Pinkel, in 1957, cultured fragments of neuroblastomas obtained from bone marrow aspirates and made the exciting observation that some of the neuroblasts matured into ganglion cells during prolonged cultivation in tissue culture.[14]

From these preliminary observations on a few samples, it appeared that some neuroblastoma cells were capable of undergoing differentiation and maturation during culture in vitro. A more detailed study of additional samples of neuroblastoma tissue was then under-

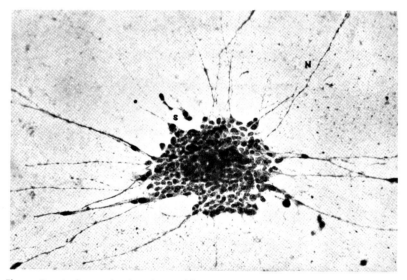

Figure 3. A clump of cultured neuroblastoma cells showing very long beaded neurites (N), after seven days growth on clotted plasma. (Courtesy of M.R. Murray and the *American Journal of Pathology*[12])

taken. Neuroblastoma cells were obtained from 13 young children and cultured in vitro for periods of one week to over a year.[7] Culture in vitro of the neuroblastoma cells resulted in differentiation and development into more mature neural elements within five months. The morphologic evidence for maturation of the neuroblastoma cells included an increase in nuclear size, development of a single large nucleolus, accumulation of Nissl ribonucleic acid substance, the formation of neurofibrils, and hypertrophy of axons (Figure 4). Explantation of a more mature-appearing neuroblastoma resulted in the rigid transformation of all the nerve cells into mature ganglion cells within 20 days. These results demonstrated that immature neuroblastoma cells obtained from young children can differentiate and mature during long-term tissue culture. These in vitro studies suggest that neuroblastoma may be the result of a biochemical defect of the host which would prevent maturation of a tumor population whose progeny have the potentialities to differentiate and mature.[7]

The growth, differentiation and maturation potentialities of neu-

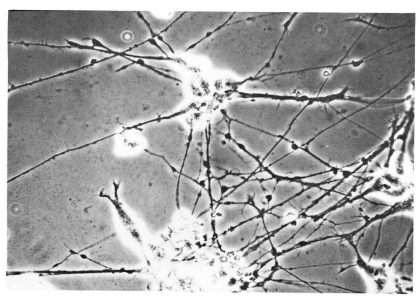

Figure 4. Clump of human neuroblastoma cells (NJB) showing outgrowth of axon fibers. These are living cells growing on glass photographed with positive phase contrast optics. The cells have been stimulated to develop long beaded neurites with mouse nerve growth factor. Some of the neurites have developed many fine spines and collateral fibers. The light areas represent aggregates of tumor cells. The cell body of one tumor cell with two large nucleoli is located in the lower right corner. (Courtesy of Dr. M.N. Goldstein)

roblastomas in plasma clot cultures were described. To facilitate further study, tumor suspensions consisting of small clumps and isolated cells from 11 children were explanted on the surface of collagen coated cover slips or directly on the surface of plastic petri dishes. The neuroblastoma cells did not spread out or migrate extensively on the surface of the collagen or plastic but formed dense aggregates. Beaded axons began to grow out 24 to 72 hours after explantation, and on continued culture the axons formed very dense intertwining networks. In those cultures containing the most immature neuroblasts, the cells on the periphery of the aggregates flattened out.[7]

Human neuroblastomas have been established as continuously multiplying cell lines (Table 1); one of these, NJB, has been in culture for many years. Electron microscope studies show that the cells of this line contain dense disorganized arrays of neurotubules in the cytoplasm which organize into parallel array in the axons. These axons are similar in morphology to those of sympathetic nerve cells. They contain dense core granules, one of the storage sites of catecholamines in adrenergic neurons. The cells of line NJB have lost their ability to store exogenous catecholamines, a property of the normal sympathetic nerve cells and of some neuroblastoma cells. NJB cells continue to multiply, differentiate, and retain the characteristic morphology of immature neuroblasts. These studies suggest that cells can be selected from immature neuroblastomas which continue to multiply and differentiate but which are unable to mature.[9]

Continuous cell lines, SK-N-SH and SK-N-MC, were established in cell culture from human metastatic neuroblastoma tissue and maintained in vitro for one to two years.[15] SK-N-SH comprises two morphologically distinctive cell types, a small spiny cell and a large epithelioid cell. SK-N-MC is composed of small fibroblast-like cells with scant cytoplasm. In monolayer culture, both cell lines form disoriented growth patterns and reach high saturation densities. Population-doubling times were 32 to 44 hours. Inoculation of 10^7

Table 1
Tissue Culture Lines of Neuroblastoma Cells

A. Human
1. NJB[1]
2. SK-N-SH[15]
3. SK-N-MC[15]
B. Murine
1. C-1300[23]

cells of both cell lines produced tumors confirmed by histopathological examination in 30 to 40 percent of cases in cheek pouches of cortisonized Syrian hamsters. SK-N-SH cells are characterized by high dopamine-β-hydroxylase activity while SK-N-MC cells have no detectable activity. However, for SK-N-MC, but not SK-N-SH, the presence of intracellular catecholamine was indicated by formaldehyde-induced fluorescence. The lines are near-diploid with several chromosomal markers; SK-N-MC cells contain double-minute chromosomes. Growth, biochemical, and cytogenetic properties confirmed that the lines comprise malignant cells of neurogenic origin.[15]

The development of successful methods of culturing human neuroblastoma cells over long durations permits the luxury of time to explore a variety of biological phenomena. Preliminary study of their cytogenetic, biochemical, and tumorigenic properties indicates that such cells retain many of their original characteristics over repeated transfers in cell culture and further supports their use as a tumor model system.[15]

The potential usefulness in cancer research of continuous cell lines established in vitro from human tumors is widely accepted. However, there are various practical requirements for their development. A fundamental one is that of providing adequate conditions for cell survival and proliferation. Another is the identification of the cultured cells as being truly derived from the diagnosed cancer.[15]

Neuroblastoma metastases have been found on bone marrow examination in as many as 50 percent of children at the time of diagnosis. Variations in cytologic characteristics of these metastases render categorical diagnosis difficult, and corroboration with other clinical data such as urinary catecholamines and, when successful, tissue culture of bone marrow aspirates is often necessary. The demonstration of biogenic amines in suspect cells found in bone marrow aspirates is an additional if not pathognomonic sign of neuroblastoma.[16] The histochemical technique for cellular localization of catecholamines and 5-hydroxytryptamine was used for visualizing catecholamine-containing cells in bone marrow smears of patients with metastatic neuroblastoma, and in neuroblastoma cells in culture derived from a metastatic site.[16]

The histofluorescence method can be used in patients with neuroblastoma to corroborate the diagnosis in those cases where the conventional stain techniques or tissue culture methods fail to differentiate it from other round cell tumors. It appears that the larger the percentage of fluorescent cells, the more nearly stationary the population of the tumor cells. Conversely, when significant discrepancies between histochemical and histofluorescent methods arise, the tumor cell population is in a rapid growth phase.[16]

Cultivation of Mouse Neuroblastoma Cells

C-1300 murine neuroblastoma arose as a spontaneous tumor of the spinal cord which has been transplanted into strain A/J mice for over 30 years. Morphologic observations indicate that culture conditions stimulate the maturation of neoplastic immature neuroblasts. Thus, the cultivated cells retain the ability of neuronal differentiation and of generating action potentials after electrical stimulation. The transplanted tumor, and the tumor cells maintained in vitro, contain choline acetylase, acetylcholinesterase and enzymes for the biosynthesis of catecholamines. Thus, this transplanted mouse tumor (C-1300) is believed to be a neuroblastoma. It has been established in tissue culture where it undergoes differentiation. The cells are able to synthesize catecholamines, as shown by the high levels of enzymes involved in their biosynthetic processes and by the conversion of tyrosine into dopamine and norephinephrine.

The high radiosensitivity of undifferentiated human neuroblastoma is well known, but the nature of the cellular changes induced by irradiation is uncertain. At present it is still uncertain whether human neuroblastoma cells are (1) destroyed by ionizing radiation or (2) are induced to differentiate or "mature" into ganglioneuroma by ionizing radiation. Experimental evidence to support the hypothesis of radiation-induced differentiation (maturation) is lacking. The availability of mouse neuroblastoma cell culture provides an opportunity to study the nature of cellular alterations produced by ionizing radiation.

Prasad showed that X-irradiation induced morphological differentiation of neuroblastoma cells which in the presence of serum undergo morphological maturation.[18] X-irradiation of mouse neuroblastoma cell culture induced axon formation as well as enlargement of cellular and nuclear size. A similar change in cellular morphology is known to occur during development of the mammalian nervous system. Morphological maturation was evident as early as 24 hours after irradiation, and by the third day most differentiated cells had matured morphologically. In the control cell population only a few of the differentiated cells matured morphologically. Did maturation of the cells result from cellular changes produced by x-irradiation or from some "factor" in the serum?[18]

6-Hydroxydopamine produces a selective destruction of sympathetic cells in newborn and young animals. Since the neuroblastoma cells are of sympathetic origin, the effect of 6-hydroxydopamine on the growth of neuroblastoma cell populations in vitro was investigated. Dopamine, and to a much greater extent 6-hydroxydopamine, reduced the growth of the mouse neuroblastoma cell population in vitro but did not induce morphological differentiation. The growth inhibition at a lower drug concentration was primarily due to inhibition of cell multiplication, which was reversible. L-Dopa, norepinephrine, epinephrine, 3,4-dihydroxyphenylacetic acid, or homovanillic acid at a similar concentration did not affect the growth of the neuroblastoma cell population in vitro.[18] The action of 6-hydroxydopamine was also explored by injecting it into mice bearing transplants of C-1300 neuroblastoma.[19] Marked tumor regression was noticeable in all cases in the first week of treatment. Histological examination performed at the end of this period showed large areas of necrosis and cell degeneration throughout the neoplastic tissue. A decrease in the effectiveness of the treatment became apparent in subsequent days, however, as the tumor increased in size.[19]

The mouse neuroblastoma provides a system for examining some neural functions and their regulation in tissue culture. Cells from this tumor express a number of differentiated neural functions in vitro. They contain enzymes, such as acetylcholinesterase, choline acetylase, catechol-O-methyltransferase and tyrosine hydroxylase, and they can generate action potentials. During active growth, in the presence of serum, the cells are mostly round and highly refractile. When serum is removed from the medium, the cells of certain clones become flatter and extend "neurites," and the specific activity of acetylcholinesterase is greatly increased.

During a study on the effects of various drugs on the expression of differentiated functions by neuroblastoma cells, it was observed that the solvent used, dimethylsulfoxide, was a potent inhibitor of neurite extension. Dimethylsulfoxide reversibly inhibits extension of neurites in mouse neuroblastoma cells in vitro at levels which do not significantly retard growth. This inhibition occurs when neurites are induced to extend either by removal of serum or by addition of dibutyryl-cyclic AMP to complete medium. Inhibition is reversed with time, however, even in the continued presence of dimethylsulfoxide in serum-free medium. At similar concentrations of dimethylsulfoxide in serum-free medium, induction of acetylcholinesterase activity is not inhibited.[20]

Inducing maturation of mouse neuroblastoma cells in vitro X-ray, dibutyryl-cyclic AMP, prostaglandin El, and inhibitors of phosphodiesterase induce morphologic differentiation in mouse neuroblastoma cells in tissue culture. This morphologic differentiation is shown by the formation of axon-like processes, and morphologic maturation, as revealed by an increase in the size of cell-body and nucleus.[21] In addition, acetylcholinesterase activity in the x-ray and dibutyryl cyclic AMP-treated cells markedly increases. Tyrosine hydroxylase is a rate-limiting enzyme in the biosynthesis of catecholamines and is present in human neuroblastoma. In patients with neuroblastoma tumors, there is generally an increased production of catecholamines in these tumors and the elevated urine-levels of dopamine and dopamine metabolites are of diagnostic value. A marked increase in tyrosine hydroxylase is demonstrated with dibutyryl-cyclic AMP-induced differentiated cells. However, additional studies with other agents indicate that the increase in tyrosine hydroxylase activity in neuroblastoma cells is not inextricably linked to morphologic changes which are presumed to reflect cellular differentiation.[21]

Dibutyryl-cyclic AMP-induced morphological differentiation of mouse neuroblastoma cells in culture requires the synthesis of new protein but not synthesis of new RNA. An appreciable increase in RNA synthesis, a slight increase in protein synthesis and a marked decrease in DNA synthesis occurs in the dibutyryl-cyclic AMP-induced differentiated cells. Tyrosine hydroxylase activity, which is barely detectable in the control neuroblastoma culture, markedly increases after treatment with dibutryryl-cyclic AMP. Sodium butyrate, which inhibits cell division without causing morphological differentiation, also increases tyrosine hydroxylase activity, but to a lesser degree.[21] X-irradiation produces inhibition of cell division and morphological differentiation similar to that observed with dibutryryl-cyclic AMP, but the tyrosine hydroxylase activity does not increase. The irradiated cells, nevertheless, retain the potential to manifest increased tyrosine hydroxylase levels upon subsequent exposure to either dibutyryl-cyclic AMP or sodium butyrate.[21]

Dopamine-β-hydroxylase is found in normal animals only in adrenal glands and in adrenergic neurons. It catalyzes the hydroxylation of dopamine to norepinephrine in the only physiologically significant pathway for the formation of this neurotransmitter. Dopamine-β-hydroxylase activity is present in mouse neuroblastoma C-1300 tumors. The activity is proportional to the weight of the tumor. Serum activity is markedly increased in mice that bear the tumors. Treatment of mice with 5-bromodeoxyuridine causes marked inhibition of tumor growth and decrease of dopamine-β-hydroxylase activity in the serum. The histochemical studies reveal that 1 to 5 percent of the cells in mouse C-1300 neuroblastoma tumors contain catecholamines and that catecholamine-containing processes terminate mainly around blood vessels of the tumor. Dopamine-β-hydroxylase is present in clonal neuroblastoma cell lines. The cell line with the greater tendency to form axon-like processes has a higher activity of this enzyme.[22]

IN VIVO STUDIES OF NEUROBLASTOMA CELLS IN MICE

The slow progress in the treatment of neuroblastomas may be attributed, in part, to the lack of a reliable animal preparation. It has been previously noted that the C-1300 murine neuroblastoma cell line differentiates into sympathetic neuron-like cells when exposed to drugs which suppress cell cycling in vitro. These biochemical and morphological investigations leave no doubt that the C-1300 line is a true neural tumor.[23]

Recently, an experimental model for studying treatment of mouse neuroblastoma was described.[23] Adult A/J mice were inoculated in the right thigh intramuscularly with one million C-1300 murine neuroblastoma cells. A palpable tumor developed in 8 to 10 days; median survival time was 22 days.[23] Radiation fractionation studies showed a dose-dependent increase in survival time. Results of radiation therapy without fractionation suggest that therapy should be started within two days postoperatively. Combination of radiation therapy and cytosine arabinoside was not significantly better than radiation therapy alone with respect to survival time, but median tumor appearance time was somewhat delayed. The results here indicate that the most effective means of delaying lethal tumor growth was radiotherapy delivered soon after inoculation. Delaying this treatment for more than two days led to a reduction in its effectiveness. These results suggest that metastases occur early in this system, as is true in human neuroblastoma. Thus, this study suggests that the murine neuroblastoma preparation may be a useful screening technique to test therapy active against human neuroblastoma and may assist in the design of optimal surgical adjuvants for this disease.

CHROMOSOMAL ABNORMALITIES IN NEUROBLASTOMA

The two predominant theories of carcinogenesis are the somatic mutation theory and the viral theory. Studies searching for common ground between these two theories have been carried out by analyzing what effects viruses have on chromosomes of the cell. Studies both in vivo and in vitro with tumor viruses and non-tumor viruses have revealed that viruses are capable of producing at least three types of change involving chromosomal material: (1) the single break; (2) a severe fragmentation of chromosome material, termed chromosome pulverization; and (3) changes in chromosome number produced by spindle abnormalities and multinucleated syncytia.[24,25,26]

The single chromosome break is felt to be the defect most likely to have mutagenic potential. This defect has been studied more extensively than the others, including attempts at elucidating the mechanism of the formation of single breaks by viruses. At the present time it would appear that there can be multiple mechanisms for induction of breaks by various agents.[25]

The induction of chromosome breaks by viruses provides a common denominator for the three classes of agents that are capable of producing cancer. X-ray and chemicals have been known to produce breaks for some time, and now viruses may be added to these two. It is felt that if the chromosome breaks are significant in the etiology of cancer, it is as an indicator system for subvisible mutations. Most cells that exhibited visible defects in the chromosomes would probably go on to die. However, these visible breaks may be indicators for subvisible mutagenic activity, similar to the way that X-ray-induced breaks indicate subvisible mutations.[25]

Cytogenetic investigation of children with cancer has not been generally rewarding. Exceptions are chronic granulocytic leukemia (Ph[1] chromosome) and neuroblastoma, where specific chromosomal changes have been found. The search for clues to the pathogenesis of human cancer through the chromosome constitution of cells has yielded a wealth of information, which is as interesting as it is perplexing. Nevertheless, in certain areas, the cytogenetic findings in human cancer have been of help in the differential diagnosis of a malignant from a benign condition (e.g., cervical cancer vs. dysplasia), in the prediction of leukemic relapse, and in the interpretation of the karyotypic changes as they relate to the causation of human neoplasia.[27]

Chromosome studies were performed on three neuroblastoma patients who had bone marrow replacement by tumor cells. They had either hyperdiploid or hypotetraploid cell lines as well as the normal diploid cell line. Either one, two, or three marker chromosomes were found in each line. Five other cases from the published data showed no more than 48 chromosomes in cells obtained from tumor tissue or effusions, and one patient had two marker chromosomes. The incidence of aneuploidy in all eight patients was 75 percent. No unique chromosomal abnormalities were associated with these cases.[28] The finding of consistent markers in these three cases suggests that although each tumor cell population has an altered genotype they are all derived from a single cell. The natural selection of certain variants probably accounts for the biological success of these tumors.[28]

Double-Minute Chromosomes

A unique and new cytogenetic finding has been seen primarily in neuroblastoma and other embryonic tumors—namely, the appearance of double-minute chromatid bodies that appear in the chromosome complement.[15,29] (Figure 5) The significance of these double-minute bodies is not known, but the fact that they occur predominantly in embryonic type tumors and that this observation is unique in cytogenetics makes it extremely interesting.

The origin of the double-minute chromosomes is uncertain. Most of these tumors have been of neurogenic origin.[27] In malignant cells, chromosomes and mitoses characteristically vary, in striking contrast to chromosomes and mitoses of normal tissues. Chromosomes in

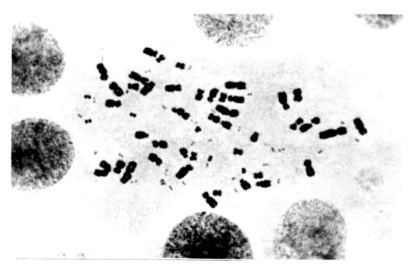

Figure 5. Metaphase preparation of cultured human neuroblastoma cells showing numerous double-minute chromosomes. (Courtesy of Dr. J.L. Biedler and Cancer Research[15])

most tumors undergo periods during which they deviate in a variety of ways from normal chromosome structure and behavior, while chromosomes in normal cells, in their natural environment, almost never deviate. When normal cells are exposed to abnormal environments, however, chromosomal variation may become frequent, and every chromosomal abnormality seen in malignant cells has also been observed in normal cells. This is probably true, too, of the remarkable phenomenon of the double-minute chromosomes, even though their cytogenetic status is not quite clear.[30] The persistence of these minute chromosomes through many mitoses indicates that they are provided with functional centromeres, even though these elude direct observation. Their whimsical behavior at anaphase and the frequent precocious separation of their chromatids show that their centromeres are less efficient than those of the normal chromosomes.[30]

Cytogenetic studies were performed on 21 children with neuroblastoma. Increased numbers of abnormal metaphases were observed in pretreatment samples of peripheral blood and bone marrow. Three bone marrows infiltrated with extrinsic cells had heteroploid cell lines with conistent marker chromosomes. Long-term survivors without evidence of active disease had chromosomal abnormalities in peripheral blood lymphocytes.[31] These findings evoke questions concerning prognosis, tumor formation, and long-term effects of radiotherapy.

SUMMARY

1. The biology of neuroblastoma cells is as fascinating and paradoxical as are the manifestations of the clinically overt tumors. Knowledge of the in vitro behavior of neuroblastoma cells is fragmentary and its clinical relevance is uncertain.

2. Nerve growth factor is elevated in the serum of some children with neuroblastoma. However, NGF is not produced by neuroblastoma cells in culture and injection of NGF into children with disseminated neuroblastomas has no effect on the malignant course of the tumor. At present, it appears unlikely that NGF or anti-NGF are causally related to growth or regression of neuroblastomas.

3. Neuroblastoma cells are capable of undergoing differentiation and maturation in vitro, especially during long-term tissue culture. Human neuroblastoma cells have been established as continuous multiplying cell lines which have been extensively studied from

the point of view of growth, biochemistry, and cytogenetics. The C-1300 mouse neuroblastoma has been also extensively studied in vitro. The various factors and stimuli that induce maturation in these cells have been reviewed.

4. In vivo, C-1300 mouse neuroblastoma cells have been studied following implantation into mice. This has been used as an experimental model for studying treatment of mouse neuroblastoma.

5. Neuroblastoma cells, both in vivo and in vitro, have shown various chromosomal abnormalities. These include multiple chromosomal breaks, aneuploidy, and double-minute chromatid bodies.

REFERENCES

1. Burdman, J., and Goldstein, M.: Long-term tissue culture of neuroblastomas. III. In vitro studies of a nerve growth-stimulating factor in sera of children with neuroblastoma. *J. Nat. Cancer Inst.* 33: 123–127, 1964.

2. Bueker, E.D.: Hypertrophy of spinal ganglion cells in chick embryos after the substitution of mouse sarcoma 180 for the hind limb periphery. *Anat. Rec.* 100: 735, 1948.

3. Cohen, S.: Nerve growth factor in mouse salivary glands. *Proc. Nat. Acad. Sci.* 46: 302, 1960.

4. Seibert, E., and Bill, A.: The chick assay test for nerve growth factor in human serum. *J. Pediatr. Surg.* 3: 170–171, 1968.

5. Waghe, M., Kumar, S., and Steward, J.K.: Nerve growth factor in human sera. *J. Pediatr. Surg.* 5: 14–17, 1970.

6. Marsden, H., and Steward, J. (Eds.): *Tumours in Children.* New York: Springer-Verlag, 1968, pp. 131–170.

7. Goldstein, M., Burdman, J., and Journey, L.: Long-term tissue culture of neuroblastomas. II. Morphologic evidence for differentiation and maturation. *J. Nat. Cancer Inst.* 32: 165–174, 1964.

8. Varon, S.: Possible involvement of nerve growth factors in neuroblastoma pathology. *J. Pediatr. Surg.* 3: 165–166, 1968.

9. Goldstein, M.: Neuroblastoma cells in tissue culture. *J. Pediatr. Surg.* 3: 166–169, 1968.

10. Bill, A.: A study of the nerve growth factor in serum of neuroblastoma patients. *J. Pediatr. Surg.* 3: 171–177, 1968.

11. Kumar, S., Steward, J.K., Waghe, M., et al.: the administration of nerve growth factor to children with widespread neuroblastoma. *J. Pediatr. Surg.* 5: 18–22, 1970.

12. Murray, M., and Stout, A.P.: Distinctive characteristics of

the sympathicoblastoma cultivated in vitro. *Amer. J. Path.* 23: 429–441, 1947.

13. Grant, H., and Pulvertaft, R.: Differential diagnosis of neuroblastoma and Burkitt's tumour. *Arch. Dis. Childh.* 41: 193–197, 1966.

14. Goldstein, M.N., and Pinkel, D.: Long-term tissue culture of neuroblastomas. *J. Nat. Cancer Inst.* 20: 675–689, 1958.

15. Biedler, J., Helson, L., and Spengler, B.: Morphology and growth, tumorgenicity, and cytogenetics of human neuroblastoma cells in continuous culture. *Cancer Res.* 33: 2643–2652, 1973.

16. Helson, L., and Biedler, J.: Catecholamines in neuroblastoma cells from human bone marrow, tissue culture and murine C-1300 tumor. *Cancer* 31: 1087–1091, 1973.

17. Prasad, K.: X-ray induced morphological differentiation of mouse neuroblastoma cells *in vitro*. *Nature* 234: 471–473, 1971.

18. Prasad, K.: Effect of dopamine and 6-hydroxydopamine on mouse neuroblastoma cells *in vitro*. *Cancer Res.* 31: 1457–1460, 1971.

19. Angeletti, P., and Levi-Montalcini, R.: Cytotoxic effect of 6-hydroxydopamine on neuroblastoma cells. *Cancer Res.* 30: 2863–2869, 1970.

20. Furmanski, P., and Lubin, M.: The effects of dimethylsulfoxide on expression of differentiated function in mouse neuroblastoma. *J. Nat. Cancer Inst.* 48: 1355–1361, 1972.

21. Prasad, K.N., Waymire, J., and Weiner, N.: A further study on the morphology and biochemistry of x-ray and dibutyryl cyclic AMP-induced differentiated neuroblastoma cells in culture. *Exper. Cell Res.* 74: 110–114, 1972.

22. Anagnoste, B., Freedman, L., Goldstein, M., et al.: Dopamine-β-hydroxylase activity in mouse neuroblastoma tumors and in cell cultures. *Proc. Nat. Acad. Sci. USA* 69: 1883–1886, 1972.

23. Arima, E., Byfield, J., Finklestein, J.Z., and Fonkalsrud, E.: An experimental model for the therapy of mouse neuroblastoma. *J. Pediatr. Surg.* 8: 757–763, 1973.

24. Brewster, D., and Garrett, J.V.: Chromosome abnormalities in neuroblastoma. *J. Clin. Path.* 18: 167–169, 1965.

25. Nichols, W.: Cytogenetic aspects of Neuroblastoma. *J. Pediatr. Surg.* 3: 143–145, 1968.

26. Mark, J.: Chromosomal characteristics of neurogenic tumors in children. *Acta Cytol.* 14: 510–518, 1970.

27. Sandberg, A.A., Sakurai, M., and Holdsworth, R.: Chro-

mosomes and causation of human cancer and leukemia. *Cancer* 29: 1671–1679, 1972.

28. Whang-Peng, J., and Bennett, J.: Cytogenetic studies in metastatic neuroblastoma. *Amer. J. Dis. Child.* 115: 703–708, 1968.

29. Cox, D., Yuncken, C., and Spriggs, A.I.: Minute chromatin bodies in malignant tumors of childhood. *Lancet* 2: 55–58, 1965.

30. Levan, A., Manolov, G., and Clifford, P.: Chromosomes of a human neuroblastoma; a new case with accessory minute chromosomes. *J. Nat. Cancer Inst.* 41: 1377–1386, 1968.

31. Wakonig-Voartaja, T., Helson, L., Baren, A., et al.: Cytogenetic observations in children with neuroblastoma. *Pediatrics* 47: 839–843, 1971.

8 Immunology of Neuroblastoma

Giora M. Mavligit, M.D.
Jordan U. Gutterman, M.D.
Evan M. Hersh, M.D.

Introduction
1. Cell-mediated immune mechanisms in neuroblastoma
2. Humoral immune mechanisms in neuroblastoma
3. Clinical parameters signifying immune activity in perspective with cell-mediated and humoral immune factors
4. Prospects of immunotherapy in neuroblastoma
Summary and Conclusions
Bibliography

The mystery surrounding growth and regression of neuroblastomas has received a great deal of attention in recent years. Unfortunately, most of the reports in the medical literature fail to make a clear distinction between immunological facts and speculations, nor do they emphasize the gap between laboratory research and studies at the clinical level. Admittedly, among the multiple components of host-tumor interactions some clinical observations can justifiably be translated into immunological parameters, but other clinical observations should be further investigated with detailed dissection of the multiple factors involved before conclusions are drawn.

Because of its bizarre clinical behavior, neuroblastoma has become a target for scientific discussion of human tumor development and host-tumor relationship of immune or non-immune nature. Neuroblastomas are also considered a model for discussion of other factors—anatomical, embryonic, and genetic—influencing the biological behavior of human tumors.

205

This review is intended to critically orient the laboratory and clinical information available in neuroblastoma. An attempt is made to view in perspective the rapidly accumulating information on tumor immunology in cancer patients and the successful initial attempts at immunotherapy of human cancer.

CELL-MEDIATED IMMUNE MECHANISMS IN NEUROBLASTOMA

It has now become widely accepted that the cellular machinery of natural defense against neoplasia consists of lymphocytes and macrophages. A growing body of evidence suggests that cellular mechanisms play a major role in the immunosurveillance of cancer.[1] The role of humoral factors will be discussed later. Owing to the pioneering work by the Hellstroms, a new dimension was given to the understanding of the immunobiological behavior of neuroblastoma in terms of host-tumor relationship.[2] These investigators have developed an in vitro assay directed to test the cytostatic or cytotoxic ability of patients' lymphocytes against neuroblastoma target cells in tissue culture (Chapter 10, Figure 5). Their exciting findings demonstrated not only a specific reactivity of patients' lymphocytes compared to controls, but also cross-reactivity between patients with neuroblastoma.[2] In other words, lymphocytes from one individual not only exerted a cytostatic or cytotoxic activity against his own tumor cells but also against neuroblastoma cells of other individuals. These observations suggest the presence of a common neuroblastoma-associated antigen shared by most tumors of this type.

If observations made in experimental animal tumors can be translated into human cancer, then the observation made by the Hellstroms makes a good case for a viral etiology in neuroblastoma. This is because oncogenic viruses invariably induce tumors which share common antigens, even regardless of their histology. Further support for environmental factors, with epidemiological repercussions, came from another important observation on mothers of children with neuroblastoma. Some of these mothers also have circulating lymphocytes capable of inhibiting the proliferation of tumor cells from their children as well as from other children with neuroblastoma.[2] Some fathers and siblings also showed similar reactions.

No difference in lymphocyte reactivity against tumor cells was found between children who became tumor-free after surgical resection, with or without ancillary radiotherapy or chemotherapy, and children whose tumor continued to progress despite such treatments.

This observation was somewhat disappointing since one would anticipate that, if cellular immune mechanisms play an important role in the control of neuroblastoma, a better prognosis should be associated with a more vigorous lymphocyte reactivity. As will be seen later, further studies of interference by humoral factors with cellular mechanisms provided an explanation for this conceptual "inconsistency." The findings of the Hellstroms have now been confirmed by a British group of investigators using similar techniques.[3] On the other hand, immunochemical studies by a French group using soluble extracts from neuroblastoma tissues failed to show the presence of tumor-associated antigens.[4]

The lack of difference between lymphocytes from tumor-bearing and from tumor-free individuals was also noted in the study of other human tumors by the microcytotoxicity assay.[5] The absence of reports using other assays of cell-mediated immunity in neuroblastoma does not permit a final conclusion. It is quite possible, however, that by using other assays such as leukocyte or macrophage migration inhibition, lymphocyte blastogenesis and skin reactions to different sources of neuroblastoma antigens (whole cells, "membranes," or 3M KCL extracts), more information would be accumulated. This information may better correlate lymphocyte-tumor cell interactions with clinical course and prognosis in these patients as it did in other human tumors.[6-8] In the absence of any single assay which can reliably reflect all the immunological parameters of host-tumor relationship, a multifaceted approach to the immunological evaluation of neuroblastoma patients should be advantageous.[9]

A different aspect of cellular immune mechanisms in neuroblastoma was emphasized by the histological demonstration of lymphocyte and plasma cell infiltration among neuroblastoma cells in tumor specimens. These studies were prompted by previous pathologic examinations of other tumors such as carcinoma of the breast.[10] In particular, in the medullary type of breast carcinoma, the presence of histiocytic or lymphoid infiltration was correlated with improved prognosis and prolonged survival; this lymphoid infiltrate was, therefore, interpreted as a sign of immune activity by the host.[11] The first such study in neuroblastoma demonstrated lymphocyte infiltration particularly in relatively well-differentiated ganglioneuroblastomas.[12] Therefore, although correlation was noted between the presence of lymphoid infiltration and survival of the patients, the relationship to the degree of differentiation of the tumor could not permit a clear distinction between the effect of each of the factors alone on the prognosis.

In a more quantitative study of lymphocyte infiltration, a positive correlation was found between the intensity of lymphocyte infiltration in the primary tumor and duration of survival of patients.[13] No difference in lymphocyte infiltration was found between infants and older children, and the presence or absence of metastases at the time of primary surgery bore no relationship to the lymphocyte infiltration in the primary tumor. It was, therefore, suggested that lymphoid infiltration in neuroblastoma may be an important factor in the control of the growth in the primary tumor, but not necessarily in preventing metastases. The mechanism by which those infiltrated lymphocytes control the growth of the primary tumor is totally unclear. Evidence from melanoma and colon carcinoma suggests that lymphocyte populations residing within those tumors are apparently anergic and do not show any sign of cytotoxicity against cultured tumor cells.[14]

The number of circulating lymphocytes in the peripheral blood at the time of diagnosis was also correlated with survival. Thus, in infants under one year of age, higher lymphocyte counts were associated with longer survival.[15]

HUMORAL IMMUNE MECHANISMS IN NEUROBLASTOMA

Antitumor Antibodies

Until recently the study of humoral immune mechanisms in human cancer was based solely on the demonstration of antitumor antibodies. The first demonstration of such antibodies relied on membrane immunofluorescence techniques in Burkitt's lymphoma and melanoma.[16,17] With the development of the colony inhibition assay by the Hellstroms,[2] it also became possible to search for cytostatic or cytotoxic humoral factors in sera from cancer patients in general and neuroblastoma patients in particular. As in the case of cytotoxic lymphocytes, a study of sera from children with neuroblastoma and their mothers revealed the presence of complement-dependent circulating antibodies with cytotoxic activity against neuroblastoma target cells.[18] The presence of cytotoxic antibodies was equally distributed between tumor-bearing patients and patients who have apparently been cured of their disease. The role of cytotoxic antibodies in the control of neuroblastoma has not been ascertained since only a small number of patients have been studied. The finding of cytotoxic antibodies in three patients who have been freed of their tumor is quite intriguing and possibly indicates an immune mechanism which may be responsible for preventing metastases.

Lewis, in his recent studies of malignant melanoma, showed the presence of complement-dependent cytotoxic antibodies in patients with early or localized disease.[19] Sequential testing of sera from individual patients not only showed disappearance of the antibodies as the disease progressed, but also that the disappearance of the antibodies preceded the appearance of metastatic tumor by several months.[20,21] This observation led to the suggestion that cytotoxic circulating antibodies may be involved in delaying or preventing blood-borne metastases. Further studies will be necessary to prove this point in neuroblastoma.

Blocking Factors

Another category of humoral factors received a great deal of attention and is currently under intensive investigation. These factors, widely known as "blocking" factors, are not necessarily antibodies. In fact, most recent evidence suggests that they are either circulating tumor antigen-antibody complexes[22] or even circulating free antigen.[23,24] Their role in the host immune response against tumor in vivo is debatable, but the evidence from in vitro studies strongly correlates with clinical parameters.[25]

In essence, "blocking" serum factors were found to interfere specifically with the cell-mediated immune mechanisms discussed above. This interference is apparently exerted at two levels: First, there may be blocking at the level of tumor target cells, where antigen-antibody complexes interact with components on the surface of the tumor cells and prevent an immune attack to be exerted by the effector lymphocytes. Second, there may be blocking at the level of the effector lymphocytes, where circulating tumor antigen apparently interacts with receptors on the surface of the lymphocytes and renders them less cytotoxic. Regardless of the active mechanisms, the end result is the same: cell-mediated immune attack against tumor cells is blocked. At the clinical level such occurrence may explain why tumors continue to grow in spite of the presence of cytotoxic lymphocytes.

Blocking serum factors in neuroblastoma could be demonstrated only in patients with progressively growing tumors. They could not be detected in tumor-free individuals or in mothers of children with neuroblastoma.[2] "Unblocking" serum factors capable of cancelling the blocking effect exerted by blocking factors were found in sera from some cancer patients who have been cured of melanoma, breast cancer, and colon carcinoma.[26] The presence of unblocking factors in sera from patients cured of neuroblastoma has not yet been reported. It is quite possible, although unproven, that serum from mothers of children with neuroblastoma may contain unblocking factors similar to the anti-melanoma unblocking factors found in sera of North American blacks.[27]

It is noteworthy that immunochemical studies by the French group failed to demonstrate either circulating neuroblastoma antigen or antibodies directed against neuroblastoma antigen in sera from their patients.[4] On the other hand, carcinoembryonic antigen (CEA) levels were found to be elevated in sera from children with active neuroblastoma. CEA levels returned to normal following successful treatment.[28] The significance of elevated CEA levels has been recently criticized in the light of its nonspecificity.[29]

CLINICAL PARAMETERS SIGNIFYING IMMUNE ACTIVITY IN PERSPECTIVE WITH CELL-MEDIATED AND HUMORAL IMMUNE FACTORS

Neuroblastoma is a tumor of childhood which appears most frequently during the first year of life. It arises from cells which originated from the neural crest and migrated during fetal life peripherally to sites of sympathetic ganglia and to the medulla of the adrenal gland. There is now evidence suggesting that neuroblastoma develops in utero and, therefore, represents a congenital embryonic malignancy.[30] The time when neuroblastoma becomes clinically apparent is a predominant prognostic factor.[31] The survival of children in whom neuroblastoma was diagnosed before one year of age is longer, and with a higher cure rate, than in children whose tumors were discovered at an older age.[32] The peak of mortality is around the fourth year of life.

Most striking, however, is spontaneous regression in neuroblastoma.[33] Spontaneous regression rarely occurs in human cancer, but is most frequent in neuroblastoma. This phenomenon is observed mostly in children whose tumors were diagnosed when the children were less than three months old. In most of the cases who showed spontaneous regression, the tumors simply disappeared. In some, there was evidence for maturation to ganglioneuroma. Even the presence of skeletal metastases, usually a grave prognostic sign, does not negate the occurrence of spontaneous regression.[34,35]

Neuroblastoma in situ is an incidental autopsy finding in infants dying of other causes before the age of three months; it occurs 40 times more often than clinically overt cases of neuroblastoma[35] (see Chapter 1). If the in situ form is either a precursor of fully developed neuroblastoma or perhaps even its abortive form, a large fraction of incipient tumors must undergo regression during the early neonatal period.

All these manifestations of vigorous host resistance against an embryonic tumor during early life have stimulated the emergence of a number of speculative immunological theories purported to explain the age-dependent cure rate in neuroblastoma. One such theory suggests that a neuroblastoma which becomes clinically manifest earlier is growing faster than the one which becomes clinically apparent later.[36] The fast-growing tumor may possess more distinct and immunologically recognizable antigens which permit a more vigorous immune response by the host with rejection of the tumor. Another theory is based on temporary differences in maturation between humoral and cell-mediated immune mechanisms in the fetus.[37] When tumor develops in the fetus, and tumor antigens are released, they sensitize both the fetal and maternal lymphocytes but only the mother can produce the antibody which may cross the placenta and form antigen-antibody complexes in the fetal circulation. These complexes may block fetal cell-mediated immune mechanisms and thus lead to further growth of the tumor. At birth, the level of maternal anti-tumor antibodies drops and blocking serum complexes may disappear, thus permitting containment and even regression of the tumor during the first few months of life. The persistence of maternal blocking factor after birth may result in neuroblastoma in situ. On the other hand, once the infant eventually becomes capable of producing significant levels of his own blocking factor, an immunological "suicide" is imminent.

PROSPECTS OF IMMUNOTHERAPY IN NEUROBLASTOMA

The principles and rules of an immunotherapeutic approach which should be applied to neuroblastoma do not seem to differ from those applicable in other human tumors. In the absence of any study of immunotherapy in neuroblastoma, any approach should be worthwhile and welcome (Table 1). However, the passive and adoptive forms of immunotherapy have, so far, been disappointing when applied to other solid tumors or leukemia.[38-41] This was either because of inefficacy or because of impracticality of the procedure. In contrast, active immunotherapy, either non-specific with immunoadjuvants such as BCG or *Corynebacterium parvum,* or specific, using tumor cells, seems rather attractive in neuroblastoma. Candidates for such therapy should have most if not all of their tumor removed prior to immunotherapy. Since cures have been observed even following incomplete resection, a case can be made for the use of adjuvant immunotherapy following surgery in neuroblastoma. The possible benefit from additional radiotherapy to the tumor bed can be offset by the general immunosuppressive effect of radiotherapy on the patient.[42] Therefore, it seems as if radiotherapy should better be saved for palliation in more advanced cases.

Since vigorous host resistance in the form of tumor regression has been noted even in the presence of bone metastases,[34,35] an immunotherapeutic approach may be justified and rational, even in the advanced stages of disseminated neuroblastoma. However, in view of the possibility of tumor growth enhancement,[43] and the well-known inefficacy of immunotherapy when given alone in the advanced state of cancer,[44] a combination of chemotherapy plus immunotherapy would be more logical. Preliminary experience with combination of chemotherapy and immunotherapy in patients with disseminated lung carcinoma, melanoma, and squamous carcinoma of the head and neck [45-47] suggests that good results might also be anticipated in metastatic neuroblastoma. Immunotherapy should be first tried in children with poor prognostic profile—that is, in children whose tumors arose in the adrenal gland and were diagnosed after one year of age. Close monitoring of the patient's immune status is mandatory during the administration of immunotherapy. Since neuroblastoma is a relatively rare tumor, collaboration between several institutions will be necessary to accumulate the information which will hopefully lead to an even higher cure rate in children afflicted with this disease.

Table 1
Classification of Immunotherapy

1. Passive—Administration of serum-containing antibodies directed against the tumor

2. Adoptive—Transfer of immunocompetent cells (transfusion of peripheral blood lymphocytes or bone marrow transplantation) or their subcellular fractions containing molecular information (transfer factor, immune RNA)

3. Active—a. Non-specific—administration of immunoadjuvants such as BCG or C. parvum
        b. Specific—vaccination with tumor cells or tumor antigens

SUMMARY AND CONCLUSIONS

Clinical and laboratory evidence now exists to indicate the presence of immunological parameters of host-tumor relationship in children with neuroblastoma. The demonstration of neuroblastoma-associated antigen and the immune responses against it forms the scientific basis for clinical trials of immunotherapy in this disease. Careful selections of suitable patients for this therapeutic approach, coupled with close monitoring of the immunological status *in vivo* and *in vitro,* would be mandatory at the outset. Immunotherapy should, therefore, be applied only in large medical centers where all these facilities are available. Wider use of this therapeutic modality by practicing physicians will have to wait for results yet to be generated.

REFERENCES

1. Mitchison, N.A.: Studies on the immunological response to foreign tumor transplants in the mouse. I. The role of the lymph node cells in conferring immunity by adoptive transfer. *J. Exper. Med.* 102: 157–177, 1955.

2. Hellstrom, I., Hellstrom, K.E., Bill, A.H., et al: Studies on cellular immunity to human neuroblastoma cells. *Int. J. Cancer* 6: 172–188, 1970.

3. Kumar, S., Taylor, G., Steward, J.K., et al: Cellular immunity in Wilms' tumor and neuroblastoma. *Int. J. Cancer* 10: 36–43, 1972.

4. Kohen, M., Buffe, D., and Burtin, P.: Étude comparative des antigènes présents dans les neuroblastomas et dans les surrénales adults et foetales. *Bull. Du Cancer* 57: 355–364, 1970.

5. Hellstrom, I., Hellstrom, K.E., Sjögren, H.O., and Warner, G.A.: Demonstration of cell-mediated immunity to human neoplasms of various histological types. *Int. J. Cancer* 7: 1–16, 1971.

6. Bull, D.M., Leibach, J.R., Williams, M.A., and Helms, R.A.: Immunity to colon cancer assessed by antigen-induced inhibition of mixed mononuclear cell migration. *Science* 181: 957–959, 1973.

7. Mavligit, G.M., Gutterman, J.U., McBride, C.M., and Hersh, E.M.: Cell-mediated immunity to human solid tumors; in vitro detection by lymphocyte blastogenic responses to cell-associated and solubilized tumor antigens. *Natl. Cancer Inst. Monogr.* 37: 167–176, 1973.

8. Bluming, A.Z., Ziegler, J.L., Fass, L., and Herberman, R.B.: Delayed cutaneous sensitivity reactions to autologous Burkitt lymphoma protein extracts. *Clin. Exper. Immunol.* 9: 713–719, 1971.

9. Mavligit, G.M., Abmus, U., Gutterman, J.U., et al: Antigens solubilized from human solid tumors; lymphocyte stimulation and cutaneous delayed hypersensitivity. *Nature* 243: 188–190, 1973.

10. Black, M.M., Opler, S., and Speer, F.: Survival in breast cancer cases in relation to the structure of the primary tumor and regional lymph nodes. *Surg. Gynec. Obstet.* 100: 543–551, 1955.

11. Bloom, H.J.G., Richardson, W.W., and Field, J.R.: Host resistance and survival in carcinoma of breast: A study of 104 cases of medullary carcinoma in a series of 1,411 cases of breast cancer followed for 20 years. *Brit. Med. J.* 3: 181–188, 1970.

12. Martin, R.F., and Beckwith, J.B.: Lymphoid infiltrates in neuroblastomas; their occurrence and prognostic significance. *J. Pediatr. Sur.* 3: 161–164, 1968.

13. Lauder, I., and Aherne, W.: The significance of lymphocyte infiltration in neuroblastoma. *Brit. J. Cancer* 26: 321–330, 1972.

14. Nind, A.P.P., Nairn, R.C., Rolland, J.M., et al: Lymphocyte anergy in patients with carcinoma. *Brit. J. Cancer* 28: 108–117, 1973.

15. Bill, A.H., and Morgan, A.: Evidence for immune reactions to neuroblastoma and future possibilities for investigation. *J. Pediatr. Sur.* 5: 111–116, 1970.

16. Klein, G., Clifford, P., Klein, E., and Stjernsward, J.: Search for tumor specific immune reactions in Burkitt's lymphoma patients by the membrane immunofluorescence reaction. *Proc. Nat. Acad. Sci.* (Washington, D.C.) 55: 1628–1634, 1966.

17. Morton, D.L., Malmgren, R., Holmes, E., and Ketchem, A.S.: Demonstration of antibodies against human malignant melanoma by immunofluorescence. *Surgery* 64: 233–240, 1968.

18. Hellstrom, I., Hellstrom, K.E., Pierce, G.E., and Bill, A.H.: Demonstration of cell-bound and humoral immunity against neuroblastoma cells. *Proc. Natl. Acad. Sci.* 60: 1231–1238, 1968.

19. Lewis, M., Ikonopisov, R., Nairn, R., et al: Tumor-specific antibodies in human malignant melanoma and their relationship to the extent of the disease. *Brit. Med. J.* 3: 547–552, 1969.

20. Lewis, M.G., Phillips, T., Cook, K., and Blake, J.: Possible explanation for loss of detectable antibody in patients with disseminated malignant melanoma. *Nature* 232: 52–54, 1971.

21. Lewis, M.G., McCloy, E., and Blake, J.: The significance of humoral antibodies in the localization of human malignant melanoma. *Brit. J. Surg.* 60: 443–446, 1973.

22. Sjögren, H.O., Hellstrom, I., Bansal, S., and Hellstrom, K.E.: Suggestive evidence that the "blocking antibodies" of tumor-bearing individuals may be antigen-antibody complexes. *Proc. Natl. Acad. Sci.* (Washington, D.C.), 68: 1372–1375, 1971.

23. Currie, G.A., and Basham, C.: Serum-mediated inhibition of the immunological reactions of the patient to his own tumor; a possible role for circulation antigen. *Brit. J. Cancer* 26: 427–438, 1972.

24. Baldwin, R.W., Embleton, M.J., and Price, M.R.: Inhibition of lymphocyte cytotoxicity for human colon carcinoma by treatment with solubilized tumor membrane fractions. *Int. J. Cancer* 12: 84–92, 1973.

25. Hellstrom, I., Sjögren, H.O., Warner, G., and Hellstrom, K.E.: Blocking of cell-mediated tumor immunity by sera from patients with growing neoplasms. *Int. J. Cancer* 7: 226–237, 1971.

26. Hellstrom, I., Hellstrom, K., Sjögren, H.O., and Warner, G.: Serum factors in tumor-free patients cancelling the blocking of cell-mediated tumor immunity. *Int. J. Cancer* 8: 185–191, 1971.

27. Hellstrom, I., Hellstrom, K.E., Sjögren, H.O., and Warner, G.A.: Destruction of cultivated melanoma cells by lymphocytes from healthy black (North American Negro) donors. *Int. J. Cancer* 11: 116–122, 1973.

28. Reynoso, G., Chu, T.M., and Holyoke, D.: Carcinoembryonic antigen in patients with different cancers. *J.A.M.A.* 220: 361–365, 1972.

29. Kraft, S.C.: Carcinoembryonic antigen revisited. *Ann. Intern. Med.* 78: 147, 1973.

30. Voute, P.A., Wadman, S.K., and Van Putten, W.J.: Congenital neuroblastoma; symptoms in the mother during pregnancy. *Clin. Pediatr.* 9: 206–207, 1970.

31. Sutow, W.W., Gehan, E.A., Heyn, R.M., et al: Comparison of survival curves, 1956 versus 1962, in children with Wilms' tumor and neuroblastoma; report of the Subcommittee on Childhood and Solid Tumors. *Pediatrics* 45: 800–811, 1970.

32. Koop, C.E.: Factors affecting survival in neuroblastoma. *J. Pediatr. Surg.* 3: 113–114, 1968.

33. Everson, T.C., and Cole, W.H.: *Spontaneous Regression of Cancer*. Philadelphia: W.B. Saunders Company, 1966.

34. Reilly, D., Nesbit, R.D., and Krivit, W.: Cure of three patients who had skeletal metastases in disseminated neuroblastoma. *Pediatrics* 41: 47–51, 1968.

35. Beckwith, J.B., and Perrin, E.V.: In situ neuroblastomas; a

contribution to the natural history of neural crest tumors. *Amer. J. Path.* 43: 1089–1104, 1963.

36. McAllister, L.: Conference on the biology of neuroblastoma. *J. Pediatr. Surg.* 3: 186, 1968.

37. Helson, L.: Regression of neuroblastoma. *Lancet* 1: 1075–1076, 1971.

38. Mathé, G.: Immunotherapy in leukemia experimental and clinical approaches. *Series Haemat.* 5: 66–86, 1972.

39. Thomas, E.D., Buckner, C.D., Rudolph, R.H., et al: Allogeneic marrow grafting for hematologic malignancy using HL-A matched donor-recipient pairs. *Blood* 38: 267, 1971.

40. Frenster, J., and Rogoway, W.M.: Clinical use of activated autologous lymphocytes for human cancer immunotherapy. (Cumley, R., and McKay, J., eds.) In *Oncology 1970.* Chicago: Yearbook Medical Publishers, 1970. (Abstracts) p. 327.

41. Brandes, L.J., Galton, D., and Wiltshaw, E.: New approach to immunotherapy of melanoma. *Lancet* 2: 293–295, 1971.

42. Jenkins, V.K., Olson, M.H., and Ellis, H.N.: In vitro methods of assessing lymphocyte transformation in patients undergoing radiotherapy for bronchogenic cancer. *Texas Rep. Biol. Med.* 31: 19–28, 1973.

43. Bansal, S.C., and Sjögren, H.O.: Effects of BCG on various facets of the immune response against polyoma tumors in rats. *Int. J. Cancer* 11: 162–171, 1973.

44. Mathé, G., Poullart, P., and Lapeyraque, F.: Active immunotherapy of L1210 leukemia applied after the graft of tumor cells. *Brit. J. Cancer* 23: 814–824, 1969.

45. Israel, L., and Halpern, B.: Le Corynebacterium parvum dans les cancers avancés. *Nouv. Presse Med.* 1: 19–23, 1972.

46. Gutterman, J.U., Mavligit, G., McBride, C., et al: Active immunotherapy (BCG) and chemoimmunotherapy (imidazole Carboxamide and BCG) for advanced malignant melanoma. In *Immunological Aspects of Neoplasia* (A collection of papers presented at the twenty-sixth annual Symposium on Fundamental Cancer Research, 1973). (In press)

47. Donaldson, R.D.: Methotrexate plus bacillus calmette-guerin (BCG) and Isoniazid in the treatment of cancer of the head and neck. *Amer. J. Surg.* 124: 527–534, 1972.

9 Ganglioneuroma

Carl Pochedly, M.D.

Introduction
1. Clinical manifestations
   a. Ganglioneuromas of the neck
   b. Ganglioneuromas of the chest
   c. Ganglioneuromas of the gastrointestinal tract
   d. Functionally active ganglioneuromas
   e. Ganglioneuromas of the CNS
2. Relation of ganglioneuromas to neurofibromas
3. X-ray findings
4. Histopathology
5. Treatment
   Summary

Ganglioneuromas usually appear later than neuroblastomas. They may be seen in children but quite often do not present until adolescence or adult life. Nearly all of these tumors arise from the adrenal glands or sympathetic nervous system.[1] Approximately one-third arise from thoracic and cervical sympathetic chains, one-third arise from the adrenals, and one-third arise from the abdominal and pelvic sympathetic chains, with which are included the main celiac and mesenteric ganglia.[1] There is no difference between the sexes in the incidence of ganglioneuroma.[2] Clinical presentation can be diverse: it can be neurological with radicular pain, paraplegia, motor disturbance, or Horner's syndrome. It can be constitutional with fever and weight loss. It can be neurovascular with vasomotor changes in an upper limb, or it can be an incidental finding on routine x-ray examination.[1]

Schweisguth reported 40 cases of intrathoracic neurogenic

tumors, 18 of which were ganglioneuromas.[3] Hamilton treated 17 children with ganglioneuromas, 13 of whom were followed up from 3 to 23 years.[4] During the same period of time 105 patients with neuroblastoma were cared for in the same clinic. Thus, the ratio of ganglioneuromas to neuroblastomas in this series was 1:6.

Ganglioneuromas are benign tumors of sympathetic ganglia. The great chain of sympathetic ganglia which extends from the base of the skull to the pelvis including the adrenal medulla, accounts for the origin of most of these tumors. Smaller sympathetic ganglia situated elsewhere occasionally give rise to such tumors. Ganglioneuroma is a histologically benign tumor composed of adult ganglion nerve cells and medullated or non-medullated nerve fibers. It is a rare tumor. Common sites of occurrence are the retroperitoneal region, the brain, and thorax. Although it grows slowly, it may attain very large dimensions and cause symptoms of pressure as it encroaches on neighboring structures. The proper treatment is surgical excision, which usually gives satisfactory results.[5]

The locations of tumors in 417 cases of ganglioneuroma are shown in Table 1. Ganglioneuromas do not often produce acute symptoms, except when they occur in the central nervous system.[6] Ganglioneuromas have been reported in the knee, eyelids, scalp, subcutaneous tissues, uterus, ovary, cervix, fallopian tube,[7] urinary bladder,[8] adrenal glands, appendix, mesentery, neck, nerve roots, cranial nerves, central nervous system, and sympathetic nervous system.[9] The common site of origin of these tumors is along the route of the great chain of ganglia extending from the base of the skull into the pelvis including the adrenal medulla, but with a few examples arising from ganglia in other locations.[2] The anatomical distribution of these tumors confirms the general impression that the commonest sources of origin are the great chains of sympathetic ganglia which extend from the base of the skull into the pelvis passing through the neck, posterior mediastinum, and the retroperitoneal regions including the adrenal medulla.[2]

Tumors composed of sympathetic ganglion cells and sheathed neurites with or without myelin have been well known for at least 104 years, since Loretz in 1870 described one which grew in the mediastinum. Numerous cases have been reported. Early attempts at complete removal of these deep-seated tumors produced much permanent disability and even mortality. These results indicated the advisability of incomplete surgery.[2] Ganglioneuromas are benign. There are no metastases, and death can rarely be attributed to the tumor itself. The lethal tumors are usually intracranial in location and are inexcisable. The patient may die of the mechanical side effects of pressure.[10]

Neuroblastoma is primarily a disease of early childhood. Approximately 70 percent of the cases occur in the first four years of life.

Table 1
Sites of Origin of 417 Cases of Ganglioneuroma.[16]

Location	Number (percent)
A. Head and Neck	
Orbit and Lids	4
Nasopharynx	1
Pharynx	2
Larynx	1
Tongue	1
Neck	34
Total	43 (10%)
B. Chest	
Mediastinum	181
Thoracic Wall	2
Cardiac Plexus	1
Total	184 (44%)
C. Abdomen	
Lumbar	59
Suprarenal	49
Mesentery	5
Peritoneum	1
Appendix	6
Intestines	3
Duodenum	1
Stomach	1
Kidney	1
Total	126 (30%)
D. Pelvis	
Posterior Pelvis	35
Ovary	6
Uterus	4
Testis	1
Spermatic Cord	1
Bladder	1
Total	48 (12%)
E. Miscellaneous	
Leg	2
Breast	1
Vulva	1
Skin	8
Generalized	3
Bone, Multiple Sites	1
Total	16 (4%)

On the other hand, ganglioneuroma is predominately a disease of adult life. Ganglioneuromas are rarely found in patients less than four years of age.[10] If the two tumors were merely different manifestations of the same disease, they should occur at various sites with the same frequency. Table 2 presents the actual percentages of occurrence of neuroblastoma and ganglioneuroma at specific sites. Although there is considerable overlapping, there are also differences in the values for the rate of occurrence at the commonest sites.[10] From the differences in anatomic characteristics, clinical behavior and the ages and sites at which the tumors occur, it is possible that the neuroblastoma and ganglioneuroma may be essentially different diseases of the same system, rather than different manifestations of the same disease.[10] This concept has been challenged by recent workers.[11,12] Thus, it is believed that ganglioneuromas and neuroblastomas are different manifestations of the same basic neoplasm of the sympathetic nervous system.

CLINICAL MANIFESTATIONS

Ganglioneuromas are usually recognized incidental to some other ailment or on a routine physical examination. Twelve patients in one series were asymptomatic and the tumor was found either on abdominal examination or on x-ray examination of the chest.[4] Five of these patients had symptoms related to the tumor, manifested respectively as diarrhea, chest pain, abdominal distention, ptosis, and an altered gait. Ganglioneuromas apparently are slow-growing tumors and often become quite large before detection. One tumor, a left posterior mediastinal mass observed in a 9-year-old girl, mea-

Table 2
Comparison of Primary Sites of Neuroblastoma and Ganglioneuroma (Percentages)[10]

Primary Site	Neuroblastoma	Ganglioneuroma
Adrenal	39 ⎫	30 ⎫
	⎬ 76	⎬ 48
Retroperitoneal	37 ⎭	18 ⎭
Mediastinum	12	38
Other	12	14
Total cases	105	109

sured 15 by 6 by 6 cm. Another ganglioneuroma which measured 20 by 40 cm and weighed 6 kg was removed from a 3½-year-old boy.[4] Ganglioneuromas are usually asymptomatic, but may give rise to signs and symptoms as a result of their interference with local function by means of the pressure caused by the expanding growth.

The development of post-neuroblastoma ganglioneuroma was described in five patients in one series. Attention is called to its importance as a disease entity and its insidious onset after many years of treatment.[13] The finding of post-neuroblastoma ganglioneuroma in these five patients again indicates that the ultimate fate of some neuroblastomas is formation of ganglioneuromas.[14] Ganglioneuromas were detected either at the sites of the primary neuroblastoma or at the sites of metastases.[13]

The clinical findings vary with the site, rate of growth, and size of the particular tumor mass. Ganglioneuromas themselves rarely produce any symptoms until they attain such size that they encroach upon neighboring structures. Small masses located in the pelvis, abdomen, or lumbar retroperitoneal area may grow for a number of years before symptoms are produced. Whereas, if growth occurs in the mediastinum or into the spinal canal, symptoms may result from relatively short growth periods.

In one case, symptoms were present from early childhood until operation at the age of 28 years. Pain in the right lower abdomen and back prevented the patient, as a child, from bearing her full weight on her right foot. However, no further symptoms were produced until the tumor growth became large enough to be palpable through the abdomen. In many instances discovery of the tumor occurs only at the time of active labor, when pelvic delivery becomes impossible because of obstruction of the vaginal outlet by the tumor mass.[9]

Ganglioneuromas are most frequently found within the thorax, in the posterior mediastinum, and chest wall. Extension of growth from the paravertebral area has been noted in a "collar-button" or "dumbbell" fashion between the intervertebral spaces and even within the spinal canal extradurally for moderate distances. It is important to note that 10 cases of ganglioneuroma in the lumbosacral area in infancy and childhood were subjectively asymptomatic. In eight cases abdominal swelling was the only objective symptom; in one, abdominal swelling had been present since birth.[9]

Tumors composed of adult ganglion cells are rare. They are usually located in the posterior aspect of the mediastinum or in the retroperitoneum. One patient was described who had a primary solitary cutaneous ganglioneuroma.[15] This patient was a one-year-old girl who developed a lesion in the skin of the right forearm. The lesion slowly increased in size and was removed when the girl was six years old. On removal, the lesion was circumscribed, partially encapsulated, and had the histopathological appearance of ganglioneuroma.[15]

Ganglioneuromas of the Neck

Bunn and King reviewed more than 400 cases of ganglioneuroma from the literature, 20 of which occurred in the cervical sympathetic chain.[16] The diagnosis is seldom made preoperatively, but suspicion of this possibility allows the surgeon to warn the patient that he may have Horner's syndrome as a postoperative sequela. This complication was noted in approximately one-half of the reported cases. Features suggestive of this tumor include a painless, slow-growing mass and respiratory distress or dysphagia.

A differentiated or mature ganglioneuroma is a benign tumor made up of sympathetic ganglion cells and sheathed nerve cells. Any of the cervical sympathetic ganglia of the neck may be involved by this tumor. It is found predominantly in adolescents, with a slight preponderance in females. It is uncommon. These tumors contain differentiated ganglion cells and neurites. The tumor is encapsulated; it does not infiltrate and does not metastasize. It may attain a large size, however, and, as the result of pressure, grow through one of the intervertebral foramina and continue to expand in the spinal canal.[17]

When these tumors originate in one of the sympathetic ganglia of the neck, Horner's syndrome is usually present. The patient has no specific symptomatology when the tumor is small, other than the awareness of the presence of this tumorous mass. As the tumor increases in size, pressure phenomena affecting the local area and other associated nerves may manifest itself in progressive difficulty in speaking, breathing, swallowing, or moving the head. The size of the tumors may be of such magnitude as to cause asphyxiation and starvation, and, if they have entered the spinal canal, paraplegia may develop.[17]

Many authors have emphasized the characteristic envelopment and displacement of adjacent vital structures by this neoplasm. Although total removal of the lesion is desirable, it should not be insisted upon at the expense of injury to vital nerves or vessels. This is of particular importance in resecting tumors that extend through intervertebral foramina into the spinal canal. Whenever this possibility exists, myelography and neurosurgical consultation are mandatory. Postoperative recurrence is rarely a problem in patients whose tumors were only partially excised. Thus, partial excision is preferred for relief of symptoms when complete excision might cause significant postoperative neurologic deficit.[16]

An example of a large ganglioneuroma of the superior cervical sympathetic ganglion is presented and its management discussed.[18] Emphasis is placed on the importance of preserving vital structures during dissection, leaving behind a small amount of tumor if necessary, since recurrence is unlikely. Another example of ganglioneuroma of the cervical spine illustrated that, although benign, a cervical ganglioneuroma may be very difficult to remove without damaging other vital structures.[19] In this case a combined posteroanterior approach to the tumor of the cervical spinal foramen was used.

Primary neoplasms of neurogenic origin arising in the lateral neck are uncommon but must be considered in the differential diagnosis of masses in this area.[20] Benign neurilemmomas, neurofibromas, and ganglioneuromas comprise the majority of these tumors and the prognosis in patients with these neoplasms is excellent. Neurogenic sarcomas are also frequently cured by local excision. Malignant neurilemmomas have a less favorable prognosis. Neuroblastomas are uncommonly seen in this area. Treatment of these tumors is essentially adequate local excision. When a nerve must be sacrificed and interruption results in permanent disability, a nerve graft, using a sensory nerve such as the great auricular, is a worthwhile procedure.[20]

Ganglioneuromas of the Mediastinum and Retroperitoneum

Ganglioneuromas occur more commonly in the mediastinum than anywhere else in the body. Scoliosis may be a late complication of ganglioneuromas in this site.[21,22] The tumors may be single or multiple.[23,24] Dumbbell ganglioneuromas of the mediastinum may cause paraplegia.[25] In a study of 40 cases of intrathoracic neurogenic tumors in children, there were 15 neuroblastomas, 7 ganglioneuroblastomas, and 18 ganglioneuromas.[3] Clinical symptoms and intratumoral calcifications were findings that favored a malignant diagnosis. Thoracic cage deformities appear related to tumor volume rather than to growth characteristics.[3] A case of ganglioneuroma arising from the 5th intercostal nerve presenting itself as a posterior mediastinal tumor treated by surgical excision was also reported.[26]

Ganglioneuromas are located most frequently in the posterior mediastinum; but they also occur in the paravertebral sympathetic ganglia and in the adrenal medulla. A case of presacral retroperitoneal ganglioneuroma was reported in a 4-year-old child.[9] Only 28 cases of lumbosacral retroperitoneal ganglioneuroma were reported in children under 16 years of age between 1870 and 1955. Thus, ganglioneuroma in the lumbosacral retroperitoneal area in infancy and childhood is relatively infrequent. However, differential diagnosis of abdominal masses in infancy and childhood should include ganglioneuroma.

In isolated reports, ganglioneuromas have been observed to occur in bone.[27] It is not known how a ganglioneuroma may originate in bone. The theoretical possibilities as to origin in that site are: (1) the tumors are primary in bone and of multicentric origin, and (2) a primary neuroblastoma metastasized to bone with maturation of the peripheral metastases. In cases of known neuroblastoma, metastatic tumors have been observed to transform into ganglioneuromas at sites of bony metastases.[28]

Retroperitoneal ganglioneuromas have been observed in dogs[29] and in rats.[30]

Ganglioneuroma of the Small and Large Intestine

Ganglioneuroma and ganglioneuromatosis are rare tumors in the gastrointestinal tract. A total of 29 cases have been reported. Sites involved are the stomach, duodenum, terminal ileum, cecum, ascending colon, appendix, transverse colon, and rectum.[31,32,33] In one case there was ganglioneuroma in the liver.[33]

Symptoms produced by the lesions depend partly on the site. Those in the more proximal parts—that is, the stomach and duodenum—caused upper abdominal discomfort or pain, sometimes related to meals, while those in the more distal parts gave rise to hemorrhage, constipation or diarrhea and in one instance acute appendicitis. The diarrhea is usually not severe, but may be intractable if the ganglioneuroma occurs in the adrenal medulla and secretes catecholamines.[34,35] There is evidently no special age incidence, though the reported examples are in adults rather than in children.[33] One case of polypoid ganglioneuromatosis of the large bowel occurred in a child.[36]

Gastrointestinal ganglioneuromas presumably originate in the plexuses of Meissner and Auerbach. Consequently, pain and hypermotility, which are among the most frequent symptoms, may be attributable to intraluminal mechanical stimulation of these polypoid ganglia with release of acetylcholine. The resultant sustained muscular contraction stimulates sympathetic sensory fibers which produce the pain.[37]

Functionally Active Intrathoracic or Abdominal Ganglioneuromas

Ganglioneuromas were considered to be non-functional until 1952 when Hawfield noted their association with chronic diarrhea, which ceased following surgery.[34] In 1957, Mason reported elevated urinary catecholamine excretion in a patient with neuroblastoma.[38] Since that time, many additional cases of neural crest tumors associated with diarrhea have been reported and reviewed.[35,39,40]

In one report 18 cases of diarrhea associated with neurogenic tumors were summarized. Of 78 children with a histologic diagnosis of ganglioneuroma or neuroblastoma at one hospital, 7 had diarrhea or hypertension as a major feature.[35] Hormonally active neurogenic tumors are usually thought to be malignant, but ganglioneuromas can also give adrenergic symptoms.[4] Of a series of 28 patients with adrenergic symptoms or with increased secretion of catecholamines or both, 14 had neuroblastoma, 8 had ganglioneuroblastoma and 6 had ganglioneuroma.[41] Hypertension was present in 15 patients, diarrhea in 12, profuse sweating in 8, palpitation in 5, pallor in 4, a rash in 3, paroxysmal attacks in 3, polyuria and polydipsia in 3, and flushing in 2.[41] Diarrhea and hypertension were both present in 3 patients. Hypertension was found in 10 patients with neuroblastoma, in 3 with ganglioneuroblastoma and in 1 with ganglioneuroma. Diarrhea was present in 6 patients with ganglioneuroma, 4 with ganglioneuroblastoma, and in 2 with neuroblastoma.[41]

The signs and symptoms associated with functioning neurogenic tumors are presumably caused by excessive production of norepinephrine and epinephrine. Hypertension, diarrhea, excessive sweating, flushing or pallor, rash, polyuria, and polydipsia are the characteristic findings associated with excess urinary excretion of catecholamines or VMA. The occurrence of Cushing's syndrome has been found in association with increased secretion of catecholamines in a few patients.[41] Considerable variation exists in the symptomatology of patients with these tumors, possibly because of variability in the predominant metabolite of the catecholamine secreted by the tumor.

Chronic diarrhea A few cases have been reported in which there was the occurrence of chronic diarrhea with abdominal distention and wasting (celiac-like syndrome) as the presenting symptoms in patients who had either a ganglioneuroma or a ganglioneuroblastoma. The diarrhea could not be attributed to other known causes and ceased immediately after surgical removal of the tumors.[42,43,44]

The mechanism of production of diarrhea is as yet unknown but it is suggested that these tumors secrete a substance which either stimulates peristalsis or alters absorption or excretion of water and/or electrolytes in the gut. The voluminous, liquid, alkaline stools in patients with neural crest tumors appear to result from rapid transit time and in massive losses of fluid and electrolytes from below the pylorus.[4] Why some but not all patients with secreting neural crest tumors develop diarrhea is not clear. Although the mechanism of the diarrhea is obscure, its prompt cessation after removal of the tumor strongly associates diarrhea with tumor. Factors such as hormone inactivation and end-organ sensitivity have yet to be evaluated. It is interesting that patients with pheochromocytomas secreting large amounts of norepinephrine do not characteristically have diarrhea.[35]

Although neuroblastomas are far more common than ganglioneuromas in children, a higher proportion of ganglioneuromas are associated with diarrhea and/or hypertension. While the reason for this is speculative, there is some evidence that the more malignant tumors have less capacity for catecholamine secretion.[35]

A functional ganglioneuroma *without* associated increased urinary VMA excretion, hypertension, fever, flushing or x-ray evidence was reported as a cause of diarrhea and failure to thrive in a four-year-old boy. The case indicated that unsuccessful efforts to determine the etiology of chronic diarrhea in children may not be complete without laparotomy.[40] Normal VMA excretion does not rule out the presence of a neurogenic tumor. Dilated colon, abnormal glucose tolerance curves, and hypokalemic acidosis are non-specific changes that may occur with any profuse, chronic diarrhea.

Ganglioneuromas in the Central Nervous System

Synonyms for ganglioneuromas in the CNS are gangliocytoma, ganglioglioma, true neuroma, glioneuroblastoma, neuroastrocytoma, ganglioma and Purkinjeoma. Ganglioneuromas may originate in the cerebral hemispheres, brain stem, pons, spinal cord, the cerebellum, and the sympathetic trunk.[45] The age of greatest incidence is in the first three decades and occurrence is rare. Intraspinal ganglion cell tumors with and without "dumbbell" extensions through intervertebral foramina are uncommon. (There are approximately 18 cases reported in the literature according to one survey.[46]) Some of the reported intraspinal ganglioneuromas may represent connective tissue tumors which have invaded the dorsal root ganglia and surrounded the normal ganglion cells.[46]

Since ganglioneuromas, other than temporal lobe lesions, are primarily meningeal, there are two possibilities as to histogenesis: (1) temporal lobe lesions arise as primary neuroblastomas and seed the pia arachnoid with subsequent maturation to ganglioneuroma or (2) the tumors represent multiple primary lesions of heterotopic neural crest origin contained within the sympathetic fibers accompanying vessels of the pia arachnoid. While the first possibility would appear to be the more likely, it does not explain the fact that the lesions which would have to be metastatic have a greater degree of collagenization, suggesting more maturation.[46]

RELATION OF GANGLIONEUROMA TO NEUROFIBROMATOSIS

Chatten and Voorhess, in their study of familial neuroblastoma, noted that a high incidence of café au lait spots was present in their reported kindred.[47] They suggested the possibility of a developmental relationship between neuroblastoma and neurofibromatosis (von Recklinghausen's disease). From subsequent studies of familial neuroblastoma, it was observed that regressive maturation of metastatic skin tumors to ganglioneuroma was followed by continued degeneration and loss of ganglion cells, so that the ganglion cells became inconspicuous.[12] At the same time, there was an increase in the neuroid connective tissue stroma of the tumors to the extent that metastatic tumors in the skin came to closely resemble neurofibromas. A striking similarity to neurofibromatosis was achieved in this kindred. Conversely, the presence of ganglion cells and/or ganglioneuromatous tissue within the neurofibromas of von Recklinghausen's disease has also been observed.[12]

The case of a child affected with neuroblastoma, ganglioneuroma and neurofibromatosis was reported. Germinal mutation is probably the cause of this coincidence. In view of the dominant inheritance of neurofibromatosis and of pheochromocytoma, the inference is made that neuroblastoma generally may be attributable to a dominant mutation which in the past has been lethal but which, as a result of the therapeutic progress, may be inherited by the offspring of survivors in the future, as has been noted for retinoblastoma.[11] This child had metastatic abdominal neuroblastoma diagnosed at five months of age. He was treated with vitamin B_{12}. Operation a year later revealed a ganglioneuroma and neurofibromas, but no neuroblastoma.

Fifty-six neurofibromas from 19 cases of neurofibromatosis were reviewed.[12] Six cases were found with ganglion cells or ganglioneuromatous elements present within neurofibromas. Seven cases of isolated ganglioneuromas were studied; the morphology of these tumors was critically compared with the neurofibromas and found to be quite similar. Ultrastructural similarities among ganglioneuroma, neurofibroma, and neuroblastoma maturing into ganglioneurofibroma are documented. Based on this experience and a review of the literature, it was theorized that neurofibromatosis may in some instances be derived from disseminated neuroblastoma or aberrantly migrating neural crest cells, particularly in the syndrome of congenital neuroblastomas with multiple regressing skin and visceral metastases.[12]

One case of neurofibromatosis had associated dumbbell ganglioneuroma of the cervical spine, which was surgically relieved by cervical spinal-cord compression. Of a series of 15 cases of dumbbell ganglioneuromas of the spine, only one was of the cervical spine. A previously reported case of ganglioneuromas of the cervical spine had associated neurofibromatosis. Only 6 cases of ganglioneuromas associated with neurofibromatosis have been reported.[45] It is concluded that dumbbell ganglioneuromas of the spine and association with neurofibromatosis occur very infrequently.[45]

X-RAY FINDINGS

Neurogenic tumors are the most common neoplasms in the posterior mediastinum in children. Ganglioneuromas are usually seen as round or oval masses in the paravertebral gutters. Their relatively superior or inferior position is of little help in the differential diagnosis of posterior mediastinal tumors.[4] Calcification is commonly present and may assume any form; it was detected by x-ray examination in 7 out of 17 patients in one series.[4]

Schweisguth suggested that intratumoral calcification is a finding which favors immaturity or at the very least a malignant tendency. It appears that presence of calcification in neurogenic tumors indicates the end stage of a mass that is growing faster than its blood supply with subsequent necrosis and calcification. This calcification has no significance in differentiating malignant from benign tumors. Its presence does help in differentiating neurogenic tumors from other posterior mediastinal masses such as duplications of the foregut or neurenteric or bronchogenic cysts.[4]

Costal deformities frequently accompany the thoracic ganglioneuromas and are usually seen as horizontal flattening, increased density, and contour irregularities of the ribs. The ribs may also be spread apart, usually at their junction with the vertebra. Such rib deformities do not serve to differentiate benign from malignant neurogenic tumors.[4]

HISTOPATHOLOGY

Ganglioneuromas were first described by Loretz in 1870. They are usually circumscribed and encapsulated, but extensions often project from the main tumor and tenaciously entwine adjacent structures or work their way into intervertebral foramina, even to compress the spinal cord on occasion.[4]

Ganglioneuromas vary in size but are always encapsulated and firm and on cut surface have a pearly-gray color (Figure 1). Calcification was evident macroscopically in 23 percent.[10] Ganglioneuromas are round to oval in shape and, although at times they reach huge dimensions, do not invade or metastasize. These tumors are derived from mature sympathetic nerve cells. Histologically, they are composed of mature ganglion cells intermixed with nerve fibrils that are twisted and irregular in appearance and without connection with an end organ. Characteristically the ganglion cells are large, round to oval in shape, and contain one or two round nuclei with prominent nucleoli (Figure 2). Cytoplasmic processes may be prominent, and at times the nerve sheaths may show microcystic changes.[6] To the pathologist the term ganglioneuroma is limited to a tumor of adult ganglion cells in a bulky matrix composed of large numbers of neurites with Schwann's sheaths, occasionally myelinated and supported in an inconspicuous fibrous framework.

These tumors consist of sympathetic ganglion cells with neurofibrillary and neural sheath tissue. The neurones vary considerably in number with scant cells rather diffusely scattered in some tumors and numerous clustered cells having the lobular arrangement of the neuroblastoma in others. The ganglion cells show variation in

230

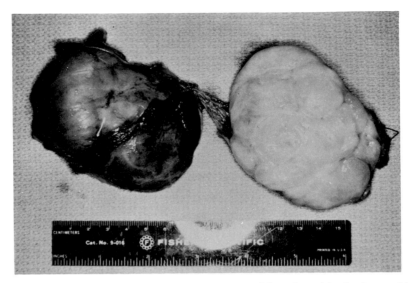

Figure 1. Cross-section of a ganglioneuroma removed from the pelvis of a 4-year-old child. The tumor is fully encapsulated and is white and lobular on cut section. (Courtesy of Dr. Martin Winnick)

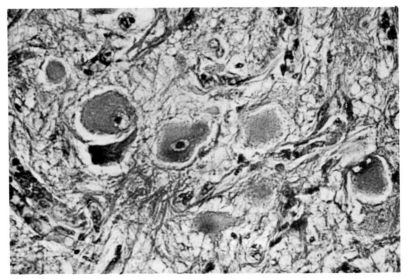

Figure 2. Photomicrograph showing histopathology of a ganglioneuroma. There are several ganglion cells, with oval nuclei and prominent nucleoli, scattered in a fibrous myxoid stroma (H and E ×400).

size with relatively normal cells and large multipolar and multinucleate forms. Swollen, degenerate, eosinophilic granular neurones may also be seen. Lymphocytic infiltration is noted in some of the tumors and the resemblance to immature neuroblasts may cause confusion. Calcification is a feature in some cases. Islands of neurofibrillary material are seen and bundles of nerve fibers are sometimes embedded in the tumor tissue. A fibrous capsule is present in some parts but this is not a constant feature, although the tumors are circumscribed and do not show invasive tendencies. Mature collagen and neurilemmal tissue are present in varying amounts and edema with separation of fibers similar to that in the nerve sheath tumors may be encountered.[6]

The mature ganglion cell is the histological hallmark of this tumor. Such cells occur in varying numbers and may be scattered singly throughout the tumor or arranged in clumps. The stroma is abundant and dense and may contain stainable neurofibrils, as well as collagenous fibers. The stroma may show considerable variation in pattern, and arrangements reminiscent of neurofibroma and neurilemmoma may be seen. It seems probable that such tumors may arise from sympathetic nerves, as well as other peripheral nerves.[10]

Ultrastructure of Ganglioneuromas

In ganglioneuroma, the most prominent features on electron microscopy are large ganglion cells and their satellites and a vast number of axons which are predominantly unmyelinated. As in neurolemmoma and neurofibroma, a basement membrane coats the plasmalemma of the tumor cells. The small osmiophilic, often membrane-bound granules observed in the cytoplasm of ganglion cells and their neural processes have been reported in a patient with peripheral ganglioneuroma and in several patients with neuroblastoma, ganglioneuroblastoma, or pheochromocytoma. These granules are morphologically similar to catecholamine granules encountered in the adrenal medulla and are presumed to contain the necessary enzymes for catecholamine synthesis.[48,49,50]

TREATMENT

Ganglioneuromas that become intimately bound up with important structures like the aorta, vena cava, or major nerve trunks may be dangerous to remove. If such a tumor is encountered, frozen sections from several representative areas of the tumor may be helpful, but it must be remembered that such sections may be misleading because of the varied histopathology of the lesion. A reasonable effort should be made at total extirpation of the tumor. However, if this is not possible, the prognosis may be better than the gross impression would seem to indicate. If the frozen section seems to indicate ganglioneuroma with reasonable accuracy, it is far wiser to remove only that part of the tumor which can be removed without endangering life or producing permanent disability, since re-operation on ganglioneuromas is rarely needed. Thus, caution should be employed in the excision of ganglioneuromas which are intimately bound to vital structures inasmuch as a long-term follow-up suggests that such tumors partially excised rarely cause further symptoms.[4]

In seven patients of one series tumor was left behind because of involvement with vital structures.[4] Reoperation was necessary only in a case of ganglioneuroma which originated in the spinal cord. Two laminectomies were carried out three years apart in this patient with complete extirpation never possible. Central ganglioneuromas are difficult to diagnose histologically because of varied morphology, and their clinical behavior differs from peripheral tumors because of the bony confines of the central nervous system. Reoperation was not needed in six patients with peripheral ganglioneuromas which were incompletely removed.[4] Two of the tumors in this series had extensions into the thoracic spinal canal which were cut off even with the bone and have remained asymptomatic for 13 and 17 years, respectively, without evidence of enlargement. There was not a single instance of a ganglioneuroma becoming a neuroblastoma.[4] X-ray therapy or chemotherapy has not been used in treating these tumors. Surgical excision is the treatment, when treatment is necessary. These tumors are extremely radioresistant.

A long-term follow-up investigation of ganglioneuroma in 17 children was carried out.[4] Two patients with histologically verified malignant neuroblastomas on subsequent biopsy had only mature ganglioneuromas. Two patients with histologically verified hepatic metastases of neuroblastoma on subsequent biopsy had no evidence of tumor, benign or malignant. The youngest patient with a ganglioneuroma in this series was three years old, whereas 78 percent of the patients with neuroblastomas were under three years of age. This finding suggests that these neurogenic tumors may start out in a primitive malignant form and later mature into a benign state.

SUMMARY

Ganglioneuromas usually appear later than neuroblastomas. They may be seen in young children, but usually they do not present until adolescence or adult life. Ganglioneuromas are benign tumors of sympathetic ganglia. The chain of sympathetic ganglia which extends from the base of the skull to the pelvis, including the adrenal medulla, accounts for the origin of most of these tumors. Smaller sympathetic ganglia situated elsewhere occasionally give rise to such tumors. About one-third of these tumors arise from the thoracic and cervical sympathetic chain and one-third arise from the adrenal medulla. The incidence ratio between ganglioneuromas and neuroblastomas is about 1:6. It is believed that ganglioneuromas and neuroblastomas are different manifestations of the same basic neoplasm of the sympathetic nervous system. Ganglioneuromas, as well as neuroblastomas, may occasionally occur in association with neurofibromatosis.

The clinical findings depend on the site, rate of growth, and the size of the particular tumor mass. Ganglioneuromas rarely produce any symptoms until they attain such size that they intrude on neighboring structures. Ganglioneuromas almost always cause excretion of excessive catecholamines in the urine, which makes it necessary for these tumors to be distinguished histologically from neuroblastomas. Occasionally, ganglioneuromas are functionally active and cause such symptoms as diarrhea, hypertension flushing, excessive sweating and other adrenergic symptoms. Since ganglioneuromas often become intimately bound up with vital structures like the aorta, vena cava, and major nerve trunks, it may be dangerous to attempt complete excision. Long-term follow-up studies have shown that even partial excision of such tumors results in cure.

REFERENCES

1. Gaches, C.: Thoracic tumors of neurogenic origin. *Guy's Hosp. Rep.* 114: 15–27, 1965.

2. Stout, A.P.: Ganglioneuromas of the sympathetic nervous system. *Surg. Gynec. Obstet.* 84: 101–110, 1947.

3. Schweisguth, O., Mathey, J., Renault, P., and Benet, J.P.: Intrathoracic neurogenic tumors in infants and children. *Ann. Surg.* 150: 29–41, 1959.

234

4. Hamilton, J., and Koop, C.E.: Ganglioneuromas in children. *Surg. Gynec. Obstet.* 121: 803–812, 1965.

5. Dargeon, H.: Neuroblastoma. *J. Pediatr.* 61: 456–463, 1962.

6. Marsden, H., and Steward, J. (eds.): *Tumours in Children.* New York: Springer-Verlag, 1968, pp. 131–170.

7. Wyman, H., Chappell, B., and Jones, R.: Ganglioneuroma of the bladder, report of a case. *J. Urol.* 63: 526–533, 1950.

8. Weber, D., and Fazzini, E.: Ganglioneuroma of the fallopian tube; a heretofore unreported finding. *Acta Neuropath.* (Berlin) 16: 173–175, 1970.

9. Steinberg, S.H.: Presacral retroperitoneal ganglioneuroma in a 4½-year-old child. *J. Pediatr.* 46: 562–572, 1955.

10. Stowens, D.: Neuroblastoma and related tumors. *Arch. Pathol.* 63: 451–459, 1957.

11. Knudson, A., and Amromin, G.: Neuroblastoma and ganglioneuroma in a child with multiple neurofibromatosis; Implications for the mutational origin of neuroblastoma. *Cancer* 19: 1032–1937, 1966.

12. Bolande, R.P., and Towler, W.: A possible relationship of neuroblastoma to von Recklinghausen's disease. *Cancer* 26: 162–175, 1970.

13. Helson, L., Grabstald, H., Huvos, A., et al.: Neuroblastoma; observations on long-term survival. *Clin Bull. Memorial Sloan-Kettering Cancer Center* 3: 3–9, 1973.

14. Goldman, R.L., Winterling, A.N., and Winterling, C.: Maturation of tumors of the sympathetic nervous system. *Cancer* 18: 1510–1516, 1965.

15. Collins, J., Johnson, W., and Burgoon, C.: Ganglioneuroma of the skin. *Arch. Derm.* 105: 256–258, 1972.

16. Bunn, N., and King, A.B.: Cervical ganglioneuroma; a case report and review of the literature. *Guthrie Clin. Bull.* 30: 5–14, 1961.

17. Conley, J.J.: Neurogenous Tumors in the Neck. *Arch. Otolaryng.* 61: 167, 1955.

18. Turnbull, A., and Caban, W.: Cervical Ganglioneuroma. *New York State J. Med.* 71: 470–472, 1971.

19. Habal, M., McComb, J.G., Shillito, J., et al.: Combined posteroanterior approach to a tumor of the cervical spinal foramen. *J. Neurosurg.* 37: 113–116, 1972.

20. Rosenfield, L., Graves, H., and Lawrence, R.: Primary

neurogenic tumors of the lateral neck. *Ann. Surg.* 167: 847–855, 1968.

21. Tachdjian, M., and Matson, D.: Orthopedic aspects of intraspinal tumors in infants and children. *J. Bone Joint Surg.* 47-A: 223–248, 1965.

22. Bulmer, J.: Scoliosis complicating ganglion cell tumors. *Brit. J. Surg.* 53: 619–624, 1966.

23. Schleetz, W., and Serfas, L.: Mediastinal ganglioneuromas in children; report of a case with bilateral thoracic ganglioneuroma. *Milit. Med.* 133: 226–230, 1968.

24. Armstrong, R., Lindberg, E., Trozler, G., et al.: Simultaneous excision of bilateral neurogenic tumors of the mediastinum. *Chest* 62: 348–352, 1972.

25. Shepard, F., and Sutton, D.: Dumbell ganglioneuromata of the spine with a report of 4 cases. *Brit. J. Surg.* 45: 305–317, 1958.

26. Padmanabhan, K., and Krishnamurti, M.V.: Ganglioneuroma of the mediastinum. *J. Assoc. Physic. India* 16: 213–215, 1968.

27. Wilber, M., and Woodcock, J.: Ganglioneuromata of bone. *J. Bone Joint Surg.* 39-A: 1385–1388, 1957.

28. Young, W.: Histopathologic study of ganglioneuroma in the mandible. *J. Oral. Surg.* 25: 327–335, 1967.

29. Beezley, D.N.: A trigeminal ganglioneuroma in a dog. *Cornell Vet.* 59: 585–593, 1969.

30. Todd, G., Pierce, E., and Clevinger, W.: Ganglioneuroma of the adrenal medulla in rats; report of 3 cases. *Path. Vet.* 7: 139–144, 1970.

31. Gemer, M., and Feuchtwanger, M.M.: Ganglioneuroma of the duodenum. *Gastroenterology* 51: 689–693, 1966.

32. Goldman, R.: Ganglioneuroma of the duodenum; relation to nonchromaffin paraganglioma of the duodenum. *Amer. J. Surg.* 115: 716–719, 1968.

33. Munro, K.: Ganglioneuromatosis of the sigmoid colon. *Brit. J. Surg.* 58: 350–352, 1971.

34. Hawfield, H., and Daisley, G.: A report of a case of functional adrenal ganglioneuroma. *Clin. Proc. Child. Hosp. District of Columbia.* 8: 98–105, 1952.

35. Rosenstein, B.J., and Engelman, K.: Diarrhea in a child with catecholamine-secreting ganglioneuroma. *J. Pediatr.* 63: 217–226, 1963.

36. Donnelly, W., Sieber, W., and Yunis, E.: Polypoid gan-

glioneurofibromatosis of the large bowel. *Arch. Path.* 87: 537–541, 1969.

37. Gleason, I., Beauchemin, J., and Bursk, A.: Polypoid ganglioneuromatosis of the large bowel. *Arch. Neurol.* 6: 242–247, 1962.

38. Mason, G., Hart-Mercer, J., Miller, E.J., et al.: Adrenaline-secreting neuroblastoma in an infant. *Lancet* 2: 322–325, 1957.

39. Sindhu, S., and Anderson, C.: Ganglioneuroma as a cause of diarrhea and failure to thrive. *Aust. Paediatr. J.* 1: 56–60, 1965.

40. Peterson, H.D., and Collins, O.D.: Chronic diarrhea and failure to thrive secondary to ganglioneuroma. *Arch. Surg.* 95: 934–936, 1967.

41. Kogut, M., and Kaplan, S.A.: Systemic manifestations of neurogenic tumors. *J. Pediatr.* 60: 694–704, 1962.

42. Green, M., Cooke, R., and Lattanzi, W.: Occurrence of chronic diarrhea in three patients with ganglioneuromas. *Pediatrics* 23: 951–955, 1959.

43. Greenberg, R.E., and Gardner, L.I.: New diagnostic test for neural tumors of infancy; increased urinary excretion of 3-Methoxy-4-hydroxymandelic acid and norepinephrine in ganglioneuroma with chronic diarrhea. *Pediatrics* 24: 683, 1959.

44. Frangonese, B., Cottafava, F., Vignola, G., et al.: Tumors of the neural crest with chronic diarrhea. *Minerva Pediat.* 21: 1699–1704, 1969.

45. Sinclair, J., and Yang, Y.: Ganglioneuromata of the spine associated with von Recklinghausen's disease. *J. Neurosurg.* 18: 115–119, 1961.

46. Wahl, R., and Dillard, S.: Multiple ganglioneuromas of the central nervous system. *Arch. Path.* 94: 158–164, 1972.

47. Chatten, J., and Voorhess, M.: Familial neuroblastoma; report of a kindred with multiple disorders, including neuroblastomas in 4 siblings. *N. Engl. J. Med.* 277: 1230–1236, 1967.

48. Rosenthal, I., Greenberg, R., Kathan, R., et al.: Catecholamine metabolism of a ganglioneuroma; correlation with electron micrographs. *Pediatr. Res.* 3: 413–424, 1969.

49. Hortnagl, H., Hortnagl, H., Winkler, H., et al.: Storage of catecholamines in neuroblastoma and ganglioneuroma; a biochemical immunologic, and morphologic study. *Lab. Invest.* 27: 613–619, 1972.

50. Razzuk, M., Urschel, H., Martin, J., et al.: Electron microscopical observations on mediastinal neurolemmoma, neurofibroma and ganglioneuroma. *Ann. Thorac. Surg.* 15: 73–83, 1973.

10 Surgical Management of Neuroblastoma

Anthony Shaw, M.D.

1. Preoperative work-up and preparation
2. Surgical approach to abdominal neuroblastomas
3. Surgical approach to mediastinal neuroblastomas
4. Surgical morbidity and mortality
5. Surgery for metastases
6. Surgery following radiotherapy and/or chemotherapy: the "second look"
7. Results of surgery

The natural history of neuroblastoma has always worked against the surgeon. In Boles's words, "This tumor spreads through the retroperitoneal space like crab grass through a blue grass lawn, extending across the midline, enveloping the great vessels and invading the intestinal mesenteries."[1] In addition to its aggressive local behavior, neuroblastoma disseminates early and widely, metastases being present in 60 to 90 percent of patients when they are first seen.[2,3,4] However, surgery plays an important role, even in the presence of disseminated disease.

PREOPERATIVE WORK-UP AND PREPARATION FOR SURGERY

An attempt must be made to delineate the extent of disease prior to the surgical attack. An obvious neoplastic mass may be a metasta-

237

tic deposit rather than the primary lesion, which itself may be small and difficult to detect. The surgeon is assisted by a roentgenographic survey including chest and abdominal films, skeletal survey, and IVP. Additional studies including bone marrow examination, inferior vena cavagram, laminograms, and liver scans may be helpful in assessing the extent of metastasis as well as in estimating the potential re-sectability of retroperitoneal lesions. Preoperative assay of urinary catecholamines, VMA and HVA, are useful as a guide to determining the completeness of tumor resection. Preoperative urinary catecholamine determinations are also useful for interpretation of serial postoperative assays of VMA and HVA in timing "second-look" operations later on.[2,5,6]

Even if only a biopsy of a large neoplastic mass is contemplated, adequate preparation for blood transfusion must be made. A large catheter threaded through an upper extremity or cervical vein (Figure 1B) allows rapid transfusion and also permits measurement of central venous pressure, a valuable guide to blood and fluid replacement, especially in the early postoperative period. An intra-arterial line may also be helpful in monitoring an infant or small child undergoing a major resection.

In pelvic neuroblastomas, an indwelling Foley catheter helps to identify the bladder, prevents bladder distention from obscuring the view of pelvic structures, and enables measurement of the urinary output. Occasionally, placement of ureteral catheters helps the sur-geon identify the ureters when they are involved or displaced by tumor. The colon and rectum must be cleansed preoperatively. A 24-hour period of nasogastric decompression of intestine often affords better access to retroperitoneal structures.

SURGICAL APPROACH TO ABDOMINAL NEUROBLASTOMAS

Most neuroblastomas arise intra-abdominally from the adrenal gland, organ of Zuckerkandl, or from the sympathetic ganglia any-where from diaphragm to pelvis. Wide exposure through a generous incision allows accurate assessment of the extent of local disease, facilitates detection of regional metastases, gives the surgeon access to the numerous blood vessels supplying and draining the tumor, and permits as complete an excision as is compatible with patient survival.

Such exposure to abdominal neuroblastomas is best achieved through a generous upper abdominal transverse incision extending

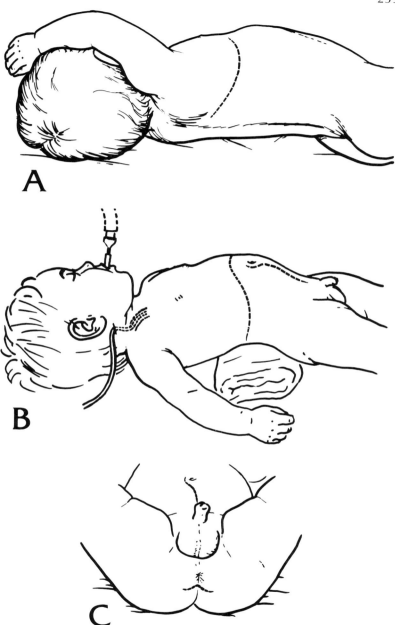

Figure 1. Anatomic diagram showing positioning of the patient and sites of incisions for mediastinal (A), abdominal (B), and pelvic (B and C) neuroblastomas. In small infants with large tumors, insertion of a jugular catheter is recommended (B).

into the flank. A kidney bridge, rolled sheet, or sandbag, under the upper-lumbar spine thrusts posterior retroperitoneal structures anteriorly and thus makes them more accessible (Figure 1). A thoracic extension of the abdominal incision may occasionally facilitate removal of a large upper abdominal lesion. Because these tumors are very vascular and friable, control of bleeding may be difficult at times. Wide exposure of the tumor and its multiple sources of blood supply is essential.

While total resection is the ideal, the surgeon must settle for partial excision or biopsy in most cases.[1,4,7-10] Because of its tendency to spread "like crab grass through a blue grass lawn," neuroblastoma is usually found to have invaded or to be intimately adherent to the liver or the major retroperitoneal or mesenteric blood vessels. A reasonable effort consistent with survival of the patient should be made to remove the tumor. Wide extension into the tissues of the renal fossa and around the vena cava and aorta makes removal hazardous; in such instances the operative procedure is best limited to removal of adequate tissue for biopsy. The tumor is sensitive to radiation, and the patient's chances for survival may be greater by such a course of action than by a hazardous attempt at complete surgical extirpation.[6] Thus, attempts to extend the resection to include portions of essential organs and vessels may result in increased morbidity and mortality without increasing the cure rate.[2,10-12] Since survival has been recorded after incomplete excision of tumor,[7,8,13,14] the surgeon must not feel compelled to undertake ultra-radical surgery with its very great risk of operative death. Paraspinal tumor invading the spinal foramina may be pursued by laminectomy at the same time as the transabdominal resection, or at a later date, perhaps following a course of radiotherapy.[11,15]

Large tumors involving aorta or vena cava or their major visceral branches are best excised using a clamp and suture-ligature technique, starting from a safe distance away from the great vessels and dissecting laterally, leaving behind only that tumor intimately adherent to them. Often the central portion of the tumor is so friable and mushy that it may be spooned out or removed by suction. Following partial excision the periphery of remaining tumor should be marked with silver clips as a guide to the radiotherapist (Figure 2).

Accurate assessment of blood loss by weighing sponges, measuring blood in suction bottles, and estimating quantities on the drapes is essential as is careful monitoring of the electrocardiogram, blood pressure, and urine output. The surgeon and anesthesiologist must not allow blood loss to outrun replacement.[16]

Pelvic neuroblastomas are best approached through a lower

abdominal transverse incision or a vertical midline incision (Figure 1B). Often a combined abdomino-perineal approach is required for extirpation of pelvic lesions[17] (Figures 1C, 3, 4). Remaining tumor should be outlined with silver clips as a guide to the radiotherapist (Figure 5).

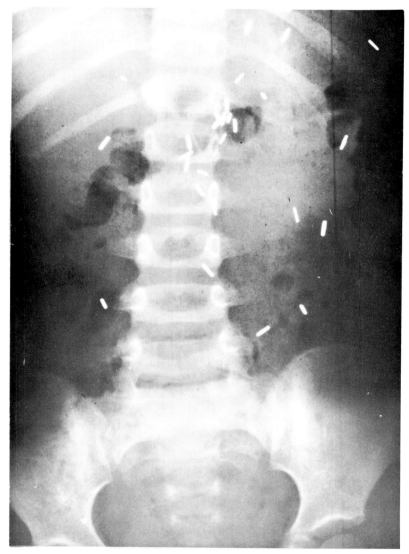

Figure 2. X-ray of the abdomen following removal of a left adrenal neuroblastoma showing silver clips marking the periphery of the excised tumor.

SURGICAL APPROACH TO MEDIASTINAL NEUROBLASTOMAS

The vast majority of thoracic neuroblastomas originate in the posterior mediastinum and often extend into the spinal foramina. The surgical approach to a mediastinal neuroblastoma should utilize the same principles as those used in removal of abdominal neuroblastomas. A posterolateral incision is preferred (Figure 1A), extending beneath the tip of the scapula and curving anteriorly under the breast to the mid-axillary line. Usually the incision is in the 4th intercostal space, but the level chosen might vary depending on the level of the tumor in the chest. Exposure can be increased by extending the incision anteriorly or dividing one or more costal cartilages above or below the interspace entered. Separate or combined thoracic and

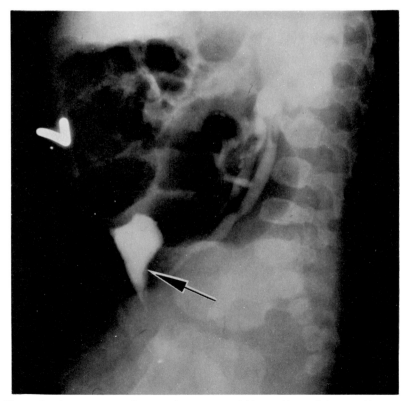

Figure 3. Intravenous pyelogram of a two-year-old boy with a pelvic neuroblastoma showing anterior and cephalad displacement of the bladder (arrow) and hydroureter due to obstruction.

cervical incisions may allow more complete removal of lesions involving the neck and mediastinum.[15,18] Care should be taken in dissection not to disturb the sympathetic system in the apex of the chest, for this may result in Horner's syndrome. On the other hand, in order to achieve a clean surgical excision, this complication should not prevent the surgeon from accomplishing a complete removal. With respect to hemostasis, the same problems exist, with the blood supply of the very vascular mediastinal neuroblastoma, as with those seen in the abdomen.

SURGICAL MORBIDITY AND MORTALITY

Surgical morbidity and mortality is related primarily to blood loss or damage to the blood supply of essential viscera. Deaths due to injury to the inferior vena cava, aorta, and superior mesenteric artery have been reported as well as deaths due to shock from uncontrollable bleeding from the tumor itself.[2,9,11] The incidence of such deaths is low in experienced hands. Koop reports no operating room deaths in a series of 134 cases managed surgically.[13] The frequency of

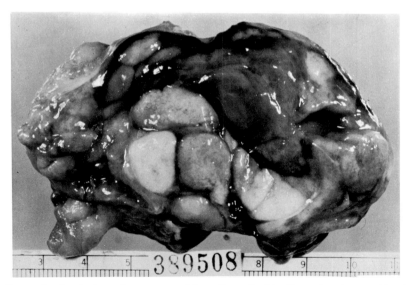

Figure 4. Surgical specimen removed from the patient in Figure 3, using combined abdominal and pelvic incisions. Although the tumor was lobular and friable, it was covered by a pseudocapsule.

postoperative mortality due to surgery (deaths under 30 days post-surgery) is difficult to assess because of the usual postoperative addition of other modalities of treatment (x-ray therapy and chemotherapy) which have their own adverse side effects. Specific complications of surgery are hard to find in the literature. A pancreatic fistula is mentioned in one report.[11] Chylothorax and brachial plexus injury have been reported as complications of excisional surgery of mediastinal and cervical neuroblastomas.[15] Horner's syn-

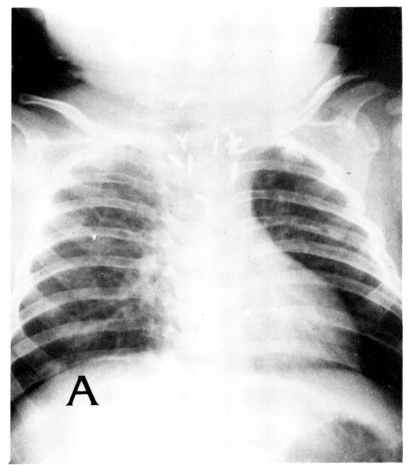

Figure 5. A: X-ray of the chest showing position of silver clips following removal of a neuroblastoma of the upper mediastinum.

drome commonly occurs after surgery of upper mediastinal and cervical neuroblastomas.[15] (See Chapter 3)

SURGERY FOR METASTASES

Two factors work against a surgical approach to neuroblastoma metastases. First, in almost all cases, metastases are widely disseminated (most commonly to liver, bone, bone marrow, and skin) and defy surgical attack. The second factor restraining the surgeon's

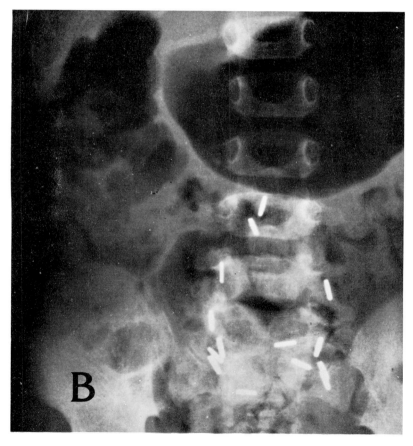

Figure 5. B: X-ray of the pelvis showing position of silver clips following removal of a lumbo-sacral neuroblastoma.

hand in metastatic lesions is the unusually high rate of curability following resection or even biopsy of the primary tumor in infants with certain types of disseminated neuroblastoma, namely, that designated as stage IV-S by D'Angio et al.[14] Thus, unlike Wilms' tumor where cure rates can be improved by an aggressive approach including excision of solitary metastases out of lung or liver or excision of contralateral kidney deposits, neuroblastoma metastases are, with perhaps rare exceptions, not in the surgeon's domain.

However, occasional successes due to aggressive surgery have been recorded. Priebe et al. reported resection of metastatic deposits in the lung of a 4-year-old girl five months post-excision and irradiation of an abdominal tumor.[11] The child was alive and well 10 years later. Fortner et al. reported excision of a "presumed" solitary metastasis of the cheek with the patient alive and well 4 years later.[9] The experience of Brown is more typical. A total right hepatectomy was performed for metastatic neuroblastoma following radiation therapy to shrink the tumor mass, but the patient died of metastatic disease one year later.[19] In general, when a "solitary metastasis" is excised with apparent cure in the absence of a demonstrable primary lesion, the diagnosis of neuroblastoma must be questioned. Some lesions, such as Ewing's sarcoma, may be difficult to differentiate from neuroblastoma histologically.[9]

SURGERY FOLLOWING RADIOTHERAPY, CHEMOTHERAPY, OR BOTH: THE "SECOND LOOK"

Irradiation therapy with or without chemotherapy given preoperatively may reduce the size of a neuroblastoma mass by 50 percent or more. Occasionally this treatment may convert an inoperable, friable, vascular tumor filling the abdominal cavity into a firm, pseudoencapsulated lesion which may be wholly or partially resectable with minimal blood loss.[2,5,9,17,19,20] Certainly it is the better part of valor for a surgeon to back away from the prospect of a massive, shocking, operative procedure and do only a biopsy. He may subsequently reoperate following reduction in size and vascularity of the tumor by radiation, chemotherapy or both. The optimal time for reoperation following biopsy and irradiation therapy has been variously estimated from three weeks to four months.[5,17,20] Such "second look" operations have also been recommended for patients whose urinary VMA levels rise postoperatively from the reduced or normal levels achieved following resection of the primary tumor.[2,5]

RESULTS OF SURGERY

Gross[8] credits Lehman[21] with the first surgical cure of neuroblastoma, an operation on a baby performed in 1917. However, 57 years after Lehman's operation, in spite of the extensive literature on the subject, the contribution of surgery to the cure rate of neuroblastoma eludes assessment for three reasons: (1) Some neuroblastomas regress spontaneously; (2) almost all neuroblastoma patients have been treated with radiotherapy, chemotherapy, or both, in addition to surgery; and (3) all published series are retrospective, with subgroups treated and classified by criteria which allow neither useful analysis nor comparison. All treatment programs have been uncontrolled, making quantitative assessment of the contribution made by surgery to the cure rate of neuroblastoma impossible.

There appears to be a correlation between cure rate and resectability in that the highest cure rates in some series have been reported in those few children in whom the primary lesions have been totally resected.[4,5,8,9,11] For the most part, children with resectable tumors have been under one year of age and constitute only from 10 to 20 percent of the patients in reported series.[4,5,8,9,11] Almost all of these have had radiotherapy and chemotherapy as well, which obscures the contribution of the surgeon.

Patients whose lesions are partially resected seem to have a better prognosis than neuroblastoma patients as a whole.[8,9] Coriell suggested that the removal of a quantity of tumor antigen could permit immune mechanisms to escape from paralysis or tolerance for the abnormal antigen.[25] By surgically reducing the number of tumor cells, the remaining neuroblastoma, whether locally invasive or metastatic, may be more vulnerable to a combination of the patient's own immune mechanisms[24] and other modalities of treatment such as radiotherapy and chemotherapy.[5]

In spite of the apparent contributions surgery has made to the cure rate, several authors have reported no cures with surgery alone.[10,26] Koop has taken the position that radiotherapy and chemotherapy do not improve survival in stage I and stage II disease.[7,13] His group has reported two-year cures with surgery alone in 16 out of 19 patients (84 percent) with complete excision of the primary lesion, 5 out of 8 (63 percent) with partial excision, and 3 out of 13 (23 percent) with biopsy alone.[7] However, it is clear that too few children had surgical resection only in recent years to compare the results with those treated with combined techniques. This may reflect an understandable reluctance of most physicians to withhold other methods of treatment of proven effectiveness. Surgery alone has been suggested or recommended for some infants with stage IV-S disease[14] and in some patients where total excision of a solitary focus has been accomplished.[4,5]

Swank et al. stated that surgical treatment seemed to play a relatively unimportant part in survival in the face of spread to lymph nodes. In their experience, only 11 patients with positive nodes out of a series of 125 cases survived.[22] Of these 11 patients, 9 were under one year of age and 8 had an extra-abdominal primary tumor, both factors being associated with improved prognosis.

Attempts to evaluate surgical treatment must take into consideration four variables, each of which has a significant effect on the natural history of neuroblastoma. Taken together, they may have a more important effect on patient survival than any single modality of treatment. These four important factors which individually affect the patient's prognosis are age, tumor type, site of the primary, and stage.

Age The prognosis in patients under the age of one year is far better than in those over one year, even where the tumor is only partially excised or where biopsy alone is performed in the presence of a disseminated disease.[3,4,8,10,13,22]

Tumor type The better differentiated tumors may tend toward regression or may be more amenable to excision.[2,5,23]

Site of primary Mediastinal neuroblastomas have a higher rate of resectability and a cure rate as high as 100 percent in those under one year of age.[3,15] The cure rate of mediastinal neuroblastoma is high in older children as well and may be a tumor type of lower malignant potential, arising from paraganglionic tissue in sensory dorsal root ganglia rather than from sympathetic ganglia.[7]

Stage As mentioned previously, the patients with metastatic tumor in the stage IV-S classification (most of whom are under one year of age) have a high cure rate.[14]

It is nonetheless true that in every clinical or pathological category of neuroblastoma there are cases which behave in a totally unpredicted fashion. (See Chapter 13)

"Second look" operations may result in increased rates of resectability but whether the cure rate is thereby increased is certainly questionable. While it often has been possible to excise much or even most of a previously inoperable lesion following radiotherapy, patients so treated usually succumb to metastatic disease within a year of surgery.[11,19,20]

REFERENCES

1. Boles, E.T.: Tumors of the abdomen in children. *Pediatr. Clin. N. Amer.* 9: 467–484, 1962.

2. Snyder, W.H., Hastings, T.N., and Pollock, W.F.: Neuroblastoma. (Benson, C., Mustard, W., Ravitch, M., et al., eds.). In *Pediatric Surgery.* Vol. II (2nd Ed.) Chicago: Yearbook Medical Publishers, 1969, pp. 1047–1051.

3. de Lorimier, A.A., Braff, K.U., and Linden, G.: Neuroblastoma in childhood. *Amer. J. Dis. Child,* 118: 441–450, 1969.

4. Wrenn, E.L., Arcari, F.A., Colodny, A.H., and Harberg, F.J.: Survey of ten years' experience of surgical fellows of the American Academy of Pediatrics. *Exhibit.* 1966.

5. Koop, C.E.: The role of surgery in resectable, non-resectable, and metastatic neuroblastoma. *J.A.M.A.* 205: 157–158, 1968.

6. Swenson, O.: *Pediatric Surgery.* (3d Ed.) Vol. I. New York: Appleton-Century-Crofts, 1969, pp. 432, 891.

7. Koop, C.E.: Neuroblastoma; two-year survival and treatment correlations. *J. Pediatr. Surg.* 3: 178–179, 1968.

8. Gross, R.E., Farber, S., and Martin, L.W.: Neuroblastoma sympathicum; a study and report of 217 cases. *Pediatrics* 23: 1179, 1959.

9. Fortner, J., Nicastri, A., and Murphy, M.L.: Neuroblastoma; natural history and results of treating 133 cases. *Ann. Surg.* 167: 132, 1968.

10. Lingley, J.F., Sagerman, R.H., Santulli, T.V., and Wolff, J.A.: Neuroblastoma; management and survival. *New Engl. J. Med.* 277: 1227–1236, 1967.

11. Priebe, C.J., and Clatworthy, H.W.: Neuroblastoma; Evaluation of the treatment of 90 children. *Arch. Surg.* 95: 538–545, 1967.

12. Komp, D.M., Marks, R.D., Shaw, A., et al.: The management of abdominal malignancy in children. *Virginia Med. Month.* 99: 1309–1314, 1972.

13. Koop, C.E., and Johnson, D.G.: Neuroblastoma; an assessment of therapy in reference to staging. *J. Pediatr. Surg.* 6: 595–600, 1971.

14. D'Angio, G.J., Evans, A.E., and Koop, C.E.: Special pattern of widespread neuroblastoma with a favourable prognosis. *Lancet* 1: 1046, 1971.

15. Filler, R.M., Traggis, T.G., Jaffe, N., and Vawter, G.: Favorable outlook for children with mediastinal neuroblastoma. *J. Pediatr. Surg.* 7: 136–143, 1972.

16. Smith, R.M.: Anesthesia for Infants and Children. (3rd Ed.) St. Louis: C.V. Mosby Company, 1968, pp. 318–320.

17. Pochedly, C., Kenigsberg, K., and Sarrafi, G.: Posterior route removal of sacral neuroblastoma with 12 month survival. *J.A.M.A.* 224: 1186–1187, 1973.

18. Pratt, C.B.: Management of solid tumors in children. *Pediatr. Clin. N. Amer.* 19: 1141–1155, 1972.

19. Brown, P.M., and Hart, J.T.: Total right hepatolobectomy for a metastatic neuroblastoma. *Minn. Med.* 49: 591–595, 1966.

20. Stanley-Brown, E.C., and Dargeon, H.W.: Second-look operation for retroperitoneal cancer in childhood. *N.Y. State J. Med.* 71: 674–676, 1971.

21. Lehman, E.P.: Adrenal neuroblastoma in infancy; 15 year survival. *Ann. Surg.* 95: 473, 1932.

22. Swank, R.L., Fetterman, G.H., Sieber, W.K., and Kiesewetter, W.B.: Prognostic factors in neuroblastoma. *Ann. Surg.* 174: 428–435, 1971.

23. Koop, C.E., and Hernandez, J.R.: Neuroblastoma; experience with 100 cases in children. *Surgery* 56: 726–733, 1964.

24. Beckwith, J.B., and Martin, R.F.: Observations on the histopathology of neuroblastomas. *J. Pediatr. Surg.* 3: 106, 1968.

25. Coriell, L.L.: Host immunity. *J. Pediatr. Surg.* 3: 124, 1968.

26. Clatworthy, H.W.: The treatment of neuroblastoma. *CA* 18: 146–150, 1968.

11 Radiotherapeutic Management of Neuroblastoma

Melvin Tefft, M.D.

1. Radiotherapy of resectable tumors
2. Consideration of radiation therapy effect on normal tissues
3. Management of patients with metastatic neuroblastoma
4. Recommendations

Recently, a staging system has been described which correlates the degree of local tumor involvement and metastatic extension to the age of the patient at diagnosis and to survival.[1] Previous reports have noted the ability of irradiation to control neuroblastoma.[2,3,4] In evaluating any therapeutic regimen, however, one must be mindful of the possibility of maturation and/or spontaneous regression of this neoplasm, even without specific therapy.[5,6,7] Reports of long-term control with surgery alone,[8,9] at times where surgery has comprised only partial excision of tumor in relatively early stages of this disease (stages I and II), and spontaneous regression in the special category of disease (stage IV-S) without systemic therapy,[10] emphasize the need for caution in establishing the efficacy of radiation therapy especially in stages I, II, and IV-S disease.

251

THERAPY OF RESECTABLE TUMORS

Total surgical extirpation of the neuroblastoma is not always possible, especially for disease more advanced than stage I, because of the tendency for early regional extension. For this reason, local irradiation has been thought to play a major role in eradicating residual neoplasm. Thus, in the case of primary neuroblastoma of the adrenal medulla, one may find localized extension to involve the ipsilateral kidney, regional retroperitoneal lymph nodes, tumor adhesions to the aorta and/or the inferior vena cava, and extension to the serosa of the bowel. Most often, the ipsilateral kidney must be removed with the main tumor mass because of close adherence.

Following surgical removal of the main tumor mass, irradiation should be directed to an area comprising the limits of tumor involvement (or tumor bed) as outlined both by radiographs and the findings at the time of surgery. In children less than one year of age, radiation doses ranging from 1,000 rads given in 6 elapsed days to 1,500 rads in 10 elapsed days may be delivered through opposed anterior and posterior portals. Doses in the range of 1,500 rads in 10 elapsed days have been found to be adequate in controlling neuroblastoma in the young child less than one year of age. This may be related to the more frequent occurrence of the sympathicoblastoma in this age group, which is a more undifferentiated and thus a more radiosensitive precursor to neuroblastoma. On the other hand, one often observes prolonged survival of children with neuroblastoma in stage IV-S, who are not given radiotherapy, and prolonged survival of children with stages I and II neuroblastoma who are treated with surgical resection alone, at times incomplete. These observations lead one to speculate that the radiotherapy given to many of these children bears little relation to the ultimate survival of the child, especially when in the very young age group.

Similar speculations have been made relative to the management of neuroblastoma arising from the paravertebral sympathetic chain, the organ of Zuckerkandl at the aortic bifurcation, or the presacral region. Because of the diffuse extension of disease at these sites, multiple sites of involvement may be found within the abdomen and the actual primary site may not be obvious at surgery, as in some cases of stage III disease. Thus, radiotherapy to a localized area probably does not affect the rate of prolonged survival in these patients.

The neuroblastoma may at times extend through the intervertebral foramina, in a dumbbell-shaped fashion, causing symptoms and signs of spinal cord compression. Emergency laminectomy may be required in such instances by a neurosurgical team. This would then be followed by laparotomy by a general surgical team to remove the retroperitoneal primary component of the mass lesion. Irradiation would then be delivered to the intra-abdominal site of involvement and would include the spinal cord level of involvement with an adequate margin both superiorly and inferiorly.

Management of intrathoracic neuroblastomas originating from (1) sympathetic ganglia in retropleural areas or in the sympathetic plexus at the root of the lung, (2) in the cervical area, or (3) in the nasopharynx (the organ of Jacobson) would be similar. Previous reports have considered neuroblastoma arising in the thoracic cavity, as compared to neuroblastoma with origin in the abdomen, to have a better prognosis by virtue of the site of origin.[11,12] The newer concept of staging of this disease raises the possibility that the prognosis of the disease is largely unrelated to the site of origin of the tumor but, rather, related to the stage of the disease. The better prognosis for intrathoracic neuroblastoma, therefore, is perhaps related to earlier stage of the disease when diagnosed in that cavity of the body, while lesions arising within the abdomen carry a worse prognosis because they are diagnosed only in the later stages of the disease process.[1] In addition, prolonged survival is often observed in patients with stage I and stage II disease treated with surgery alone, as well as in patients with stage IV-S disease who were not given concomitant radiotherapy and chemotherapy. In view of these various observations, the efficacy of combined therapy, including radiotherapy and chemotherapy, must now be re-evaluated.

Using the combined approach of surgery to the local tumor site, followed by postoperative radiotherapy and often with concomitant chemotherapy, the overall 2-year survival rate of children less than one year of age has been reported to be approximately 76 percent. Recurrences after this period are rare.[13] Whether survival of babies with neuroblastoma in any way relates to the postoperative management (radiotherapy and chemotherapy) is, at this time, unclear.

Children of more than one year of age present a greater challenge in terms of tumor control. If the older child fails to demonstrate evidence of bone dissemination by x-ray examination, combined aggressive management proceeds as outlined for the young child without dissemination. After surgery, in many centers, radiotherapy is delivered in higher doses along the following formula:

2,400 rads in 2½ weeks—two to three years of age
3,000 rads in 3 weeks—three to five years of age
3,500 rads in 3½ weeks—five to nine years of age
4,000–4,500 rads in 4 to 4½ weeks—nine years of age or
older

Those who follow this practice thus deliver higher doses to the older child whose tissues are more tolerant to the effects of irradiation and whose prognosis is generally poor.

However, it should be emphasized that the age of the patient is one of two determinant prognostic factors. The older child tends to have the more advanced disease at diagnosis. But stage I neuroblastoma, in the older child, appears to carry a relatively good prognosis, although not so good as in the younger child. Whether or not a child with stage IV-S disease would have the same prognosis at an older age as a child under one year of age is speculative because of its rarity. Unique immune mechanisms may play an important role in regression of the tumor in children with stage IV-S disease less than one year of age.[14]

More frequently in children over one year of age, a neuroblastoma may be encountered which cannot be surgically excised totally because of fixation to surrounding vital structures such as the inferior vena cava or aorta. Irradiation, with or without concomitant chemotherapy, may cause such masses to regress to the point that later total extirpation, within two to four months, may be possible. In certain selected cases, therefore, long-term control of previously inoperable tumors may be attained by preoperative irradiation.

The ganglioneuroma is a benign tumor which is resistant to radiotherapy and not ordinarily subjected to treatment other than surgical removal if possible. A child who presents with a mixed neuroblastoma and ganglioneuroma, a not uncommon presentation, should be treated in a manner similar to that which has been outlined for a child with pure neuroblastoma.

CONSIDERATIONS OF RADIATION THERAPY EFFECT ON NORMAL TISSUE

The doses quoted are considered to be within the limits of tolerance of various normal structures, such as the growing epiphyseal centers of the vertebral bodies as they are subtended in volume to encompass tumor involvement. Severe vertebral body deformities and resulting scoliosis may be minimized by careful attention to the relationship of dose, dose rate, and age of the patient. Radiation damage of growing bone is inversely related to the age of the patient.[15]

Scoliosis may occur on the basis of two factors:

1. Those *intrinsic to the disease*—thus, neurogenic involvement by the tumor because of direct extension into the spinal canal may compromise vascular structures and muscular innervation
2. Those *secondary to treatment,* including:
    (A) asymmetrical irradiation of the vertebral growth centers, which may be minimized by irradiation delivered symmetrically to the epiphyseal centers of the vertebral bodies (Figures 1 and 2)
    (b) extra-osseous soft tissue effects, due to fibrosis and contracture of soft tissues on the affected side, which may follow the combination of surgery and radiation therapy.

Radiation doses in this range should lead to negligible effects on the spinal cord[16,17] and bowel. Care is taken to carefully shield all uninvolved tissue from direct irradiation. If the contralateral kidney does not lie within an area of known tumor involvement, it is meticulously excluded from the direct radiation beam. With supervoltage technique and subsequent excellent collimation, secondary irradiation to the contralateral kidney should be insignificant. If the kidney does lie within a field of known tumor involvement, as in the case of irradiation to a liver grossly enlarged due to metastases, then the kidney or kidneys must be spared from direct irradiation as much as possible by external shielding, or careful beam direction using lateral portals.

External shielding using heavy metal blocks of four half-value-layers attenuation is introduced into the posterior radiation therapy portal, such shielding beginning with the first day of radiation therapy. Contribution of irradiation from the unshielded anterior portal, transmission through the lead shield from the posterior portal, and side scatter should all be considered in calculating the total dose to the renal tissue. Such a total dose should not exceed 1,600 rads in three to four weeks elapsed time.[18] If, because of the position of the residual tumor, the blocks lead to underdosage of major portions of the tumor, it might be elected to deliver the first 1,000 rads using opposed anterior and posterior portals, without renal shielding. At that level of dose, however, shielding must be used both on the anterior and posterior portals such that transmission and side scatter contribution, together with the 1,000 rads delivered by the unshielded beams, does not exceed the total dose to the renal tissue of 1,600 rads in three to four weeks.

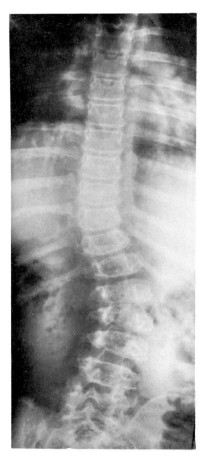

Figure 1. Anteroposterior view of the thoracolumbar spine seven years following radiation therapy. The age of the child at the time of irradiation was two years and irradiation was directed to the right hemiabdomen. There is marked scoliotic deformity of the spine with some degree of retardation of growth of the epiphyseal growth centers on the right half of the vertebral bodies. The combination of asymmetrical irradiation of vertebral bodies, plus contracture of soft tissues in the right hemiabdomen have led to this degree of morbidity. The other factors, such as "pelvic tilt" from irradiation of the right pelvis may have contributed also. (Courtesy of *Frontiers of Radiation Therapy and Oncology*[15])

However, implicit in the discussion of shielding renal tissue, is the possibility of shielding a cylinder to tumor-bearing tissue immediately adjacent to the shielded kidney. Since renal tolerance cannot be exceeded, hopefully other modalities, including a "second look" laparotomy (the latter to remove the residual tumor underdosed due to the renal shielding), might be effective in controlling tumor that must, by necessity of renal shielding, receive less than the optimum doses quoted above.

It may be possible to protect the ovaries by repositioning them either in the midline low in the pelvis or at the level of the iliac crest to exclude them from the portals that must be used to encompass residual tumor, depending on the site to be irradiated. Metallic clips should be placed around the ovaries for localization referable to the radiation therapy portal.[19] (Figure 3)

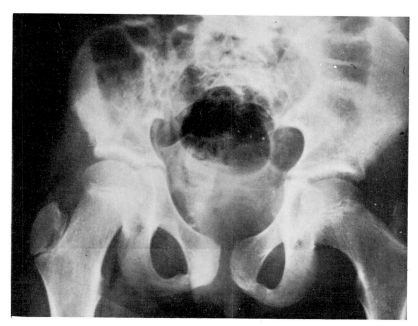

Figure 2. Anteroposterior view of the pelvis in same child as described in Figure 1. There is hypodevelopment of the irradiated right iliac bone as compared to the unirradiated left side, seven years following delivery of 3,000 rads at age two years. (Courtesy of *Frontiers of Radiation Therapy and Oncology*[15])

MANAGEMENT OF PATIENTS WITH METASTATIC NEUROBLASTOMA

The metastatic spread of the neuroblastoma follows three routes: direct regional extension along fascial planes, lymphatic extension to regional and distant lymph node echelons, and hematogenous dissemination to bone and soft tissue. Indeed, all three modes of extension may be observed in an individual patient.

Patients with metastatic neuroblastoma, who exhibit cord compression, may be managed by high-dose, rapid-fraction irradiation, without the need of intervention by a neurosurgical team to forestall cord compression,[20] if the degree of cord embarrassment is not great. Further management of such patients, with respect to laparotomy for removal of the primary tumor, as described above, would depend on the stage of disease. Thus, a child with stage III neuroblastoma, for instance, might be amenable to laparotomy for subtotal tumor removal. A child with stage IV neuroblastoma would be managed by radiotherapy for the local problem of cord compression and, thereafter, by systemic chemotherapy.

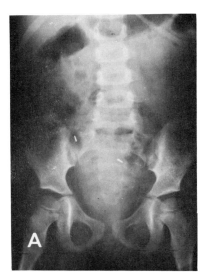
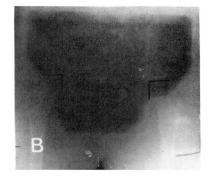

Figure 3. **A:** Anteroposterior film of the abdomen showing silver clips placed on the right and left ovaries respectively. Both ovaries have been relocated to the positions demarcated by the silver clips. **B:** Radiation therapy portal for treatment of this child entails irradiation of the pelvic contents and, necessarily, includes irradiation of the left ovary. However, as can be noted, the right ovary, demarcated by the silver clip, is just outside the portal for radiation therapy.

As previously noted in stage IV-S neuroblastoma, liver involvement at diagnosis per se, especially in a child under one year of age, does not seem to affect the prognosis significantly. Thirty-five patients under one year of age were admitted to the Children's Hospital Medical Center, Boston, between the years of 1946 and 1966. Twenty-seven were surviving free of disease after two years or more. Of this total number, 26 children had tumors originating in intra-abdominal sites; 9 of these latter had liver lesions at diagnosis, and 6 survived two years or more from diagnosis.[13] In these patients, radiation therapy was delivered to the liver in doses quoted above (1,500 rads in 10 elapsed days to children under one year of age) and an alkylating agent was given on a regular schedule for approximately two years in most patients. Later reports now suggest the possibility that such combined therapy is unrelated to ultimate prognosis and, therefore, is excessive.[1,10]

On the other hand, children with stage IV disease, including radiographic evidence of bone metastases, may require irradiation. In such cases, radiotherapy may be administered with palliative intent only. The prognosis for a child with radiographic evidence of bone destruction, irrespective of age, is far worse than that of a child with bone marrow infiltration but without radiographic evidence of bone destruction (stage IV disease vs. stage IV-S disease).[1]

Children who exhibit radiographic evidence of bone dissemination have a high mortality rate, more than 90 percent, regardless of the approaches of therapy to either the primary site or the systemic treatment administered. Indeed, only isolated instances of prolonged survival of children with radiographic bony dissemination have been recorded. These patients have usually been in the younger age group and many did not have aggressive therapy.[21] Supposedly, factors other than the treatment given have been of major importance in such cases.[14] From our own experience,[13] based on a series of 220 children over one year of age at diagnosis, 30 percent of all such children have radiographic evidence of bone metastases at the time of diagnosis, and the overall survival is about 18 percent.

In the cases with widespread dissemination, therefore, radiotherapy is administered with palliative intent and directed to control local symptoms. These local symptoms include pain, bowel or bladder obstruction (in patients with intra-abdominal primary tumors, intra-abdominal metastases, or both, respiratory distress (in patients with intrathoracic primary neoplasms or extensions into the thorax), and symptoms of cord compression (in patients with intraspinal extension from metastatic disease to vertebral bodies or paravertebral soft tissues).

At times, it has been thought appropriate to remove the main mass of the primary tumor even in patients with widespread dissemination. In this way, rapid relief of local symptoms can be obtained and lower doses of irradiation might be effective when fewer cells are present, especially the hypoxic component. However, our own experience indicates that removal of the "bulk" mass, especially in those with stage IV disease, has no relation to overall survival.[9,11,12] Those stage IV patients who have had surgical extirpation of their tumor, followed by high dose irradiation and systemic chemotherapy, showed no improvement in overall survival despite such aggressive management.

Palliative doses of radiotherapy vary from 200 rads, in one treatment, to 600 rads in three elapsed days in the average patient. However, as many as 2,000 rads in five days may be required for relief of bone pain, symptoms and signs of localized or diffuse intracranial metastases, diminution in size of unsightly scalp masses, and control of intra-abdominal tumor. In the latter instance, when large areas of the abdomen must be included in the portal for palliative radiation therapy, the daily dose must be adjusted to take into account the volume subtended. Control of symptoms and reduction in the size of masses may be dramatic and of great importance in patient comfort.

RECOMMENDATIONS

The radiotherapeutic management of neuroblastoma is difficult to assess at the present time. The role of radiation therapy, on the basis of past experience, has been described. However, in view of the present understanding of the survival patterns in early stages of disease, and in the special category of stage IV-S disease (especially in patients under one year of age), one hesitates to relate directly the use of radiation therapy to the local tumor site for local control and ultimate survival.

Radiotherapy causes secondary effects on normal tissues, including the effects on growing bone, such as the vertebral spinal column, the physiologic disturbance of liver[22] and lung,[23] and possibly secondary oncogenic disturbances following radiation therapy.[24] Because of these adverse side effects of radiotherapy, hopefully, there

will come a time when radiation therapy may be definitively excluded from the management of certain patients with neuroblastoma.
However, at this time, it is suggested that radiotherapy be employed
in all patients other than those very young patients who have had
total extirpation of the primary tumor (stage I). Radiotherapy is used
in all other patients in stages I, II and III, the total dose being adjusted
to the age of the patient. Care must be taken to exclude as much
normal tissue as is possible from the radiation beam, and tolerance of
normal tissue should not exceed the doses cited.

Radiotherapy might be withheld from patients with stage IV-S
disease and the patient followed carefully. For example, should the
liver be involved as part of the stage IV-S presentation, treatment is
not given unless the liver size fails to show evidence of regression or
at least stabilization. Irradiation is then delivered in relatively low
dosage, such as 1,200 rads in eight days, in the hope that regression
might thus be initiated and then proceed to complete resolution.

REFERENCES

1. Evans, A.E., D'Angio, G.J., and Randolph, J.: A proposed
staging for children with neuroblastoma. *Cancer* 27: 374–378, 1971.

2. Perez, C.A., Vietti, T.J., Ackerman, L.V., et al.: Treatment of
malignant sympathetic tumors in children: clinicopathological correlation. *Pediatrics* 41: 452–462, 1968.

3. Seaman, W.B., and Eagleton, M.D.: Radiation therapy of
neuroblastoma. *Radiology* 68: 1–7, 1957.

4. Wittenborg, M.H.: Roentgen therapy in neuroblastoma.
Radiology 54: 670–688, 1950.

5. Dyke, P.C., and Mulkey, D.A.: Maturation of ganglioneuroblastoma in ganglioneuroma. *Cancer* 20: 1343–1349, 1967.

6. Goldman, R.L., Winterling, A.N., and Winterling, C.C.:
Maturation of tumors of the sympathetic nervous system. *Cancer* 18:
1510–1516, 1965.

7. Farber, S.: Neuroblastoma. *Amer. J. Dis. Child.* 60: 749–
750, 1940.

8. Koop, C.E., and Hernandez, J.R.: Neuroblastoma: Experience with 100 cases in children. *Surgery* 56: 726–733, 1964.

9. Koop, C.E. and Johnson, D.G.: Neuroblastoma: An Assessment of therapy in reference to staging. *J. Pediatr. Surg.* 6: 595–
599, 1971.

10. D'Angio, G.J., Evans, E.A., and Koop, C.D.: A special pattern of neuroblastoma associated with a favorable prognosis. *Lancet* 1: 1046–1949, 1971.

11. Gross, R.E., Farber, S., and Martin, L.W.: Neuroblastoma sympatheticum; A study and report of 217 cases. *Pediatrics* 23: 1179–1191, 1959.

12. Filler, R.M., Traggis, D.G., Jaffe, N., and Vawter, G.F.: Favorable outlook for children with mediastinal neuroblastoma. *J. Pediatr. Surg.* 7: 136–143, 1972.

13. Tefft, M., and Wittenborg, M.H.: Radiotherapeutic management of neuroblastoma in childhood. *J.A.M.A.* 205: 159–160, 1968.

14. Hellstrom, I., Hellstrom, K.E., Bill, A.H., et al.: Studies on cellular immunity to human neuroblastoma cells. *Int. J. Cancer* 6: 172–188, 1970.

15. Tefft, M.: Radiation effect on growing bone and cartilage. *Frontiers of Radiation Therapy and Oncology* 6: 289–311, 1972.

16. Boden, G.: Radiation myelitis of the cervical spinal cord. *Brit. J. Radiol.* 21: 464–469, 1948.

17. Pallis, C.A., Louis, S., and Morgan, R.L.: Radiation Myelopathy. *Brain* 84: 460–479, 1961.

18. Mitus, A., Tefft, M., and Fellers, F.X.: Long term follow-up of renal functions of 108 children who underwent nephrectomy for malignant disease. *Pediatrics* 44: 912–921, 1969.

19. Nahhas, W.A., Nisce, L.Z., D'Angio, G.J., and Lewis, J.J. Jr.: Lateral ovarian transposition. *Obstet. Gynecol.* 38: 785–788, 1971.

20. Tefft, M., Mitus, A., and Schultz, M.D.: Initial high dose irradiation for metastases causing spinal cord compression in children. *Amer. J. Roentgenol.* 106: 385–393, 1969.

21. Reilley, D., Nesbit, M.E., and Krivit, W.: Cure of three patients who had skeletal metastases in disseminated neuroblastoma. *Pediatrics* 41: 47–51, 1968.

22. Tefft, M., Mitus, A., Vawter, G.F., and Filler, R.M.: Irradiation of the liver in children; review of the experience in the acute and chronic phases and in the intact normal and partially resected. *Amer. J. Roentgenol.* 108: 365–385, 1970.

23. Phillips, T.L., and Margolis, L.: Radiation pathology and the clinical response of lung and esophagus. *Frontiers of Radiation Therapy and Oncology* 6: 254–273, 1972.

24. Tefft, M., Vawter, G.F., and Mitus, A.: Secondary primary neoplasms in children. *Amer. J. Roentgenol.* 103: 800–822, 1968.

12 Chemotherapy of Neuroblastoma

John T. Truman, M.D.

1. Early trials of chemotherapy
2. Results of recent studies
3. Treatment according to probability of cure
4. Summary and conclusions

The chemotherapy of neuroblastoma has been a confusing and disappointing problem over the past quarter-century. It is *confusing* because of the difficulty in differentiating beneficial chemotherapeutic effect from the benign natural history of the tumor in certain infants; it is *disappointing* because of the failure to improve the overall cure rate. At best the mean survival of older children with metastatic disease is presently 18 months,[1] roughly equal to the survival in childhood leukemia a decade ago.

Cure for the large number of children who are more than one year of age at the time of diagnosis and who have metastatic disease is still anecdotal in 1975. This situation has not changed since Harvey Cushing reviewed the biopsy material from a 21-month-old boy who survived a paravertebral neuroblastoma with possible cerebellar metastases in 1911, and went on to have a successful laminectomy with removal of a benign ganglioneuroma in 1921.[2] The mechanism

263

of cure for the infant less than one year of age is as poorly understood now as it was 40 years ago, although cures are distinctly more predictable than they were when Lehman reported the successful removal of an adrenal neuroblastoma from an 11-month-old in 1916[3] and noted his continuing freedom from tumor in 1932.[4]

EARLY TRIALS OF CHEMOTHERAPY

The chemotherapy of neuroblastoma (Table 1) began with the use of nitrogen mustard during the mid 1940s, when two children showed transient responses of several weeks' duration and survivals of 10 and 16 months.[5] The value of alkylating agents continued to be shown with the demonstration of partial remissions in five out of nine patients receiving triethylene phosphoramide[6] and three out of five patients receiving nitromin.[7]

The advent of cyclophosphamide with its greater ease of administration facilitated larger studies with results which have contributed to its remaining a mainstay of present-day chemotherapy. A beneficial effect was first noted in 1961,[8] and by 1964 Thurman demonstrated a response in 19 out of 24 patients with disseminated disease.[9] Of these, 10 had a "good response," but 2 of the 3 with remissions of greater than 16 months were under one year of age. The dosage schedule used was 5 mg/kg given intravenously daily for 10 days, and continued orally at 2.5 mg/kg/day thereafter. Leukopenia occurred in 42 percent, gastrointestinal symptoms in 46 percent, hyperpigmentation in 19 percent, and hemorrhagic cystitis in only

Table 1
Drugs That Have Been Effectively Used in Chemotherapy of Neuroblastoma

1. Drugs of historical interest
   Nitrogen mustard
   Triethylene Phosphoramide
   Nitromen

2. Drugs in current use
   Cyclophosphamide
   Vincristine
   Daunorubicin
   Adriamycin

3. Promising new agents
   Acetylenic carbamate
   Imidazole carboxamide
   Ifosphamide

one child. No attempt was made to show that this therapy improved the cure rate, as only two children in the over one year group still showed response at 13 and 16 months. Presumably, however, the overall survival was prolonged.

Vincristine was first shown to be effective against neuroblastoma in 1961,[10] and by 1966 Windmiller[11] demonstrated a response in 3 out of 13 patients with disseminated disease. This was confirmed by Selawry[12] in 1968 with responses in 18 out of 33 patients, 4 with complete remissions and 5 with partial remissions. The mean duration of response was 3.5 months; the age of the 4 long-term responders was not recorded.

Combination chemotherapy with cyclophosphamide and vincristine was first reported by James[13] in 1965 showing a response in nine out of nine patients, with seven being complete, three of the children being older than two years at onset. Further data from the same institution reported by Pinkel[14] in 1968 analyzed the outcome with this older age group and showed a median survival of 13 months in six patients with metastatic disease. This was a clear improvement over the 6-month median survival of an analogous group of children who were not treated with cyclophosphamide and vincristine.[14] Nevertheless, the final outcome remained the same in both series, with all children expiring. Of five children below the age of two years, however, four were living without evidence of disease for one to five years. The dosage schedule used was vincristine 1.5 mg/m^2 alternating at weekly intervals with cyclophosphamide 300 mg/m^2 for one year given intravenously.

Less encouraging results using vincristine and cyclophosphamide were then published from the three major pediatric cooperative chemotherapy study groups. From the Children's Cancer Study Group A, Evans[15] reported responses in only 6 out of 22 children over one year of age with metastatic disease. These responses lasted only seven months. Similar poor results were obtained from a later larger study.[16] From the Southwest Cancer Chemotherapy Study Group, Sullivan[17] reported responses in only 8 out of 21 children (all ages). These responses lasted a median of only three months.

From the Acute Leukemia Group B, Sawitsky[18] reported responses in 26 out of 48 children (all ages). The median survival time for responders was 427 days compared to 126 days for nonresponders, an increment of ten months. The overall median survival was eight months which improved significantly on the untreated survival time of only four months.[19] However, with the exception of two children, age three months and fifteen months at onset, all patients died. This comprehensive study compared various regimens of vincristine and cyclophosphamide: sequential vs. concurrent, and alternate week combined therapy with high vs. low dosages. No differences were noted among any of the protocols except the toxicity was least with low dose cyclophosphamide. This dosage schedule called for vincristine 1.5 mg/m² plus cyclophosphamide 300 mg/m² given together every other week.

RESULTS OF RECENT STUDIES

Interest in the role of daunorubicin was raised by Tan's report[20] of responses in 6 out of 15 children older than one year of age, though no response lasted longer than five months. A similar response rate of 40 percent was confirmed by Samuels,[21] though not by Sutow,[22] who showed only a minor anti-tumor effect in 3 out of 29 patients. Helson[1] added daunorubicin to the combination of vincristine and cyclophosphamide and achieved a mean survival of 18 months in 11 children over two years of age and 9 children under two. Of those over two years, only two failed to show some response, and although all patients ultimately died, these figures are the best to date. The dosage schedule is as follows:

1. Vincristine 2.0 mg/m² on days 1, 8, and 33
2. Cyclophosphamide 1,000 mg/m² on days 1 and 33
3. Daunorubicin 45 mg/m² on days 15, 17, and 19
4. Rest 3 to 10 weeks depending on age and stage

Currently this regimen has shown the best results, although it cannot be recommended for general use because of the investigational status of daunorubicin, which has not yet been cleared by the Federal Drug Administration (FDA).

The search for more effective chemotherapeutic agents has been disappointing. Conventional agents such as methotrexate, 6-mercaptopurine, and actinomycin-D have only occasionally shown any effect and have been abandoned. Newer agents which have shown some promise are acetylenic carbamate,[23] imidazole carboxamide,[24] adriamycin,[25] and ifosfamide.[26] It is doubtful, however, if any of these individually will be of highly predictable value. The search for a specific agent will thus continue. More effective combinations of the agents already at hand are being sought, and will be the subject of future publications from the various cooperative study groups and larger chemotherapy centers. For example, the Southwest Cancer Chemotherapy Study Group is currently investigating a combination of prednisone, vincristine, cyclophosphamide, actinomycin-D, and daunorubicin.[24] In a similar fashion Evans[24] has suggested a program of non-cell-cycle specific agents to increase the percentage of dividing cells and thus enhance the subsequent use of cell-specific agents.

TREATMENT ACCORDING TO PROBABILITY OF CURE

An equally urgent and unresolved question is whom to treat or not to treat with chemotherapy when the prognosis is often unpredictable. Much order has been brought to this chaotic problem by the proposal of a new staging system which recognizes a special stage IV-S category which has remarkably good prognosis.[27,28] This staging system was outlined in Chapter 1, Figure 4. By classifying 134 children from the Children's Hospital of Philadelphia and 112 children from the Children's Cancer Study Group A (CCSGA), Beslow and McCann were able to construct two-year survival curves which reflect the influence of age and stage on outcome.[29] (This is shown in Chapter 10, Figure 4.) It is worth noting that these curves were drawn by matching the Philadelphia cases between the years 1947 and 1967 with the CCSGA cases between 1966 and 1968. Even though the Philadelphia cases were treated in a much less vigorous fashion, with less radiation therapy and less chemotherapy, the data suggested that therapy appeared to have little effect upon ultimate survival, at least up to 1968.

The decision to begin chemotherapy could be based on the above survival probabilities, although no firm rules have been established as yet. It seems reasonable to state that a child who has less than a 50 percent chance of cure should receive maximum chemotherapy. Risks are taken and the suffering of the child is considerable, but the probability is high that his life will be prolonged, and the possibility exists that his chance of cure will be increased—though this latter point has not been proved. Thus, the Helson regimen,[1] outlined above, could be used, or a combination of vincristine plus cyclophosphamide. A readily administered schedule is as follows:

1. Vincristine 1.5 mg/m² given intravenously every week for 8 doses

2. Cyclophosphamide 300 mg/m² given intravenously every week for 8 doses, cyclophosphamide is then continued at the same dose orally for two years.

Children who have less than a 50 percent cure probability are those with stage II disease and over two years of age, stage III disease and over one year of age, or stage IV disease at all ages.

Children who have a very high probability of cure should not receive chemotherapy because of the unpredictable adverse side effects. How high a probability should be accepted, likewise, remains to be defined, and perhaps should be resolved by each physician according to his personal philosophy and experience. It seems reasonable to select a figure of 90 percent probability of cure. In this case children who should not receive chemotherapy would be those with: stage I disease up to age one year, stage II disease identified at birth, or stage IV-S disease up to age three months.

There then remains a category of children whose prognosis is neither excellent nor poor, and who have a 50 to 90 percent probability of cure. There are no data to prove that chemotherapy will be of value, although most chemotherapists are cautiously optimistic that it will. Certainly it is of vital importance in this gray area to do no harm; thus any program of chemotherapy must be given with caution as to the immediate and long-term effects. Vincristine may be a better choice than cyclophosphamide because it is less suppressive of both the bone marrow and immunologic defense mechanisms. Cyclophosphamide has the added potential hazard of long-term effects on the male gonads.[30,31] A reasonable dosage schedule for vincristine is 1.5 mg/m² given intravenously every week for eight doses. Children who have a 50 to 90 percent cure probability are those with stage I disease and over one year of age, stage II disease beyond the neonatal period to two years of age, and stage IV-S with bone marrow involvement. Stage IV-S without bone marrow involvement presents a very interesting problem for which a strong argument has been made by D'Angio that no chemotherapy be given.[28] Out of 25 cases reviewed, the two-year survival was 84 percent. Out of 20 infants only two died, both from infection secondary to chemotherapy-related leukopenia. It thus appears preferable to observe the natural history of stage IV-S disease (without bone marrow involvement), and withhold chemotherapy unless the disease continues to advance in spite of surgery and radiotherapy.

An interesting historical post-script concerns the use of vitamin B₁₂ in the treatment of neuroblastoma. This was first reported in detail by Bodian in 1959.[32] Bodian's hypothesis was that vitamin B_{12} might hasten the maturation of neuroblastoma to ganglioneuroma, or otherwise facilitate physiologic tumor lysis. Further data[33] on the original group of patients showed no improvement over those who did not receive vitamin B_{12}, and it appeared that those children who had responded were primarily infants in whom natural regression could be predicted in a similar percentage. A similar failure of vitamin B_{12} to improve upon the natural remission rate was reported by Sawitsky.[34]

SUMMARY AND CONCLUSIONS

In no other childhood tumor is accurate staging at the onset more important because of the tendency of neuroblastoma to undergo spontaneous regression. The choice of chemotherapeutic agents must be made on the basis of achieving maximum anti-tumor effect, as well as causing the least harm. Currently the most effective drugs are cyclophosphamide and vincristine, plus daunorubicin where available. Hopefully, a balanced treatment program tailored to age and stage will result in improved survival statistics by recognizing the relative advantages of endogenous versus exogenous tumor lysis.

REFERENCES

1.   Helson, L., Vanichayangkul, P., Tan, C.C., et al.: Combination intermittent chemotherapy for patients with disseminated neuroblastoma. *Cancer Chemother. Rep.* 56: 499, 1972.

2.   Cushing, H., and Wolbach, S.B.: The transformation of a malignant paravertebral sympathicoblastoma into a benign ganglioneuroma. *Amer. J. Path.* 3: 203, 1927.

3.   Lehman, E.P.: Neuroblastoma; with report of a case. *J. Med. Res.* 31: 309, 1917.

4.   Lehman, E.P.: Adrenal neuroblastoma in infancy; 15 year survival. *Amer. Surg.* 95: 473, 1932.

5.   Jacobson, L.O., Spurr, C.L., Barron, E. et al.: Nitrogen mustard therapy. *J.A.M.A.* 132: 263, 1946.

6.   Farber, S., Appleton, R., Downing, V., et al.: Clinical studies on the carcinolytic action of triethylene phosphoramide (TEPA). *Cancer* 6: 135–146, 1953.

7. Farber, S., Toch, R., Sears, E.M., and Pinkel, D.: Advances in chemotherapy of cancer in man. *Advances in Cancer Res.* 4: 2, 1956.

8. Kontras, S.B., and Newton, W.A.: Cyclophosphamide therapy of childhood neuroblastoma. Preliminary report. *Cancer Chemother. Rep.* 12: 39, 1961.

9. Thurman, W.G., Fernbach, D.J., and Sullivan, M.P.: Cyclophosphamide therapy in childhood neuroblastoma. *N.Engl. J. Med.* 270: 1336, 1964.

10. Selawry, O.S., and Hananian, J.: Vincristine treatment on cancer in children. *J.A.M.A.* 183: 741, 1963.

11. Windmiller, J., Berry, D.H., Haddy, T.B., et al.: Vincristine sulfate in the treatment of neuroblastoma in children. *Amer. J. Dis. Child.* 111: 75, 1966.

12. Selawry, O.S., Holland, J.F., and Wolman, I.J.: Effect of vincristine on malignant solid tumors in children. *Cancer Chemother. Rep.* 52: 497, 1968.

13. James, D.H., Hustu, W., Wrenn, E.L., and Pinkel, D.: Combination chemotherapy of childhood neuroblastoma. *J.A.M.A.* 194: 123, 1965.

14. Pinkel, D., Pratt, C., Holton, C., et al.: Survival of children with neuroblastoma treated with combination chemotherapy. *J. Pediatr.* 73: 928, 1968.

15. Evans, A.E., Heyn, R.M., Newton, W.A., and Leikin, S.L.: Vincristine sulfate and cyclophosphamide for children with metastatic neuroblastoma. *J.A.M.A.* 207: 1325, 1969.

16. Leikin, S., Evans, A., Heyn, R., and Newton, W.A.: The Impact of chemotherapy on advanced neuroblastoma; survival of patients diagnosed in 1956, 1962, and 1966–68 in Children's Cancer Study Group A. *J. Pediatr.* 84: 131–134, 1974.

17. Sullivan, M.P., Nora, A.H., Kulapongs, P., et al.: Evaluation of vincristine sulfate and cyclophosphamide chemotherapy for metastatic neuroblastoma. *Pediatrics* 44: 685, 1969.

18. Sawitsky, A.: Vincristine and cyclophosphamide therapy in generalized neuroblastoma. *Amer. J. Dis. Child.* 119: 308, 1970.

19. Bodian, M.: Neuroblastoma. *Arch. Dis. Childh.* 38: 606, 1963.

20. Tan, C., Tasaka, H., Yu, K-P, et al.: Daunomycin, an antitumor antibiotic in the treatment of neoplastic disease. *Cancer* 20: 333, 1967.

21. Samuels, L.D., Newton, W.A., and Heyn, R.: Daunorubicin therapy in advanced neuroblastoma. *Cancer* 27: 831, 1971.

22. Sutow, W.W., Fernbach, D.J., Thurman, W.G., et al.: Daunomycin in the treatment of metastatic neuroblastoma. *Cancer Chemother. Rep.* 54: 283, 1970.

23. Pratt, C.B., and Wang, J.J.: Acetylenic carbamate in childhood cancer. *Cancer* 27: 109, 1971.

24. Evans, A.E.: Treatment of neuroblastoma. *Cancer* 30: 1595, 1972.

25. Acute Leukemia Group B protocol #7141. Unpublished data.

26. Acute Leukemia Group B protocol #7341. Unpublished data.

27. Evans, A.E., D'Angio, G.J., and Randolph, J.: A proposed staging system for children with neuroblastoma. *Cancer* 27: 374, 1971.

28. D'Angio, G.J., Evans, A.E., and Koop, C.E.: Special pattern of widespread neuroblastoma with a favorable prognosis. *Lancet* 1: 1046, 1971.

29. Breslow, N., and McCann, B.: Statistical estimation of prognosis for children with neuroblastoma. *Cancer Res.* 31: 2098, 1971.

30. Fairley, K.F., Barrie, J.U., and Johnson, W.: Sterility and testicular atrophy related to cyclophosphamide therapy. *Lancet* 1: 568, 1972.

31. Kumar, R., Biggart, J.D., McEvoy, J., and McGeown, M.G.: Cyclophosphamide and reproductive function. *Lancet* 1: 1212, 1972.

32. Bodian, M.: Neuroblastoma. *Pediatr. Clin. N. Amer.* 6: 449, 1959.

33. Langman, M.J.S.: Treatment of neuroblastoma with vitamin B_{12}. *Arch. Dis. Childh.* 45: 385, 1970.

34. Sawitsky, A., and Desposito, F.: A survey of American experience with vitamin B_{12} therapy in neuroblastoma. *J. Pediatr.* 67: 99, 1965.

13 Prognosis: The Biological Vagaries of Neuroblastoma

Carl Pochedly, M.D.

Introduction
1. Criteria for definition of cure
2. Spontaneous regression
3. Factors that affect prognosis
   a. Age and stage at diagnosis
   b. Presence of metastases
   c. Location of the primary tumor
   d. Degree of histological differentiation of the tumor
   e. Immunological status
   f. Therapy
4. Late recurrence of tumor and other problems in prolonged survivors
   Summary and conclusions

Neuroblastoma has a sinister reputation because widespread metastases often are present at diagnosis or develop soon thereafter. There can be no doubt that the outlook for patients with neuroblastoma is very grave. For example, in the Memorial Center series of 135 cases only 14 patients, or 10.4 percent, showed prolonged survival.[1] There are many factors which may help determine prognosis in children with neuroblastoma (Figure 1). The factors which appear to give a favorable prognosis are:

1. Onset or diagnosis at less than one year of age
2. Absence of metastases or limitation to regional lymph nodes
3. Primary tumor located extra-abdominally
4. Partial or total resectability of the primary tumor
5. Histological differentiation of the tumor

273

In one series, 41 patients had three or more of these prognostically favorable factors; of these, 27 (66 percent) showed prolonged survival.[2]

CRITERIA FOR DEFINITION OF CURE

The clinical course of neuroblastoma is much more accelerated than that of many adult tumors. Survival beyond an interval of time when most incurable patients would have died has been used to gauge treatment efficacy. Thus, for neuroblastomas, as for several childhood neoplasms, 14 months[3,4] to 24 months[5] has been used rather than the five-year period common in adult cancer statistics. Collins[6] proposed another method based on the assumption that there is a constant rate of tumor cell division. He thus defined a period of

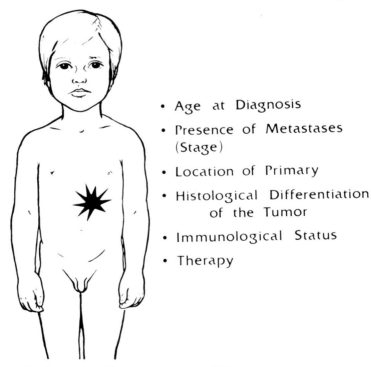

- Age at Diagnosis
- Presence of Metastases (Stage)
- Location of Primary
- Histological Differentiation of the Tumor
- Immunological Status
- Therapy

Figure 1. Factors that affect prognosis in the child with neuroblastoma. "Location of the primary" affects prognosis in that extra-adrenal tumors are usually diagnosed before distant metastases have occurred. "Immunological status" is still an ill-defined concept.

risk beyond which recurrence would be unlikely. This was defined as an interval of time equal to the age of the patient at diagnosis plus nine months, the latent period allowing for a theoretical possibility that the tumor grew from the moment of conception and through fetal life. In comparative studies, the two-year survival rate seems to give data similar to that derived from the Collins "period of risk," and may be used as a definition of prolonged survival.[7]

SPONTANEOUS REGRESSION

It is well known that neuroblastomas undergo spontaneous regression more commonly than any other human cancer, most often by disappearance of the neoplastic cells and rarely by maturation into benign ganglioneuromas.[8,9] Spontaneous regression may even occur after metastasis to bone.[10] Dramatic responses to x-ray therapy or chemotherapy, or both, in cases of immature and clinically inoperable tumors are not rare. Maturation to ganglioneuroma is also observed at the sites of metastases.

A three-month-old girl presented with a massive abdominal tumor, arising from the right lumbar region. Microscopic examination of a biopsy specimen showed a typical neuroblastoma. Although no treatment was given, spontaneous regression occurred and resulted in maturation of the tumor to a small ganglioneuroma found at necropsy examination at the age of ten years. Death was due to urinary infection due to a persistent neurogenic bladder.[11] This is one of many examples of spontaneous disappearance of neuroblastoma with maturation to ganglioneuroma.[12-17] In addition, symptomatic ganglioneuromas may occur in children showing prolonged survival following successful therapy of a neuroblastoma.[18] The possibility of maturation of a neuroblastoma into a ganglioneuroma is one of the most intriguing features of this tumor. Maturation of neuroblastomas may occur in those originating either in the adrenal gland or in extra-adrenal sites.

On the other hand, a neuroblastoma showing histologic evidence of this transformation, even in a major proportion of its volume, may still progress to widespread metastases and death.[19] A neuroblastoma which transformed into a ganglioneuroma was well studied by the use of large histological sections. This technique allowed the observation of the actual transformation of one element into the other. Despite extensive therapy and despite the presence of large areas of maturation, the child died with widespread neuroblastoma metastases. There is a need to study such cases in detail, in order to elucidate the factors involved in the intriguing question of maturation of neuroblastomas.[19,20]

Spontaneous regression and maturation into benign tumor are part of the extraordinary biological behavior of neuroblastoma.[21] The reasons for spontaneous regression of this tumor remain speculative, but there can be no doubt that it exists. Laboratory evidence of tumor-host interaction is being accumulated, but it remains to be shown why children with this syndrome develop especially potent mechanisms for tumor rejection, if factors of this kind are indeed responsible for tumor disappearance.[22]

FACTORS THAT AFFECT PROGNOSIS

Age and Stage at Time of Diagnosis

The age of the patient at the onset of symptoms or at diagnosis is generally accepted as one of the most important factors in assessing prognosis of neuroblastomas. Thus, the younger the patient, the better the chance of survival (Figure 2). In addition, the frequency of incidental (in situ) neuroblastomas in children under three months of age far exceeds the clinical occurrence of these tumors.[23,24] The vast majority of these tumors must disappear or mature to benign forms with age.

It is common experience that children less than two years old have a better survival rate than older patients, but the reason for this is not known. The over-all survival rate is inversely proportional to age. In patients less than one year old the survival rate is 60 to 82 percent; in those between one and two years old the survival rate is 20 to 31 percent; and in children over two years old only 5 to 13 percent survive.[9,25,26,27] In another series, 50 percent of children who showed prolonged survival were under two years of age and one-third were less than one year of age at the time of diagnosis.[2] The number of survivors drops steadily as children get older and a child over eight years of age at time of diagnosis rarely shows prolonged survival.

It should be emphasized that age and stage are independent variables in assessing prognosis in neuroblastoma. Therefore, survival rate for stage I tumors is higher than for cases with a more advanced stage at time of diagnosis, even for infants. But age under one year is associated with high survival rates regardless of location of the primary tumor or degree of histological differentiation of the tumor.[2] The preponderant influence of age presents an interesting paradox for which an adequate explanation is lacking. It seems well established that spontaneous "maturation" to more benign forms is a function of the increasing age of the cells. Although cell maturation apparently occurs more and more completely with advancing age, spontaneous regression is virtually unknown in tumors appearing after the age of two years.

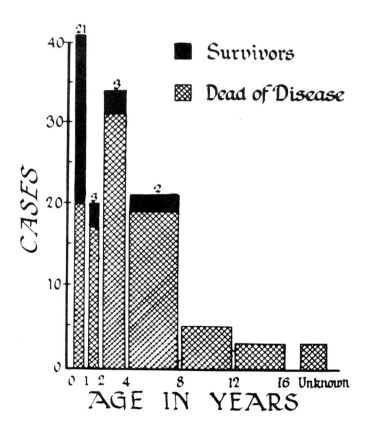

Figure 2. Graph showing the relation of age at diagnosis and prolonged survival of children with neuroblastoma. (Courtesy of Dr. R. Swank and *Annals of Surgery*[2])

Except for patients with stage IV-S disease, the prognosis for the youngest children is proportional to the stage at diagnosis. The prognosis for older children is poor because of the very frequent presence of metastases. In Horn's series[28] the average age of the children showing prolonged survival was 7.5 months at the time of diagnosis while the average age of the fatal cases was 32 months at the time of diagnosis. Similar average ages for fatal and surviving cases at the time of diagnosis were reported in other series.[29] Spontaneous regression occurs in about 1 percent of cases, but it is extremely rare for spontaneous regression to occur in a tumor that first appeared in a child older than two years of age. Neuroblastomas which appear after the age of four years are associated with a much worse prognosis than those appearing before the age of two years.[29]

The relationship of age to prognosis in children with neuroblastoma was studied by Sutow in 292 patients.[30] The patients were arbitrarily divided into two age groups: those two years or younger at the time of diagnosis and those over two years of age. Prognosis was measured in terms of survival for 14 months or longer following diagnosis. Forty percent of children less than two years of age with neuroblastoma survived for at least 14 months irrespective of therapy and other factors. In contrast to this, only 7.5 percent of children over the age of two years survived 14 months or longer.[30] In another series the prolonged survival rate for 67 infants less than one year old was 60 percent; for 29 children between one and two years old it was 21 percent; for 78 children two to six years old it was 10 percent; and for the 38 children over seven years old only 8 percent showed prolonged survival.[7] These data clearly indicate that the occurrence of prolonged survival is related to age. Chances of prolonged survival were definitely good among those two years of age or younger and definitely poor in the older age group.

From statistical evaluation of survival data of children with neuroblastoma, two conclusions seem justified: (1) prognosis is poor among the older age group because metastases are nearly always present at the time of diagnosis and (2) age and stage are independent factors in assessing prognosis. Age less than one year and/or stage I disease carry a high survival rate.

Presence of Metastases (Special Features)

Metastatic spread is found at the time of diagnosis in 55 to 70 percent of children with neuroblastoma. Bone, liver, and lymph nodes are the most frequent sites of metastases. Eleven survivors with lymph node metastases were studied in one series. Nine were under a year of age. Eight had extra-abdominal primary lesions, and eight had metastases confined to lymph nodes. Surgical treatment seemed to play a relatively unimportant part in survival in the face of lymph node metastases. Six survivors had had only biopsy of the primary tumor, while the other five had partial or complete removal of the primary lesion.[2] There were only three survivors among 40 children with neuroblastoma who had hepatic metastases at surgery. No patient with pulmonary, renal, or cranial metastases survived.[2]

Bone metastases Metastases to bone are associated with a very poor prognosis, especially in children over one year old.[10] In one series, 20 patients had x-ray evidence of osseous metastases and only two showed prolonged survival. Eighteen of these had negative bone marrow aspirates. Of 37 other cases with positive bone marrow smears as well as bony metastases by x-ray, only one patient survived.[2]

Presence of tumor cells in the bone marrow and x-ray evidence of cortical involvement of bone both imply a very poor prognosis.[31] In one series, 50 cases had positive bone marrow smears and none survived.[32] Others have reported occasional survivors after proof of marrow metastases. Fifty-one patients in Swank's series had positive bone marrow smears, three of whom survived.[2] On the other hand, 23 out of 69 patients with negative bone marrow smears survived.

It is important to emphasize the difference between bone marrow smears positive for "tumor cells" and x-ray evidence of bone involvement.[33] Evans and Hummeler pointed out that "positive" bone marrow smears (stage IV-S) may not mean the presence of true neuroblastoma cells. Instead, what appear to be neuroblasts in these cases may actually be sheets of normal lymphoblasts (immunoblasts). Thus, there may be a vast difference in prognostic significance between the finding of abnormal bone marrow cytology and the finding of skeletal lesions on x-ray examination.

While the prognosis is poor when there are bony metastases, it is by no means always hopeless; even in the presence of local extension of the tumor or presence of multiple bony metastases prolonged survival may still occur.[1] Long-term survival with disseminated skeletal metastases due to neuroblastoma was reported by Reilly et al. who added their 3 cases to 10 others who survived longer than two years after the development of metastatic osseous lesions.[20] A review of the cases did not reveal a specific treatment regimen which could have accounted for the prolonged survival. The presence of skeletal involvement, therefore, should not indicate a hopeless prognosis.[20,34,35]

Neuroblastoma metastases in bone of patients with prolonged survival may show any of three patterns of evolution: There may be either (1) complete disappearance of neuroblastoma, (2) maturation of neuroblastoma to the less anaplastic ganglioneuroma, or (3) persistence of nonproliferating, metastatic osseous foci of neuroblastoma.[35]

Complete disappearance of osseous metastases was reported by Reilly and co-workers who described two infants presenting with metastatic neuroblastoma, but who were found to be free of tumor up to nine years following radiotherapy.[20] *Maturation* of neuroblastoma in soft tissue into ganglioneuroma has been well documented, but transformation of osseous metastases into ganglioneuromas has been reported infrequently. Kissane described a two-year-old child with a primary posterior mediastinal tumor metastatic to the ribs and vertebrae.[36] X-ray therapy was given to those sites with good response. The patient died of an unknown cause four years later and was found to have a ganglioneuroma in the posterior mediastinum with no evidence of bony metastases. In another case, a 6-month-old boy had a diagnosis of neuroblastoma established on the basis of a biopsy of a swelling over the left orbit. Subsequently, he was found to have a left-sided abdominal mass and multiple widespread bone involvement. The patient died of gastric hemorrhage at 22 years of age. At post-mortem examination, a ganglioneuroma was found in the retroperitoneal space at the site of a right adrenal gland. Other sites of ganglioneuroma were in one of the vertebrae and in a lymph node, indicating evidence of previous neuroblastoma metastases.[37]

Persistence of *non-proliferating* neuroblastoma in sites of bony metastases was shown by a 3-year-old child. He had extensive resection of an abdominal tumor and irradiation of the tumor bed despite the presence of a lesion in the roof of the left acetabulum. Subsequently, osteolytic defects developed in the entire vertebral axis, the ribs, the calvarium, and in the pelvic bones. Nine years later, at 12 years of age, the patient was asymptomatic in spite of evidence of widespread bony metastases. It would seem that in this particular child the neuroblastoma was in equilibrium with the host. Uncontrolled widespread growth of tumor occurred later.[35]

Two unfavorable prognostic signs, older age at onset and the presence of multiple bony metastases, appeared to be overcome for a long period of time in a patient who survived 17 years after diagnosis. A good host-tumor relationship was postulated by the authors.[39] Another patient was noted to have skull metastases at the age of 6 months which were treated by irradiation of the head. At the age of 17 months, partial resection of an abdominal mass was followed by abdominal radiotherapy. At the age of 24 months, an ulnar metastasis was identified and treated locally by irradiation. The patient remained asymptomatic for 6 years after diagnosis.[32]

Relation of metastases to survival The clinical behavior of most types of cancer has justified the assumption that the presence or absence of local and distant metastases influences survival. Wittenborg presented data to show that in neuroblastoma specifically there is a significant decrease in the rate of two-year survivals among those patients with demonstrable metastases at time of diagnosis as compared with the survival rate among those with no demonstrable metastatic lesions.[30]

In another study, pooled data were examined to evaluate, first, the relation of age to the incidence of metastases and, second, the relation of metastases to survival rate.[30] Not all the published reports contained satisfactorily detailed clinical information. It was assumed, however, that, unless specifically stated, reasonably similar diagnostic procedures had been instituted in all patients. From a total of seven studies data on 138 patients were tabulated. These figures indicated that a majority (73 percent) of the children already had evidence of metastases when first seen. The distribution of patients with metastases between the two age groups appeared to be at random. The occurrence of skeletal metastases, however, did show a significant relationship with age. The probability that the age distribution of skeletal metastases occurred by chance alone is extremely small. These data, therefore, indicate that at the time of diagnosis skeletal metastases were found significantly more often among the older age group than among those two years of age and younger.[30]

Survival is strongly influenced by the patient's age, stage, and perhaps by the degree of cell differentiation. Breslow and McCann analyzed data on 246 children with neuroblastoma.[27] Ninety-two percent of infants with Evans' stage I disease survived, tumor-free, two years from diagnosis, compared with only 3 percent of those over two years of age with stage IV disease. More than 50 percent of patients in their study had stage IV disease and, irrespective of age, only 6 percent survived two years without disease.

Variants of a linear logistic model were used to statistically analyze two-year survival proportions for these 246 children treated for neuroblastoma. The statistical analysis showed that age and stage of disease at diagnosis are both important factors in determining chances for survival, even after adjusting for the effects of the other (Figure 3). Estimation of prognosis is faciliated by curves relating the probability of survival to age (up to 5 years) for each of 5 stages.[27] The purpose of this study was to illustrate the joint effect on chances for survival of the two most prominent factors, age and stage of disease, by means of a detailed statistical analysis of a relatively large series of cases. This analysis permitted an assessment of the effect of extent of disease, while adjusting for, and at the same time getting at, the effect of age.[27] The plots of survival probability against age presented in Figure 3 offer a convenient means of estimating prognosis in neuroblastoma. They represent the best estimates possible from the two available series of data.[27]

The analysis by Sutow failed to show that stage of disease, as indicated by presence or absence of metastases, had a statistically

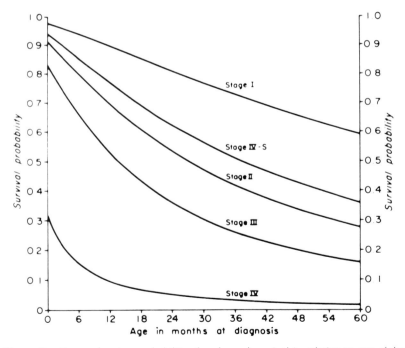

Figure 3. Curves showing probability of prolonged survival in relation to age of the child and stage of the neuroblastoma at the time of original diagnosis. (Courtesy of Dr. N. Breslow and *Cancer Research*[27])

significant effect on prognosis among patients two years or older at diagnosis. However, Breslow and McCann concluded that stage is important regardless of the age of the child at diagnosis. They believe that this discrepancy is due mainly to the fact that survival for the group of children with non-metastatic disease aged two years or older was about twice as high in their study.[27] However, the trend in the data of Sutow[38] was clearly in the direction of improved survival for those without metastatic disease. In view of the small number of patients in this category (about 40 in each study), the discrepancy may be more apparent than real.[27] Thus, age and stage both play important roles in determining prognosis, even after adjusting for the other factor.

It is important to note that children less than one year old, with distant metastatic neuroblastoma, may have a survival rate as high as 46 percent.[7] These infant survivors had primary tumors arising from the retroperitoneum, mediastinum, and unknown sites, and the metastases were confined to the liver or subcutaneous tissues. Of the 21 infants who died of distant metastases, three apparently had hepatic metastases only, and the other patients had intracranial, skeletal, or pulmonary metastases. There were two patients less than two years old with distant metastases whose tumors matured to ganglioneuroma, but they subsequently died of recurrent and metastatic neuroblastoma beyond the Collins period of risk.[7]

Two of 59 patients, with remote metastases in the two- to six-year-age group, were alive beyond the two-year interval after treatment. These patients had hepatic and bony metastases from mediastinal primary origin, and they were still alive without active disease at the end of Collins' period of risk.[7] Although the incidence of regional and distant metastases was less in the infant age group, compared to children older than two years, the prognosis in all stages of the disease is better in the infant age group.

Frequent prolonged survival in stage IV-S Children with widespread neuroblastoma are generally thought to have a poor prognosis. However, certain patterns of organ involvement, almost invariably lethal in other neoplastic diseases, are associated with a good prognosis with neuroblastoma. Specifically, very young patients with multiple nodules in the skin or the liver, or even presence of tumor cells in the bone marrow, have a surprisingly high rate of prolonged survival.[22]

In one study, 25 out of 234 children fulfilled the criteria given for stage IV-S (see Chapter 1). Twenty-one out of 25 of these patients (84 percent) survived for two years or longer. Several interesting facts emerge:

1. Most of the children with this constellation of findings were under 13 months of age (20 out of 25)
2. Of the 67 infants in the whole series 20 (30 percent) were in stage IV-S
3. The probability for prolonged survival is extremely good in infants with stage IV-S disease, especially when compared with survival for children with stages III and IV.[22]

The improved prognosis of patients in stage IV-S is apparently not related in any way to therapy. In fact, radiation therapy and chemotherapy may not be necessary in the management of these children.[22]

The unexpectedly high rate of prolonged survival of children with stage IV-S neuroblastoma makes one ask if these lesions are truly metastastic foci. The distribution of neuroblastoma foci in tissues not expected to produce a neuroblastoma favors their being metastases rather than multifocal sites of primary involvement. The frequent identification of free-floating tumor cells and clumps in the bone marrow of children with neuroblastoma indicates that neoplastic cells are circulating throughout the body, and supports the contention that the lesions represent metastases. It is nonetheless possible that the tumors represent multiple independent foci of disease. There are no known specific anlage in the skin or liver, but two possible mechanisms for the independent development of neuroblastoma in these sites can be postulated. First, there might be an abnormal distribution of neural-crest cells during embryonic life. Alternatively, the cells might undergo abnormal differentiation—for example, a primordial cell of neural-crest origin destined to become a skin melanoblast could aberrantly shift to a nerve-cell pattern of differentiation.[22]

The favorable response to therapy of children with stage IV-S neuroblastoma also may depend on unknown intrinsic factors of the host toward the tumor. Surgical excision of the tumor with adjunctive use of radiotherapy may aid in immunologic rejection by the host.[25] It is possible that an immune reaction from the organism against the tumor exists and that surgery or x-ray therapy may favorably alter the immunologic rejection of the tumor. On the other hand, enhanced anti-neuroblastoma immunity of the host, perhaps even initiated by the diffuse metastatic disease, rather than any therapy, may be responsible for the increased survival rate.[26]

Location of the Primary Tumor

The anatomic site of the primary tumor is another variable of prognostic importance in neuroblastoma (Figure 4). Production of symptoms or development of mass in readily apparent areas could lead to earlier diagnosis. It is also conceivable that the anatomic location affects the ease and degree of therapeutic attack on the tumor. It is doubtful that there are true differences in malignant behavior among neuroblastomas arising in different parts of the body. Stage, not location of the primary tumor, determines prognosis.[9]

Adrenal and non-adrenal abdominal neuroblastomas In the abdomen, where most neuroblastomas occur, Gross found 25 percent survival in adrenal tumors and 32 percent survival in extra-adrenal

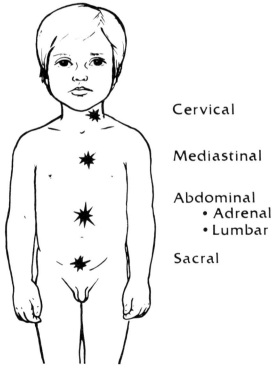

Cervical

Mediastinal

Abdominal
  • Adrenal
  • Lumbar

Sacral

Figure 4. Prognosis of neuroblastoma varies depending on the site of origin of the primary tumor. Adrenal or upper abdominal tumors have fewer prolonged survivors than neuroblastomas originating in the neck, chest, or pelvis. This observation is due to the fact that non-abdominal neuroblastomas are usually diagnosed before distant metastases have occurred.

primaries.[5] Similarly, Lingley observed 29 percent survival with adrenal neuroblastomas and 50 percent survival with extra-adrenal primaries.[39] Young observed no survivors in eight children with adrenal primaries, but three out of five with "lumbar" tumors survived.[40] However, since it is often impossible to distinguish adrenal from extra-adrenal abdominal neuroblastomas as to anatomic origin, these reports must be interpreted with caution.[2]

Non-abdominal neuroblastomas Patients with non-abdominal lesions have a much higher rate of prolonged survival than those with abdominal neuroblastomas. In one series, four out of five patients with cervical neuroblastomas survived, although only one of the tumors was completely excised. Eleven out of 16 patients with mediastinal neuroblastoma survived although only nine of the tumors could be completely excised. In another series, 9 out of 19 cases of cervical and mediastinal neuroblastoma survived.[9] All four patients with pelvic primary tumors survived, although only one had complete excision. On the other hand, only 8 of 89 children with abdominal neuroblastomas survived. Five of these survivors had complete tumor excision and six were under a year old at diagnosis.[2] The increased rate of survival in non-abdominal neuroblastomas is due to the fact that non-abdominal neuroblastomas are usually diagnosed before metastases have occurred.

Anatomic site of the primary tumor seems to have an effect on the course of neuroblastomas unrelated to age of the patient and the histologic pattern of the tumor. The primary sites with least evidence of spread at the time of the initial examination are the neck and the pelvis. Perhaps neuroblastomas in the neck are more likely to be circumscribed and, hence, completely removable and likely to be discovered earlier. As for those in the pelvis, which also seem to have a better prognosis, the reason may be that they tend to cause urinary obstruction and, hence, are also diagnosed and treated earlier. At any rate, prolonged survival following treatment of a neuroblastoma occurs most often when the tumor arises in sites other than in the abdomen.

The results of one study, however, did not support this conclusion. To investigate the relationship between tumor site and survival, the incidence of prolonged survivors in 230 children was tabulated for two anatomic divisions: "abdomen" and "extra-abdomen." It was concluded that the incidence of prolonged survivors was not significantly related to whether the primary tumor arose abdominally or extra-abdominally.[30] Subsequent studies[17,40] seem to have refuted this conclusion.

Mediastinal neuroblastomas A better prognosis has been observed in patients with mediastinal primaries, but once again the major influence may be age, since most of the survivors tend to be in the younger age group. Also there is a tendency for mediastinal tumors to be less undifferentiated; some investigators have been able to relate prognosis to the degree of histopathological differentiation.[41]

The site of origin of the primary tumor has been considered a factor that might influence survival in patients with neuroblastoma. In several reports, neuroblastomas arising in the mediastinum and neck appeared to be less malignant than those arising in the abdomen. In a recent series the results of treatment of 27 children with mediastinal neuroblastoma at one cancer center were reviewed by Filler et al.[17] The data derived from this series indicated that a neuroblastoma that arises in the mediastinum usually can be successfully treated.[17]

The most striking finding in this study of mediastinal neuroblastoma is the very low mortality rate that was observed. Although survival did decrease with the patient's age at diagnosis, this decrease was not nearly so striking as that seen in patients having neuroblastomas originating at other sites. No deaths occurred in 14 children with mediastinal neuroblastoma under one year of age, or in 19 children under two years. In children over two years of age, the survival rate was 50 percent. Overall survival of the 27 children in this series was 85 percent. Comparative survival statistics with 340 cases of neuroblastoma (all sites) seen at the same center during the same time period was 62 percent for children under one year of age, 16 percent for children over one year, 7 percent for children over two years, and 26 percent for the entire series.[17]

Survival in this series of children with mediastinal neuroblastoma is higher than that generally reported in other published series. In three combined series[3,7,42] the rate of prolonged survival was 37 out of 65 or 57 percent. Since the criteria for diagnosis of mediastinal neuroblastoma, the age of the patients, the presence of bone metastases at diagnosis, and treatment are not generally available in these reports, it is difficult to decide which factors might have been responsible for these differences in survival. However, one point of agreement deserves emphasis: In two series in which data are available, a total of 26 infants with mediastinal neuroblastoma under one year of age have been treated with 100 percent survival.[7,17] Thus, age less than one year is a very favorable prognostic factor. Evans' carefully studied series also confirmed these findings.[9]

Other than increasing age, the only clinical finding that seemed to affect prognosis adversely in Filler's series was the presence of bone metastases. Four out of five children with either microscopic or radiographic evidence of bone metastases at diagnosis succumbed. But other children with large primary tumors, cervical and axillary lymph node metastases, epidural space metastases, Horner's syndrome, and erosion of ribs and thoracic vertebra all survived despite incomplete excision of the mediastinal tumor.[17]

A high rate of radiocurability despite the local aggressiveness and extension of neuroblastoma is often observed in extra-adrenal tumors. Even huge tumors with extradural invasion of the spinal canal can be controlled. A 100 percent radiocurability in 13 cases of extra-adrenal neuroblastoma was reported by King et al.[10] Their cure rate in adrenal neuroblastoma was only 10 percent. In extra-adrenal neuroblastomas in children less than one year old, the rate of prolonged survival approaches 100 percent.[40]

In another series, de Lorimier compared the survival for 33 patients with mediastinal neuroblastomas with survival of patients with retroperitoneal primary tumors.[7] In the age group under one year, all 12 mediastinal cases survived, whereas only 22 of 45 retroperitoneal cases (49 percent) survived. For patients older than one year, the survival rate for mediastinal origin was 19 percent, whereas the survival rate for retroperitoneal origin was 6 percent. However, the difference in the survival for these two sites of origin beyond infancy was not significant, since nearly all of the tumors then were stage IV. When all age groups combined were compared, the survival rate for mediastinal neuroblastomas was 48.5 percent, and for retroperitoneal neuroblastomas it was 20 percent.[7]

But these reports should not be interpreted as meaning that neuroblastomas in extra-adrenal locations are biologically different from primary adrenal tumors. It is roughly correct to say that site of the primary tumor is an important fact in assessing prognosis. But the facts are that most extra-adrenal neuroblastomas are less than stage IV on presentation and occur in younger patients. If one corrects for the lower stage and younger age, survival of extra-adrenal neuroblastomas obey the same principles as adrenal neuroblastomas. To say that extra-adrenal neuroblastomas are less malignant than adrenal neuroblastomas is like saying that the corner of Elm and Chestnut Streets in Littletown is safer for pedestrians than Times Square. But if someone gets hit by a fast-moving car, he will be equally dead in Littletown or New York. Thus, extra-adrenal neuroblastomas have a good prognosis, as long as they are not stage IV ("hit by a car"). Stage IV neuroblastoma of the mediastinum is just as malignant as stage IV neuroblastoma of the adrenal.[9]

Causes of the apparent lesser malignancy of extra-abdominal neuroblastomas One can only speculate on the possible reasons for the better prognosis in extra-abdominal neuroblastomas. It is true that earlier diagnosis is more likely in extra-abdominal neuroblastomas because the tumors occur in sites where physiological functions are more quickly disturbed, and the patient is brought earlier for medical attention. But even where the diagnosis has been delayed, cure can still be obtained in extra-abdominal neuroblastomas. This raises the question of the factors involved in dissemination of the tumor with clinical appearance of metastases shortly after diagnosis. Extra-abdominal neuroblastomas show less of this tendency.[43]

It is tempting to ascribe this favorable survival rate to the therapy that is employed. However, it is well known that a malignant neuroblastoma might "mature" into a benign ganglioneuroma; thus, spontaneous maturation and/or regression occurs at a rate much higher in patients with neuroblastoma than with any other tumor. Likewise, the more benign behavior of extra-abdominal neuroblastoma, as compared to abdominal neuroblastoma, may in part be due to an increased rate of spontaneous maturation and/or regression, but there is no evidence for this.

Histological review of all pathologic specimens in one series revealed that none of the patients with mediastinal neuroblastoma died whose tumor was classified as a ganglioneuroblastoma.[17] However, two of the three children with poorly differentiated neuroblastomas succumbed, confirming the suggestion that tumors with the least differentiation have the worst prognosis. Substantial numbers of "mitoses" that were common in tumors of children under one year of age were an ominous prognostic sign in children over two years of age. The presence of lymphocytes in the tumor did not necessarily indicate a favorable outcome, and in nine survivors (oldest three years of age) lymphocytes were essentially absent in the histopathologic specimens.[17]

It has been suggested that upper mediastinal neuroblastomas may originate at sites other than in sympathetic ganglia. Those mediastinal tumors with a major intraspinal component possibly arise from sensory dorsal root ganglia. It seems likely that a tumor originating in the dorsal ganglia, in contrast to one from sympathetic ganglia, would not release excessive quantities of catecholamines. In this regard, only 2 of 11 patients with mediastinal neuroblastoma in one series had increased quantities of VMA in the urine.[17] In comparison, over 70 percent of the children with abdominal neuroblastoma were found to excrete increased quantities of VMA. A tumor originating in a sensory ganglion also might be expected to produce segmental sensory disturbances. Another suggested site of origin for mediastinal neuroblastoma is paraganglionic tissue, which is abundant near the aortic arch and adjacent to the sympathetic ganglia in the embryo. Since many mediastinal neuroblastomas are found in close relation to the aortic arch, it is possible that they originate from this paraganglionic tissue. Paraganglionic tumors in the adult are seldom highly malignant, and catecholemine production in them is only occasionally demonstrated.[17] However, the vast majority of mediastinal neuroblastomas are located posteriorly and appear to arise in sympathetic ganglia.

Degree of Histological Differentiation of the Tumor

Neuroblastomas represent an important challenge to the pathologist. No other tumor has so high a rate of spontaneous regression, which may occur even in the presence of metastases. Yet neuroblastomas are also capable of extreme malignancy. It is important for the histopathologist to try to identify morphological correlates of these various biological expressions.[44]

Histological maturation of neurogenic tumors is related to prognosis or prolonged survival. It is well known that neuroblastomas constitute a histopathological spectrum characterized by varying degrees of maturation of tumor cells toward mature, predominantly neural, elements. At one end of the spectrum are tumors composed only of cells so incompletely differentiated that distinction from other small-celled neoplasms may be difficult or impossible. At the other end are ganglioneuromas, composed solely of mature cell types. Between these extremes are those tumors characterized by (1) uniform partial differentiation, (2) focal partial differentiation, or (3) focal complete differentiation. These partially differentiated tumors, particularly the latter, are termed ganglioneuroblastomas.[44]

Attempts to relate survival to histology of the tumor have been disappointing. The general rule is that the lesions at the benign end of the malignancy scale do better, but there are frequent exceptions. Ganglioneuromas behave in a benign fashion. However, there is a lack of precise information concerning the effect of lesser degrees of maturation on prolonged survival of children with neurogenic tumors. In particular, it is unclear to what extent the degree of histological maturation correlates with other favorable prognostic indicators, such as age of the patient, and site of the primary tumor on prolonged survival. However, there is no convincing evidence that the more favorable outcome in young infants, and in tumors of extra-abdominal origin, is related to higher degrees of histological maturation.

Pathologists have emphasized the variability in the histologic appearance of different areas within the tumors in neuroblastomas. Classification of tumors on the basis of histological characteristics has been attempted. These data were examined by Sutow to see whether or not such classifications could be correlated with prognosis as measured by survival in children with neuroblastoma.[30]

Early studies showed that the occurrence of tumors of different histological characteristics was unrelated to age.[30] On the other hand, there was a marked difference in the distribution of prolonged survivors among the differentiated and undifferentiated tumor groups in patients two years of age and younger. A much greater number of prolonged survivors were found among those with differentiated tumors and significantly fewer survivors were found among those with undifferentiated types of tumors.[30]

In a more recent series, Beckwith and Martin studied 53 cases who either died with a diagnosis of neuroblastoma or were free of tumor at least two years after this diagnosis was established.[44] These two groups were thus classified as "non-survivors" and "survivors." A system of histologic grading based upon degree of maturation was devised which distinguished sharply between those neoplasms without evidence of differentiation and those with early attempts at neurogenesis.[44] Those with more advanced degrees of maturation were categorized according to whether differentiating or undifferentiated elements predominated based upon an estimate of the surface area of available sections occupied by differentiating and undifferentiated cells respectively (Table 1).[44]

Table 1
Criteria for Histological Grading of Neuroblastomas[44]

Grade I	—Predominantly differentiated, or over 50 percent differentiating elements.
Grade II	—Predominantly undifferentiated, or 5 to 50 percent differentiating elements.
Grade III	—Slightly differentiated, or under 5 percent differentiating elements.
Grade IV	—Undifferentiated, no recognizable neurogenesis.

Beckwith and Martin noted a direct relationship between histological differentiation of the tumor and prolonged survival.[44] In the most undifferentiated tumors (grade IV), survival was 4 percent, while well-differentiated tumors (grade I) gave 100 percent survival. There was a questionable relationship between histologic grade to age, there being only a slight tendency for fewer grade IV tumors to occur in the younger age group. Despite a suggestive tendency for tumors in the first year of life to show evidence of maturation, this difference was insufficient to account for the much better prognosis seen in the younger age group. Tumors arising in the adrenal tend to be undifferentiated. This may in part relate to the poor prognosis observed for adrenal neuroblastomas in most series.[44,45] Grading tumors from I to IV in malignancy, Fortner had only one survivor in 65 patients with undifferentiated tumors.[32] In another series there was 31 percent prolonged survival with well-differentiated tumors, and 9 percent prolonged survival with undifferentiated tumors.[2]

It is possible that neuroblastomas are not solely neoplasms of sympathetic ganglia but may on occasion arise from certain other neural-crest derivatives, such as dorsal root ganglia, parasympathetic ganglia, paraganglia, and perhaps even Schwann cells.[44] This may also account for observed differences in histological appearance and differences in prognosis (biological behavior).

In summary, these studies demonstrate an apparently important effect of histological differentiation upon prognosis. Differences in degree of maturation probably do not account for the more favorable outcome of neuroblastomas in infancy. Adrenal primary tumors are usually undifferentiated, which may account for the relatively poor prognosis of adrenal neuroblastomas.

Immunological Status

The peculiar behavior of this tumor, both clinically and in vitro, has caused speculation on the possibility of immunological control. Thus, Burnet referred to spontaneous regression of in situ neuroblastomas in infants as an example of immunological surveillance.[46] A small nodule of tumor cells recognized by the immune mechanism as foreign could be destroyed by the ordinary process of homograft rejection.[2] The role of surgical treatment might even be immunological; thus, the surgical removal of a quantity of tumor antigen could permit immune mechanisms to escape from paralysis or tolerance for the abnormal antigen.[47] The immune status of children with malignant tumors is difficult to assess, since many have received radiation therapy and/or chemotherapy with immunosuppressive drugs. Basically, the most important determinant of survival in neuroblastoma may well be the effectiveness of the host's resistance.

Martin and Beckwith found the degree of lymphoid infiltrate roughly correlated with differentiation of neuroblastomas.[48] Survivors had tumors with more lymphoid invasion, suggesting a host response. Lauder and Aherne studied the significance of lymphocytic infiltration in a retrospective series of 23 primary neuroblastomas. The degree of lymphocytic infiltration was estimated and scored in 5 categories. A significant positive correlation was found between lymphocytic infiltration and survival both in infancy and in childhood. It was found, unexpectedly, that the presence of metastases did not invalidate the correlation between lymphocyte score and survival.[49] It did not appear that such infiltrates are a special feature of relatively well-differentiated ganglioneuroblastomas. The better survival rate did not seem to be due necessarily to a higher degree of differentiation. In spite of the poor degree of differentiation in all of Lauder and Aherne's cases, it was still possible to demonstrate a correlation between the intensity of lymphocytic infiltration and the survival time of the patient. This correlation may in part be due to a tumor-specific lymphocytotoxicity, such as that demonstrated in vitro by the colony inhibition test in neuroblastomas.[50] It is suggested that lymphocytic infiltration of the tumor is an important factor in retarding and even reversing tumor growth, but not necessarily in preventing metastasis. Metastases are potentially able to regress in the same way as the primary tumor, presumably by the same lymphocytotoxic mechanisms.[49]

In addition, Bill and Morgan suggested a prognostic correlation between the total lymphocyte count in the peripheral blood and survival.[51] Those under a year of age who were cured had a statistically higher number of lymphocytes than did those who succumbed. While survivors over one year of age also had higher total lymphocyte counts than the children who died, it was not statistically significant.[51] Prognostically, therefore, lymphocyte count elevation is not as reliable or accurate as the other factors discussed above.[2]

Evidence for immune mechanisms against the tumor in neuroblastoma patients includes:

1. The finding of infiltrates of lymphocytes in the tumors from patients who later showed prolonged survival

2. The finding of higher peripheral lymphocyte counts in prolonged survivors
3. Presence in tissue culture of a lethal immune reaction by the lymphocytes of neuroblastoma patients against the tumor cells
4. A less constant lethal immune activity by the plasma against tumor cells in tissue culture
5. Demonstration of an unfavorable immune factor which is a humoral "blocking antibody."[51]

Hellstrom found that lymphocytes from neuroblastoma patients exhibit a cell-bound immunity lethal against neuroblastoma cells in tissue culture, as demonstrated by the colony inhibition test (Figure 5). The cytotoxic effect of plasma is similar but less consistent. This is presumed to be due to an antibody.[50,52]

Thus, in favor of the child with neuroblastoma will be his small lymphocytes, which are cytotoxic against the tumor in vitro. This has been true in 86 percent of the cases in one series.[26] An additional factor in his favor is a humoral cytotoxic antibody, on which there are fewer data, but which can be demonstrated in some patients. A factor acting against the patient's survival is obviously the degree of malignancy of his tumor, which may spread and cause his death, and which is also the stimulus for his immune responses. Another recently recognized factor against the patient is the so-called blocking antibody in the serum that differentiates patients who are dying from the ones who survive. Patients with active, progressive disease seem to produce blocking antibodies that prevent the lymphocytes from working against the tumor cells. The patients who are cured do not have this blocking antibody. The presence or absence of this factor separates those who have persisting tumor from those who are cured.[26]

Thus, the prognosis of patients with neuroblastoma may be assessed in part by the extent of infiltration of lymphocytes in the tumor itself.[48] In addition, the lethal potential of the child's lymphocytes and plasma against the tumor can be measured by the colony inhibition test. The lymphocyte count at diagnosis should also be taken into account, and it may be followed during treatment, particularly in children under two years of age.[51] (Table 2)

Treatment

The impact of treatment on the course of the individual child with neuroblastoma is hard to assess. The extent of the disease when

Table 2
Immunological Factors that Affect Prognosis in
a Child with Neuroblastoma

Favoring Survival	Against Survival
Lymphoid infiltrate in tumor	Degree of malignancy of the tumor
Increased lymphocyte count of blood	Presence of blocking antibody
Anti-neuroblastoma antibodies	
Anti-neuroblastoma lymphocytes	

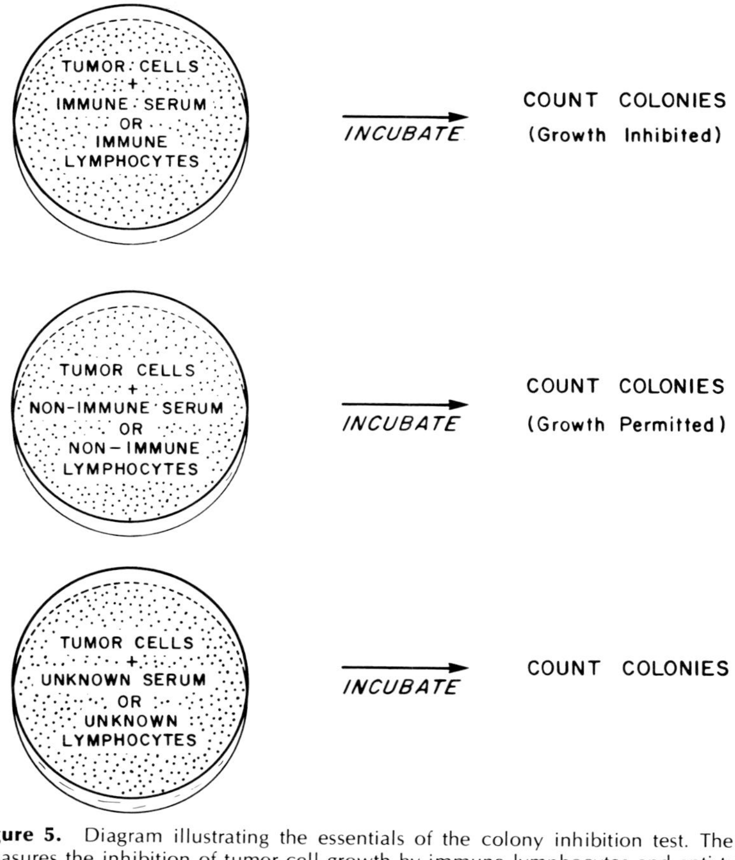

Figure 5. Diagram illustrating the essentials of the colony inhibition test. The test measures the inhibition of tumor-cell growth by immune lymphocytes and anti-tumor antibodies. By comparing the growth-inhibiting effects of the unknown lymphocytes or serum with immune lymphocytes or serum, the anti-tumor characteristics of the unknowns may be measured. (Courtesy of *American Family Physician*[52])

it is discovered is a major determinant of the type and extent of treatment that is given.[2] The comparison of results in one series with another is often difficult.

Neuroblastomas are highly peculiar in their response to treatment. Regression may occur spontaneously. It may also occur after incomplete surgery,[53] or radiation therapy, or following administration of various drugs (vincristine, cyclophosphamide, nitrogen mustard, and other alkylating agents). The mode of action of all of these agents is only partially understood. Survival rates are high following total excision of localized neuroblastomas. But survival often occurs after only partial excision of the tumor, regardless of what adjunctive treatment is employed. Maturation of the tumor into a benign ganglioneuroma may occur; but it is possible that the processes of regression and maturation are distinct and unrelated, both from each other and from prior therapy. It is also possible that the child's defenses are capable of being stimulated by a variety of agents and that the defense mechanism may be more efficient when the tumor is in the embryological stage of its existence.[43] These factors need to be considered in assessing the results of therapy.

Effects of treatment on survival Because of the relatively high rate of spontaneous regression in neuroblastomas, there are divergent opinions as to the effects of surgery, x-ray therapy, and chemotherapy in producing prolonged survival. Controlled studies using the various modalities of therapy individually have never been done. Only combination therapy is used. Koop went so far as to say that the addition of x-ray therapy and chemotherapy had no effect on survival, even when these modalities were used on patients with advanced disease.[54,55] He later modified this to say that x-ray therapy was useful only in patients with stage III disease.[26] On the other hand, Lingley[39] argued that x-ray therapy was the most important form of therapy in patients with regionally contained neuroblastoma.

Gross considered x-ray therapy to be extremely important, starting treatment the day of surgery.[5] Tefft and Wittenborg reported survival of 27 out of 35 patients under one year of age who were treated with combined surgery and x-ray therapy.[56] The same combination, however, afforded only 18 percent survival in patients over one year of age in their experience. There were no totally resectable lesions in the series of 35 reported by Young, but there were 9 survivors.[40] It was concluded that x-ray therapy is the most important modality in achieving the high cure rate in extra-adrenal neuroblastomas. All 9 survivors had extra-adrenal tumors, which have been associated with survival of 50 percent or better in other series.[2]

In another series, there were 77 patients who had unresectable neuroblastomas. Six had biopsy only, with no treatment and no survivors. The remaining 71 were treated with surgery, x-ray therapy, and chemotherapy; only 6 of these were two-year survivors.[2] Forty-eight patients in this series, who were resectable, had partial or complete excision of the primary tumor. Twenty-three of the 48 survived—almost half. Fifteen of the 23 survivors were under a year of age; none of the other 8 had metastases beyond the regional lymph nodes.[2]

Radiotherapy was used on a series of 93 patients.[2] It was the sole treatment in 32 patients. Of the 5 survivors, all were under one year of age and only 1 had an abdominal primary lesion. Sixty-one patients had x-ray therapy plus surgery and/or chemotherapy with 19 survivors; 13 of the 19 survivors were under one year old. Thirteen had extra-abdominal primary sites and 1 had an undetermined primary tumor. All 5 with abdominal primary tumors had partial or complete excision of the tumor. Eighteen of the 19 total survivors underwent major resection of the primary lesion. Thirteen of the 19 had no metastases, and 3 had lymph node metastases only. All but 1 of these survivors had more than one "favorable factor," so it is not clear what role x-ray therapy played in causing prolonged survival.[2]

Koop stated that if the stage of the tumor is accurately assessed, patients with stage I and II tumors require no radiation therapy, whereas those with stage III tumors benefit from postoperative radiation.[26] Survival in stage II is at least as good in this group with residual tumor and no radiotherapy as for the radiated group.

Prolonged survivals have been reported with almost every combination of surgery and x-ray therapy. Most adrenal neuroblastomas are so invasive locally that total surgical excision is impossible, but there is some reason to believe that the prognosis is directly related to the degree of excision even when it is known to be incomplete. If biopsy alone is done, less than 10 percent of patients survive, but after a wide but incomplete excision, nearly half of the cases may show prolonged survival.[28]

Chemotherapy A nationwide questionnaire survey was conducted by Sutow and his co-workers. Data regarding diagnosis, treatment, and clinical course were obtained in 84 cases of neuroblastoma diagnosed in 1956, and on 142 cases of neuroblastoma diagnosed in 1962.[38] The frequency and extent of x-ray therapy and surgery used in treatment of children with this tumor seemed comparable between 1956 and 1962. The age distributions of patients were also comparable between 1956 and 1962. The frequency and

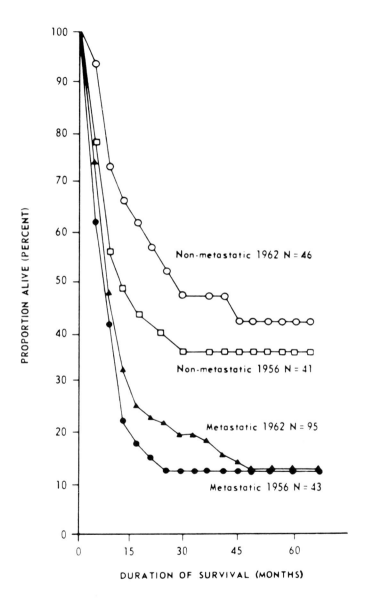

Figure 6. Graph showing survival curves of children with neuroblastoma originally diagnosed in 1956 compared with those diagnosed in 1962. (Courtesy of Dr. W. Sutow and *Pediatrics*[38])

intensity of chemotherapy increased markedly from 1956 to 1962 in patients with neuroblastoma. By 1962 the clinical use of vincristine and cyclophosphamide in patients with solid tumors was common. Analysis of the data on patients in this study showed that there were no statistically significant differences in survival of children with neuroblastoma first seen in 1956 as compared with those diagnosed in 1962 (Figure 6). The survival pattern of children with or without metastasis had not changed. Since radiation and surgical aspects of neuroblastoma management were considered to have been similar during the two study periods, it was concluded that the addition of new anti-neoplastic drugs and the increased use of chemotherapy in 1962 had not improved the survival of children with neuroblastoma.[38]

Comparison of the survival curves for children with both metastatic and non-metastatic neuroblastoma in 1956 and 1962 showed no significant difference. However, there is a possible increase in the median survival time for nonmetastatic neuroblastomas treated in 1962 as compared with 1956. Thus, although the two-year survival is not different statistically, the shift of the curve to the right is impressive (Figure 6). Increasing age and the presence of metastases were deleterious prognostic factors in each of the two time periods. Survival among children under two years of age, and particularly among those younger than one year of age, was significantly better than that in older children when the disease was non-metastatic. This difference was not present when the patients had metastases. In all age categories, survival in children with metastatic disease was significantly inferior to survival among children without metastases.[38]

The role of chemotherapy is exceedingly difficult to assess in terms of survival, since many authors report remissions or objective responses rather than survival. Also, most patients treated with chemotherapy have unresectable tumors, and many receive radiotherapy as well. Enthusiasm for drug therapy increased after James reported five survivors in nine consecutive unresectable neuroblastomas.[57,58] Subsequent reports from other centers have been less optimistic.[2] Currently, a cyclic regimen of vincristine and cyclophosphamide is widely used. The response to vitamin B_{12} seems no greater than the natural rate of spontaneous tumor regression.[59]

In one series, 52 patients had chemotherapy, the drugs used being those in vogue at the time of treatment.[2] Fifteen had chemotherapy alone, and all died. Thirty-seven had chemotherapy plus surgery and/or x-ray therapy, and four survived. Two of these four prolonged survivors underwent total excision of thoracic primary lesions and had no metastases. The other two were under one year of age; one with an adrenal primary lesion had complete excision, the other with an undetermined primary lesion had only lymph node biopsy. These last two prolonged survivors are remarkable in that one had cortical bone metastasis and the other had a positive marrow aspirate (possibly stage IV-S). Thus, only 2 of 52 patients may have had remissions attributable to chemotherapy. But both of these were infants, who are known to have a high rate of spontaneous regression of neuroblastomas. Thus it is difficult to attribute prolonged survival to chemotherapy even in these two cases.

Even though one cannot reach definite conclusions regarding relative merits of different types of therapy, examination of available data permits certain generalizations:

a. Prolonged survivals (two years or more) have followed the use of either surgery alone or radiation therapy alone
b. Prolonged survivals without radiation therapy have resulted from complete excision of tumor, partial excision of tumor, or even simple biopsy of tumor
c. Though infrequent, prolonged survivals have occurred in children over the age of two years and in children with skeletal metastases, irrespective of age
d. Children under the age of two years with neuroblastoma had significantly higher survival rate, regardless of type of treatment, than did the children over the age of two years.[30]

It may be concluded that the available data fail to demonstrate that treatment as currently given has any influence on two-year survival, despite the fact that radiotherapy and chemotherapy each lead to tumor shrinkage in some patients. However, recent studies suggest that chemotherapy is useful in stage III neuroblastomas.

Further investigation of the biological behavior of this unique tumor as well as the continued evaluation of new and improved methods of treatment must be pursued in order to improve the outlook for patients with this potentially curable neoplasm.[41]

LATE RECURRENCE OF TUMOR AND OTHER PROBLEMS IN PROLONGED SURVIVORS

Despite the many variables which are known to affect the prognosis of neuroblastoma, specific criteria have been previously listed to define a cure. Two reported patients died of neuroblastoma after a prolonged, asymptomatic period when they would have been considered cured by most currently accepted criteria.[60] One child who had a retroperitoneal neuroblastoma diagnosed at three days of age responded well to therapy but relapsed and died 6½ years later. Another child who had a sacral neuroblastoma diagnosed at 19 months of age also responded well to therapy but relapsed and died 9 years later.[60] Both of the above patients appeared to be free of tumor for at least two years, and therefore "cured" according to the accepted criteria for definition of cure. Furthermore, because of young age and extra-adrenal location of tumor, both would have been expected to have a favorable prognosis. Although one patient had metastases, the tumor was diagnosed at birth. The second patient was under two years of age at the time of diagnosis and had no evidence of metastases.[60]

The number of late deaths from neuroblastoma after a prolonged remission is certainly small. However, the fact that they do occur is of great importance to the physician who must responsibly manage these children and counsel their parents. The use of the term "cure" when discussing individual patients may be inadvisable, although the parents may be assured that late recurrences are very rare.[60]

In one study prolonged survival of infants with neuroblastoma was accompanied by additional morbidity from recurrence of tumor or from adverse effects of therapy in 12 of 19 patients.[18] These factors need to be taken into account when planning treatment of neuroblastoma for patients in good prognostic categories. The development of post-neuroblastoma ganglioneuroma is described in 5 patients; attention is brought to its importance as a disease entity, and its insidious onset many years after treatment.[18] The finding of post-neuroblastoma ganglioneuroma in these 5 patients again indicates that the ultimate fate of some neuroblastomas is the formation of ganglioneuromas.[61] Ganglioneuromas were detected either at the sites of the primary tumor or at the sites of metastases.

SUMMARY AND CONCLUSIONS

From a study of pooled data on cases of neuroblastoma the relationship of various factors (age, stage, site of primary tumor, metastases, histological differentiation, and therapy) to prognosis for prolonged survival was evaluated. Age over two years, presence of skeletal metastases, and histological undifferentiation of the tumor were associated with poor survival rates. The most important of these seem to be the patient's age at diagnosis and the extent of the disease (stage), although some children with widespread disease (stage IV-S) appear to have a particularly good prognosis. No differences in therapeutic effectiveness among x-ray therapy alone, surgery alone, and combined surgery plus x-ray therapy were noted. It is difficult to evaluate the influence of chemotherapy on survival in patients with neuroblastoma but it has not been of great significance.

The unique biological characteristics of this tumor require further study in the hope of providing more effective therapy.

REFERENCES

1. Dargeon, H.W.: Problems in the prognosis of neuroblastoma. *Amer. J. Roentgenol.* 83: 551, 1966.
2. Swank, R., Fetterman, G.H., Sieber, W., and Kiesewetter, W.: Prognostic factors in neuroblastoma. *Ann. Surg.* 174: 428–435, 1971.
3. Koop, C.E., and Hernandez, J.: Neuroblastoma; experience with 100 cases in children. *Surgery* 56: 726–733, 1964.
4. Koop, C.E.: Factors affecting survival in neuroblastoma. *J. Pediatr. Surg.* 3: 113, 1968.
5. Gross, R.E., Farber, S., and Martin, L.W.: Neuroblastoma sympatheticum; a study and report of 217 cases. *Pediatrics* 23: 1179, 1959.
6. Collins, V.P., Loeffler, R.K., and Tivey, H.: Observations on growth rates of human tumours. *Amer. J. Roentgenol.* 76: 988, 1956.
7. de Lorimier, A., Bragg, K., and Linden, G.: Neuroblastoma in childhood. *Amer. J. Dis. Child.* 118: 441–450, 1969.
8. Greenfield, L.J., and Shelley, W.M.: The spectrum of neurogenic tumors of the sympathetic nervous system; Maturation and adrenergic function. *J. Nat. Cancer Inst.* 35: 215–226, 1965.
9. Evans, A.E., D'Angio, G.J., and Randolph, J.: A proposed staging for children with neuroblastoma. *Cancer* 27: 374–378, 1971.
10. King, R.L., Stonaasli, J.P., and Bolande, R.P.: Neuroblastoma: Review of twenty-eight cases and presentation of two cases with metastases and long survival. *Amer. J. Roentgenol.* 85: 733–747, 1961.
11. Eyre-Brook, A., and Hewer, T.F.: Spontaneous disappearance of neuroblastoma with maturation to ganglioneuroma. *J. Bone Joint Surg.,* 44B: 886–890, 1962.

12. Cushing, H., and Wolback, S.: Transformation of malignant paravertebral sympathicoblastoma into benign ganglioneuroma. *Amer. J. Path.* 3: 203, 1927.

13. Fox, F., Davidson, J., and Thomas, L.B.: Maturation of sympathicoblastoma into ganglioneuroma. *Cancer* 12: 108–116, 1959.

14. Everson, T.C., and Cole, W.H.: *Spontaneous Regression of Cancer*. Philadelphia: W.B. Saunders Co., 1966.

15. Dyke, P.C., and Mulkey, D.A.: Maturation of ganglioneuroblastoma to ganglioneuroma. *Cancer* 20: 1343–1349, 1967.

16. Wilkerson, J.A., Van de Water, J.M., and Gaepfer, H.: Role of embryonic induction in benign transformation of neuroblastomas. *Cancer* 29: 1335–1342, 1967.

17. Filler, R., Traggis, D., Jaffe, N., and Vawter, G.: Favorable outlook for children with mediastinal neuroblastoma. *J. Pediatr. Surg.* 7: 136–143, 1972.

18. Helson, L., Grabstald, H., Huvos, A., et al.: Neuroblastoma; observations on long-term survival. *Clin. Bull. Memorial Sloan-Kettering Cancer Center* 3: 3–9, 1973.

19. Alterman, K., and Schueller, E.: Maturation of neuroblastoma to ganglioneuroma. *Amer. J. Dis. Child.* 120: 217–222, 1970.

20. Reilly, D., Nesbit, M.E., and Krivit, W.: Cure of three patients who had skeletal metastases in disseminated neuroblastoma. *Pediatrics* 41: 47–51, 1968.

21. Pochedly, C.: The broad clinical spectrum of neuroblastoma. *Postgrad. Med.* 51: 79–85, (April) 1972.

22. D'Angio, G.J., Evans, A., and Koop, C.E.: Special pattern of widespread neuroblastoma with a favorable prognosis. *Lancet* 1: 1046–1049, 1971.

23. Beckwith, J.B., and Perrin, E.V.: In Situ Neuroblastoma; A Contribution to the Natural History of Neural Crest Tumors. *Amer. J. Path.* 45: 1089, 1963.

24. Guin, G.H., et al.: Incidental Neuroblastoma in Infants. *Amer. J. Clin. Path.* 51: 126, 1969.

25. Varkarakis, M., Bhonaleph, T., Albert, D., et al.: Current status of prognostic criteria in neuroblastoma. *J. Urol.* 109: 94–97, 1973.

26. Koop, C.E., and Johnson, D.G.: Neuroblastoma; an assessment of therapy in reference to staging. *J. Pediatr. Surg.* 6: 595–600, 1971.

27. Breslow, N., and McCann, B.: Statistical estimation of prognosis for children with neuroblastoma. *Cancer Res.* 31: 2098–2103, 1971.

28. Horn, R.C., Koop, C.E., and Kiesewetter, W.: Neuroblastoma in childhood; clinicopathologic study of 44 cases. *Lab. Invest.* 5: 106, 1956.

29. Benson, C., Mustard, W., Ravitch, M., et al. (eds.): *Pediatric Surgery*. (Vol. II). Chicago: Year Book Medical Publishers, 1962, pp. 874–885.

30. Sutow, W.: Prognosis in neuroblastoma of childhood. *Amer. J. Dis. Child.* 96: 299–305, 1958.

31. Marsden, H., and Steward, J. (eds.): *Tumors in Children*. New York: Springer-Verlag, 1968, pp. 131–166.

32. Fortner, J., Nicastri, A., and Murphy, M.L.: Neuroblastoma: natural history and results of treating 133 cases. *Ann. Surg.* 167: 132, 1968.

33. Evans, A., and Hummeler, K.: The significance of primitive cells in marrow aspirates of children with neuroblastoma. *Cancer* 32: 906–912, 1973.

34. McGoldrick, K., and Lanzkowsky, P.: Prolonged survival in neuroblastoma with multiple skeletal metastases and bone marrow infiltration. *Acta Paediat. Scand.* 59: 711–714, 1970.

35. Vogel, J., Coddon, D., Simon, N., and Gitlow, S.: Osseous metastases in neuroblastoma; a 17-year survival. *Cancer* 26: 1354–1360, 1970.

36. Kissane, J.M., and Ackerman, L.V.: Maturation of tumors of the sympathetic nervous system. *J. Fac. Radiol.* 7: 109–114, 1955.

37. Vesfeldt, J.: Transformation of sympathicoblastomas into ganglioneuroma with a case report. *Acta Path. Microbiol. Scand.* 58: 414–428, 1963.

38. Sutow, W., Gehan, E., Heyn, R., et al.: Comparison of survival curves, 1956 versus 1962, in children with Wilms' tumor and neuroblastoma. *Pediatrics* 45: 800–811, 1970.

39. Lingley, J.F., Sagerman, R.H., Santulli, T.V., and Wolff, J.A.: Neuroblastoma; management and survival. *New Engl. J. Med.* 277: 1227, 1967.

40. Young, L., Rubin, P., and Hanson, R.: The extra-adrenal neuroblastoma; high radiocurability and diagnostic accuracy. *Amer. J. Roentgenol.* 108: 75–91, 1970.

41. Finklestein, J., and Gilchrist, G.: Recent advances in neuroblastoma. *California Med.* 116: 27–36 (March), 1972.

42. Priebe, C., and Clatworthy, H.W.: Neuroblastoma; an evaluation of 90 children. *Arch. Surg.* 95: 538–545, 1967.

43. Kelly, F.: Prognosis in extra-abdominal neuroblastoma. *Acta Radiol.* 6: 100–194, 1967.

44. Beckwith, J.B., and Martin, R.F.: Observations on the Histopathology of Neuroblastoma. *J. Pediatr. Surg.* 3: 106–108, 1968.

45. Ackerman, L., and del Regato, J.: *Cancer, Diagnosis, Treatment, and Prognosis.* St. Louis: C.V. Mosby Company, 1962, pp. 911–921.

46. Burnet, F.M.: Immunological aspects of malignant disease. *Lancet* 1: 1171–1174, 1967.

47. Coriell, L.L.: Host immunity. *J. Pediatr. Surg.* 3: 124, 1968.

48. Martin, R.F., and Beckwith, J.B.: Lymphoid infiltrates in neuroblastoma: Their occurrence and prognostic significance. *J. Pediatr. Surg.* 3: 161, 1968.

49. Lauder, I., and Aherne, W.: The significance of lymphocytic infiltration in neuroblastoma. *Brit. J. Cancer* 26: 321–330, 1972.

50. Hellstrom, K., and Hellstrom, I.: Immunologic defense against cancer. *Hospital Practice* 5: 45–61 (January), 1970.

51. Bill, A., and Morgan, A.: Evidence for immune reactions to neuroblastoma and future possibilities for investigation. *J. Pediatr. Surg.* 5: 111–116, 1970.

52. Pochedly, C.: The child with neuroblastoma. *Amer. Fam. Physician* 5: 74–79 (February), 1972.

53. Koop, C.E., Kiesewetter, W.B., and Horn, R.C.: Neuroblastoma (abdominal) survival after major surgical insult to tumor. *Surgery* 38: 272, 1955.

54. Koop, C.E.: The role of surgery in resectable, nonresectable and metastatic neuroblastoma. *J.A.M.A.* 205: 157, 1968.

55. Koop, C.E.: Neuroblastoma: Two year survival and treatment correlations. *J. Pediatr. Surg.* 3: 178, 1968.

56. Tefft, M., and Wittenborg, M.H.: Radiotherapeutic management of neuroblastoma in childhood. *J.A.M.A.* 205: 195, 1968.

57. James, D., Hustu, O., Wrenn, E.L., and Pinkel, D.: Combination chemotherapy of childhood neuroblastoma. *J.A.M.A.* 194: 123, 1965.

58. Pinkel, D., Pratt, C., Holton, C., et al.: Survival of children with neuroblastoma treated with combination chemotherapy. *J. Pediat.* 73: 928, 1968.

59. Sawitsky, A., and Desposito, F.: A survey of American experience with vitamin B_{12} therapy of neuroblastoma. *J. Pediat.* 67: 99, 1965.

60. Konrad, P., Singher, J., and Neerhout, R.: Late death from neuroblastoma. *J. Pediat.* 82: 80–82, 1973.

61. Goldman, R.L., Winterling, A.N., and Winterling, C.C.: Maturation of tumors of the sympathetic nervous system; Report of long-term survival in two patients, one with disseminated osseous metastases, and review of cases from the literature. *Cancer* 18: 1510–1516, 1965.

INDEX

A

Abdominal neuroblastoma, 1, 2,
41, 49, 59, 74-81, 238-242,
285-286
    Diagnosis, 75
    Functionally active, 79-81
    Hutchison type, 2, 74
    Pepper type, 1, 74
    Radiographic findings, 76-79
    Surgery, 238-242
    Symptoms, 74-75, 79-81
Adenopathy, mediastinal, 69
Adrenal neuroblastomas, 3, 59,
63-64, 165, 171, 285-286,
292-294
Adrenergic metabolites, 79-81
Age, and neuroblastoma, 2,
18-19, 47, 211, 227, 253,
276-278, 281
    Prognosis, 276-278
    Response to therapy, 253
Animals, neuroblastoma in,
27-28, 194-197
    Mouse, 194-197
Anti-nerve growth factor, 21, 185
Autonomic nervous system,
156-160
    Embryological development,
    157-160

B

Biochemical diagnosis, 133-135
Biology of neuroblastoma cells,
181-203
    Chromosomal abnormalities,
    197-200
    In vitro behavior, 189-197
    In vivo (mice), 197
    Nerve growth factor, 182-189
Biopsy, 238
Bladder compression, 82
Blocking factors, 209-210, 294
Bone diseases, 107-109
    Local, 107-108
    Systemic, 108-109

Bone lesions, see **Skeletal lesions**
Bone metastases, see **Skeletal
    system**
Brain metastases, 35-41, 103
    Bone involvement, 37-38
    Calvarium, 38, 41, 103
    Cerebrospinal fluid, 37
    Cushing's syndrome, 41, 80
    Dural metastases, 41
    Incidence, 37
    Intracranial pressure, 38
    Localization, 37
    Meninges and venous sinuses,
    37
    "Scalp" nodules, 38
    Widened cranial sutures, 40
    Wieberdink hypothesis, 38
Burkitt's tumor, 177

C

Calcification, 62, 69, 75, 77, 78,
163-164, 228-229
Calvarium, 38, 41, 103
Catecholamines, 2, 5, 6, 25, 47, 49,
81, 115-154, 160, 171, 238,
289-290
    Assay, specific procedures,
    121-124
    Chromatographic technique,
    123, 126
    Diagnosis of neuroblastoma, 2,
    6, 25, 63, 109, 120-135
    Effect of drugs and diet on
    testing, 124-125
    In pregnant women, 5, 135
    Metabolism, 117-119, 142-143
        Destruction, 118
        Enzymes and cofactors,
        table, 144
        Metabolic pathways, 119
        Metabolites and
        precursors, table, 144
        Synthesis, 117, 142
    Normal values, 125-133
    Prognosis and, 136-142

307

Catecholamines *(cont.)*
  Screening tests, 120-124
    Urinary spot test,
      ("Dipstick test"), 25,
      120
    VMA "test strip," 120
  Therapy and, 136
Celiac-like syndrome, 80
Cells, neuroblastoma, biology of,
  181-203
  Chromosomal abnormalities,
    197-200
  In vitro behavior, 189-197
    In vivo (mice), 197
    Nerve growth factor,
      182-189
Central nervous system, 35-58,
  103, 226-227
  Ganglioneuroma, 226-227
  Neuroblastoma, 35-58
    Brain metastases, 35-41,
      103
    Cerebellar
      encephalopathy, 48-51
    Olfactory, 46-48
    Periorbital metastases,
      41-46, 103
    Primary intracranial, 36-37
    Spinal cord compression,
      51-54
Cerebellar encephalopathy,
  48-51
  Etiology, 50-51
  Myoclonic encephalopathy, 48
  Opsoclonus, 48, 49
  Therapy, 49-50
Chemotherapy, 49, 247, 263-271,
  297-300
  Adriamycin, 266
  And prognosis, 297-300
  Cure probability, 268
  Cyclophosphamide, 264-266
  Daunorubicin, 264, 266
  Ifosfamide, 266
  Imidazole carboxamide, 266
  Survival curves, 267
  Vincristine, 264-269
Chest neuroblastoma, 65-73
  Catecholamines, 66
  Diagnosis, 66, 67, 69-73

  Importance of distinguishing
    between primary and
    metastatic, 74
  Intrathoracic neurogenic
    tumors, 66
  Location, 65-67
  Paralysis, 68
  Pleural tumor, 67
  Radiographic findings, 69-73
    Paravertebral widening,
      69-71
  Scoliosis, 68, 255-256
  Symptoms, 65-69
Chromaffin system, 159, 160-162
Chromatography, 123, 126
Chromosomal abnormalities,
  197-200
  Aneuploidy, 199
  Double-minute chromosomes,
    199-200
Cultivation, neuroblastoma, in
  vitro, 189-197
  Human, 189-194
    Continuous cell lines,
      192-193
    Growth, differentiation,
      and maturation,
      191-192
    Histofluorescence,
      193-194
    Plasma clot technique, 190
    Tissue culture, 192-193
  Mouse, 194-197
    C-1300 murine, 194
    Inducing maturation,
      196-197
Cure, definition, 274-275
Cushing's syndrome, 41, 80

D

Diarrhea, 79-81, 226
Diagnosis, 2, 3-5, 66, 67, 98-109,
  120-135, 155, 177-178, 193-194,
  223
  And catecholamines, 2, 6, 25,
    63, 109, 120-135
  Biochemical, 133-135
  Bone-marrow smears, 95-97

Flank masses, differential, 75
Histofluorescence, 193-194
Histological differential,
    177-178
Neck masses, 223
Radiographic findings, 69-73,
    76-79, 98-106
Scanning techniques, 109-111
Skin blanching, 6
Spinal cord compression, 53-54
Dibutyryl-cyclic AMP, 196
Differentiation, histological,
290-292
DOPA (3,4-dihydroxy-
phenylalanine),
116, 117, 133
Dopamine, 116, 117, 118, 125,
127, 128, 131, 133
Dopamine-beta-hydroxylase, 132
Dosage, radiation, 252, 253-254
"Drooping lily" deformity, 75
"Dumbbell" tumors, 51, 53, 54,
61, 66, 68, 221, 228, 253
Dural mestastases, 41

E

Ecchymosis, 42, 44, 45, 46
Embryological development of
autonomic nervous system,
157-160
    Chromaffin system, 159
    Neural crest, 15-17, 26, 115,
    157
    Neural tube, 158
    Sympatheticoblast, 158
    Sympathogon, 158
Embryonic development and
neuroblastoma, 16-18, 157-160
Epinephrine, 117, 118, 125, 127,
128, 130
Esthesioneuroepithelioma, 47
Esthesioneuroma, 47, 48
Etiology, 27
Ewing's tumor, 106, 108, 177
Exophthalmos, 44, 46
Eye, 38
    Periorbital metastases,
    41-46, 103

F

Fetal neuroblastoma, 5-6, 9-11,
211
    And fetal circulation, 9-11, 211
    Placental involvement, 5
"Floating teeth," 64

G

Ganglioneuroblastoma, 66, 69,
116, 162, 170-173, 289, 290
    Age, 171
    Granules, 173
    Histology, 170-171
    Location, 171
Ganglioneuroma, 26, 27, 28, 66,
69, 79, 116, 135, 162, 173-177,
217-233, 254
    Age and, 173, 217
    Clinical manifestations,
    217-220, 227
        Primary sites, 220
        Symptoms, 217-227
    Ganglion cell, 176
    Histology, 173-177, 229-231
    In central nervous system,
    226-227
    Intestine, 224-226
    Intrathoracic, functionally
    active, 225-226
    Location, 174, 218-219
    Lymphocytic infiltration, 176
    Mediastinum and
    retroperitoneum, 223-224
    Neck, 222-223
    Origin, 217-219
    Post-neuroblastoma, 221
    Relation to neurofibromatosis,
    227-228
    Treatment, 231-232
    X-ray findings, 228-229
Genetic mechanisms, 27
Grading, histologic, 167

H

Head, neuroblastoma of, 35-58
    Brain metastases, 37-41

310

Head, neuroblastoma of *(cont.)*
  Cerebellar encephalopathy,
    48-51
  Olfactory, 46-48
  Periorbital metastases, 41-46
  Primary intracranial, 36-37
Hepatic metastases, 7-8, 13, 77
Histogenesis, of neuroblastoma,
  155-162
  Anatomy and physiology of
    central nervous system,
    156-157
  Chromaffin cells, 160-161
  Embryological development of
    autonomic nervous system,
    157-160
  Neural crest differentiation, 161
  Primitive sympathetic
    neuroblasts, 160
Histologic grading, 167-170
  Maturation, 167
  Prognosis and, 167-170
Histopathology of
  neuroblastoma, 165-170,
  177-178, 289-291
  And prognosis, 167, 290-292
  Histologic grading, 167-170,
    291
  Maturation, 167
  Rosettes, 155, 165
  Tumors resembling
    neuroblastoma, 177-178
Horner's syndrome, 51, 53, 61, 68,
  222, 244-245
"Hour glass" tumors, 51 (see also
  "Dumbbell" tumors)
Humoral cytotoxic antibody, 294
Hutchison type, 2, 74
HVA (homovanillic acid), 116,
  122, 124-125, 126, 127, 133,
  134, 137-138, 143
Hydrocephalus, 39
Hypertension, 79-81

I

Immunology of neuroblastoma,
  18-20, 205-216, 292-294
  And prognosis, 292-295

Cell-mediated immune
  mechanisms, 208-210
Clinical parameters, 210-211
  Spontaneous regression,
    210
Humoral immune mechanisms,
  208-210
  Anti-tumor antibodies,
    208-209
  Blocking factors, 209-210
Immunosuppressive drugs, 293
Immunotherapy, 211-213
Immunosuppressive drugs, 293
Immunotherapy, 211-213
  Classification, 212
Infancy, neuroblastoma in, 1-34
  And fetal circulation, 9-11
  Diagnosis, 2-5
  Fetal, 5-6, 9-11, 211
  Location of primary tumors and
    metastases, 3-4
  Peculiarities of, 6-20
In situ neuroblastoma, 18, 20,
  22-26, 211, 276
  Oncogenetic significance,
    24-25
Intestines, ganglioneuromas of,
  224-225
Intracranial metastases, 37-41
Intracranial neuroblastomas,
  primary, 36-37
Intraspinal lesion, 53
Intrathoracic neurogenic tumors,
  217, 225-226
In vitro neuroblastoma cells,
  189-197 (see also Cultivation)
In vivo neuroblastoma cells, 197
  (see also Cultivation)
Irides, heterochromia of, 46, 61

L

Laparotomy, 257
Leukemia, 106, 109, 177
Lymphocytes, 18, 176, 293-294
  And prognosis, 293
  Infiltration of ganglioneuroma,
    176
Lymphosarcoma, 106, 177

M

Mandible, 45, 63-65
Management, of neuroblastoma,
 237-271, 294-300
 And prognosis, 294-300
 Chemotherapeutic, 237-250
 Immunotherapeutic, 211-213
 Radiotherapeutic, 251-262
 Surgical, 237-250
Marrow invasion, 96, 279
Mass, 4, 74-75
 Flank, differential diagnosis of,
  74
Maturation, 165, 171, 174,
 191-192, 196-197, 277, 279,
 290-292
 And prognosis, 290-292
 Induced, in vitro, 196
  Dibutyryl-cyclic AMP, 196
Maxilla, 45, 63
Mediastinum, neuroblastoma,
 65-67, 223-224, 242-243
 Anterior, 67
 Ganglioneuromas, 223-224
 Posterior, 65
 Superior, 65
 Surgery, 242-243
Metastases, 1, 3-4, 6-8, 13, 35-36,
 62-63, 65, 77, 93-111, 245-246,
 258-260, 278-284
 Blood-borne, theory of, 65
 Bone marrow demonstration of,
  95-97
  And diagnosis, 95-97
 Brain, 35, 36, 37-41
 Dural, 41
 In infant, 1, 3-4, 6
 In neonate, 3-4
 Liver, 7-8, 13, 77
 Location, 93-95
 Mandible, 45, 63-65
 Maxilla, 45, 63
 Neck, 62-63
 Periorbital, 41-46
 Prognosis, 278-284
  Linear model, 281-282
 Radiotherapy, 258-260
 Scanning techniques, 109-111
 Skeletal, 93-111, 259, 279-281

 Spinal cord, 35, 36
 Subcutaneous, 6
 Surgery, 245-246
 Xygoma, 45
MHPG
 (3-methoxy-4-hydroxyphenylethyl-
  eneglycol, 122, 124-125, 127,
  128, 133, 134,
  137-139
Morbidity, surgical, 243-245
Mortality, 243-245, 287
 Surgical, 243-245
Myoclonic encephalopathy, 48

N

Neck, 60-65
 Metastatic neuroblastomas,
  62-65
  Theory of blood-borne
   metastases, 65
 Symptoms, 60-63
Neonate, and neuroblastoma, 1,
 6, 37
 And metastases, 1, 3-4, 6
Nerve growth factor, 20-22,
 182-189
 Anti-NGF, 21, 185
 Clinical studies of levels, 186
 Role in pathogenesis, 184-185
 Use in treatment, 188-189
Neural crest, 15-17, 115, 157, 161
Neuroblastoma,
 Abdominal, 1, 2, 41, 49, 59,
  74-81, 238-242, 285-286
 Adrenal, 1, 3, 59, 63-64, 165,
  171, 285-286, 292-294
 And age, 2, 18-19, 47, 211,
  227, 253, 276-278, 281
 Catecholamine metabolism, 2,
  5, 6, 25, 47, 49, 81, 115-154,
  160, 171, 238, 289-290
 Cells, 95, 181-203
 Description, 155-156, 162,
  163-170
  Gross pathology, 162-170
  Histopathology, 165-170
 Development of, 15-17
  Stages, 13-14, 252-254,
   276-278

Neuroblastoma *(cont.)*
    Extra-abdominal, 289-290
    Diagnosis, 2, 2-5, 67, 98-109,
       133-135, 155, 177-178,
       193-194, 223
    Fetal, 5-6, 9-11, 211
    Head and central nervous
       system, 35-38
    Histogenesis and pathology,
       155-180
    Immunology, 18-20, 205-216,
       292-294
    In animals, 27-28, 194-197
    In infancy, 1-34
    In neonate, 1, 6, 37
    In situ, 18, 20, 22-26, 211, 276
    Intrathoracic, 71, 79-81
    Management, 237-271
    Metastases, 1, 3-4, 6-8, 13,
       35-36, 62-63, 65, 77,
       93-111, 245-246, 258-260,
       278-284
    Neck, chest, abdomen, and
       pelvis, 59-91
       Abdomen, 74-81
       Chest, 65-73
       Neck, 60-65
       Pelvis, 81-83
    Non-proliferating, 280
    Olfactory, 46-48
    Origin, 3, 16-18, 59-60, 115,
       160-162, 289
    Prognosis, 3, 13, 73, 81, 116,
       167-170, 212, 248, 273-306
    Regression, 11-14, 18-22,
       275-276
    Skeletal system, 93-113
Neuroblasts, 156, 160
    Primitive sympathetic
       (sympathogonia), 160
Neurofibroma, 26, 27
Neurofibromatosis, 227-228
Nissl granules, 174, 176
Norepinephrine, 117, 118, 125,
   127, 128, 129, 133

O

Olfactory neuroblastomas, 46-48
Opsoclonus, 48, 49, 83

Orbital metastases, 41-46, 103
Origin, 3, 16-18, 59-60, 115,
   160-162, 289
    Of ganglioneuroma, 218-219
    (see also **Embryonic origin**
    and **Location**)
Osteogenic sarcoma, 108
Osteolytic metastases, 98-100
Osteomyelitis, 108
Ovaries, 257

P

Papilledema, 44
Paralysis, 67
Paraplegia, 51, 68
Pathology, of neuroblastoma,
   162-178
    Gross pathology, 163-165
    Histopathology, 165-170
       Histologic grading, 167
    Major variants, 162
Pelvic neuroblastoma, 81-83, 238,
   240, 241
    Symptoms, 82-83
       Bladder compression, 82
       Opsoclonus, 83
Periorbital metastases, 41-46
    Clinical picture, 43-46
    Ecchymosis, 42, 44, 45, 46
    Exophthalmos, 44-46
    Heterochromia of irides, 46
    Incidence, 43
    Papilledema, 44
    Pathology, 46
Periosteal reaction, 98-99
Pepper type, 1, 74
Pheochromocytoma, 26, 115,
   116, 120, 135, 142, 160-161, 227
Prognosis, 3, 13, 73, 116, 167-170,
   248, 273-306
    And catecholamine
       metabolism, 136-142
    Cure criteria, 274-275
    Factors influencing, 273-274,
       276-300
       Age and stage, 13-16,
        18-19, 248, 267-278,
        281

Histological features,
167-170, 248, 290-292
Immunological status,
292-294
Location of primary tumor,
3, 248, 285-290
Metastases, 3, 278-284
Treatment, 294-300
Late recurrence of tumor,
300-301
Spontaneous regression,
275-276
Ptosis, 61

R

Radiographic findings, see **X-ray findings**
Radiotherapeutic management,
49, 247, 251-262, 288, 296-297
And prognosis, 296-297
And staging system, 251
Effect on normal tissue,
254-258, 260
Dosage, 252, 253-254,
255
Repositioning ovaries, 257
Scoliosis, 255-256
Shielding, 255-257
Metastatic neuroblastoma,
258-260
Resectable tumors, 251-254
Regression, 11-14, 18-20, 275-276
And nerve growth factor, 20-22
Spontaneous, 275-276
Reticuloendotheliosis, 108
Rhabdomyosarcoma, embryonal,
177
Rosettes, 155, 165, 169

S

Sacral neuroblastoma, 81-82
"Scalp" nodules, 38
Scanning techniques, 109-111
Selenium-75 methionine, 109
Scoliosis, 68, 255-256
Selenium-75 methionine, 109
Skeletal lesions, 93-111
Course of, 104-106

Incidence, 97
Location, 97-98
Solitary, 98
Skeletal system, neuroblastoma of, 93-113
Bone-marrow demonstration of
metastases, 95-97, 279
Bone lesions, 97-98
Course of, 104-106
Detecting occult metastases by
scanning techniques,
109-111
Differential diagnosis of x-ray
findings, 106-109
Disappearance of metastases,
280
Location, 93-95
Prognosis and metastases,
279-281
X-ray appearance, 98-106
Skin lesions, nodular, 6
Skull involvement, 37 (see also
Skeletal metastases)
Spinal cord compression, 51-54
"Dumbbell" tumors, 51
Diagnosis, 53-54
Horner's syndrome, 51
Paraplegia, 51
Spinal cord dysfunction, 52, 53
Symptoms, 51-54
Spinal cord metastases, 35, 36
Staging of neuroblastoma, 13-14,
252-254, 276-278
And surgery, 247-248
Prognosis, 276-278
Stage I, 13, 247, 252-254
Stage II, 13, 247, 252-254
Stage III, 13
Stage IV, 13, 260
Stage IV-S, 13, 18, 20, 248,
252-254, 259, 278, 279,
283-284
Supraclavicular (Virchow's) node,
62
Surgical management, 49,
237-250
Abdominal neuroblastomas,
238-242
Exposure, 238
Pelvic, 240-241

314

Surgical management *(cont.)*
  And prognosis, 297
  Following radio- or
    chemotherapy, 246
  Mediastinal neuroblastoma,
    242-243
  Metastases, 245-246
  Morbidity and mortality,
    243-245
  Preparation, 237-238
  Results, 248-249
Survival, 281-284, 296-300 (see
  also **Prognosis**)
Sympathetic ganglia, 54, 59
Sympathetic nervous system, 52,
  156-157
Sympatheticoblast, 158
Sympathogon, 158
Symptoms, 2, 4-5, 6, 36, 38-41,
  43-46, 47-49, 51-53, 59-63,
  66-69, 74, 79-81, 82-83, 217-227
Sweating, 79

T

Thoracotomy, 52
Therapy, 136, 211-213, 237-300
  (see also **Management**)
Treatment, 237-300 (see also
  Management)
Tumors, 3, 4, 18, 20, 22-26, 51, 53,
  54, 66, 69, 71, 76, 77, 106-108,
  177-178, 223-224, 253, 285-290,
  300-301
  Abdominal, 4, 238-242,
    285-286
  Brain, 35
  Burkitt's, 177
  "Dumbbell," 51, 53, 54, 66,
    68, 71, 221, 228, 253
  Ewing's, 106, 108, 177
  Histologically similar to
    neuroblastoma, 177-178

In situ, 18, 20, 22-26, 211, 276
Intrathoracic neurogenic, 66
Late recurrence, 300-301
Location, 3, 218, 285-290
    And prognosis, 3, 285-290
Mass, 4, 75
Mediastinal, 65-67, 223-224,
  287-288
Non-abdominal, 286
Pleural, 67
Wilms', 4, 69, 76, 77, 106-107

V

Virchow's (supraclavicular) node,
  62
VMA (vanillylmandelic acid), 116,
  120, 122, 124-125, 126, 127,
  123, 134, 137-138, 142

W

Wieberdink hypothesis, 38
Wilms' tumor, 4, 67, 69, 75, 77,
  106-107

X

X-ray findings, 69-73, 76-79,
  106-109
    Bone metastases, 98-103, 259,
      279
    Calcification, 69, 76, 77, 78
    Differential diagnosis of,
      106-109
    Ganglioneuromas, 228
    Paravertebral widening, 69-71
X-ray therapy, see **Radiotherapy**
Xygoma, 45

Z

Zuckerkandl, bodies of, 59,
  82, 159